Progress in Drug Research

Founded by Ernst Jucker

Progress in Drug Research

Systems Biological Approaches in Infectious Diseases

Vol. 64

Edited by
Helena I. Boshoff and Clifton E. Barry III

Birkhäuser Verlag
Basel · Boston · Berlin

Editors

Helena I. Boshoff
Clifton E. Barry III
Tuberculosis Research Section
Laboratory of Immunogenetics
National Institute of Allergy and Infectious Diseases
Rockville, MD 20852
USA

Library of Congress Cataloging-in-Publication Data

Systems biological approaches in infectious dieseases / edited by Helena J. Boshoff and
Clifton E. Barry, III.
p. cm. – (Progress in drug research vol. 64)
Includes bibliographical references and index.
ISBN-13: 978-3-7643-7566-9 (alk. paper)
ISBN-10: 3-7643-7566-3 (alk. paper)
I. Communicable diseases–Epidemiology–Mathematical models. 2.
Drugs–Design–Mathematical models. I. Boshoff, Helena J., 1968- II. Barry, Clifton E.,
1963-

ISBN 10: 3-7643-7566-3 Birkhäuser Verlag, Basel – Boston – Berlin
ISBN 13: 978-3-7643-7566-9

Part of Springer Science+Business Media
Printed on acid-free paper produced from chlorine-free pulp. TCF
Cover design and layout: Micha Lotrovsky, CH-4106 Therwil, Switzerland
Printed in Germany

ISBN 10: 3-7643-7566-3 e-ISBN: 3-7643-7567-1
ISBN 13: 978-3-7643-7566-9

9 8 7 6 5 4 3 2 1 www.birkhauser.ch

Contents

Foreword

The much-lamented "innovation gap" often referenced by current authors with respect to drug discovery in the pharmaceutical industry is a sure sign that an era has passed. The reductionist view of disease as the direct consequence of isolated errors of metabolism that could be explained and understood as simple enzyme alterations is a thing of the past. Likewise the naïve view that the system-wide consequences of small molecule interventions could be predicted through simple *in vitro* assays has become obsolete. Infectious diseases, representing an evolved and complex evolutionary conflict between two life-forms, have been at the vanguard of embracing systems biology concepts due to the obvious failure to cure such diseases by simply studying an invading parasite's physiology in a test tube. Driven by a virtual renaissance in technology the simple approaches of the previous era have given way to a vast new array of integrative sciences aimed at modeling and understanding the complex and dynamic interactions that characterize real human diseases. Although still struggling for granularity these integrative sciences share a common vision – erasing the differences between disciplines and embracing complexity in tools that offer glimpses of whole biological systems and mesh seamlessly with infinite chemical space.

Rather than focus this book on the tools, approaches, successes and failures of the old era we challenged our contributors to look forward and project the tools that will become indispensable to the new era – the tools that would turn this "innovation gap" into an "innovation leap". The "omic" sciences are one prime example of the integrative approach to infectious disease. With hundreds of genome sequences of organisms from all branches of the tree of life literally at our fingertips, transcriptomics, proteomics and metabolomics are proving to be only the first wave of large, complex datasets that are now being augmented by protein interaction networks, reverse protein arrays, the protein-DNA interactome, etc. The magnitude of these datasets has challenged experimental, mathematical and computational scientists who are banding together around the emerging discipline of "Systems Biology". Systems biology aims towards nothing less than the complete reconstruction of the biological complexity of living organisms in chemically and mathematically defined terms. Complete models for simple prokaryotes are within our grasp and models of complex multi-cellular organisms will emerge within our scientific careers and these models will have a profound impact on drug discovery.

Systems biology at present is defined by the tools employed to generate large-scale datasets. There remains a gap between those tools that have been reduced to practice and give reproducible, reliable datasets with information that allows us to model part of the system, for example transcriptomics, and tools that have critical information but cannot currently provide robust datasets such as metabolomics. Transcriptomics has been applied widely in infectious disease research and has already resulted in significant insights with therapeutic consequences. Metabolomics, however, is the frontier between analytical chemistry and biology, and the tools required for the simultaneous identification and quantitation of all the relevant small molecules in even a simple prokaryote are still being developed. Metabolomic analyses, however, have the potential to inform many aspects of the drug discovery pipeline from target identification to biomarkers of response to therapy. As the complexity of the link between transcription, translation and metabolic flux has expanded, so too have the models required to explain and interpret such data.

The information emerging from measurements and models of host-pathogen systems also requires bridging another gap between chemists with a desire for simple isolated enzyme assays and biologists with a desire for complex whole-cell based assays. Chemical genetics is one element of such a bridge and is on the verge of becoming a core large-scale technology. "Reverse chemical genetics" is perhaps the more intuitive approach where a candidate target is screened for small molecule ligands that are then used to examine the influence of target interruption in a whole-cell context. "Forward chemical genetics", however, is arguably a more powerful approach for target identification in anti-infectives programs. In this approach small molecules are directly screened for a desired phenotypic effect followed by identification of the relevant protein target in the pathogen or in the host – an exercise that minimizes the "biological uncertainty" associated with target selection. More and more often decreasing biological uncertainty involves an intense integration of the full suite of "omics" technologies. The approach is a natural complement of traditional genetic approaches since it directly asks the therapeutically relevant interruption of protein function question in an appropriately complex system.

In a sense what all of these large-scale biology approaches are pushing towards is accurate information in highly disease-relevant environments in an effort to choose smarter targets and minimize the risk of drug development. While this is a direction that the pharma industry has been evolving towards in many ways, systems biology is pushing the fringe of what is possible. The future of many development compounds is dramatically affected by their performance at a systems level. Nowhere is this more acute than in the area of predictive toxicology where current guidelines specify increasing numbers of standard assays. The number of *in vitro* toxicology examinations that are mandatory is increasing and this trend is likely to continue. As these tests grow increasingly sophisticated (e.g. whole rabbit heart screening for cardiac toxicology assessment) they are increasingly being informed by systems biology data, and in the future toxicogenomics is likely to play a large role in preclinical development.

We think that the impending "innovation leap" in anti-infectives therapeutics development lies squarely within the sort of interdisciplinary, integrative efforts described within the systems biology framework in this book. Every step of the drug-development pathway will benefit directly from assays and models that do not make reductionistic assumptions to make predictions but rather are based upon embracing biological complexity to gain true insight into the consequences of therapeutic strategies as early as possible.

July, 2006

Helena I. Boshoff
Clifton E. Barry III

Progress in Drug Research, Vol. 64
(Helena I. Boshoff and Clifton E. Barry III, Eds)

Systems biology and its impact on anti-infective drug development

By Michael P. Stumpf[1],
Brian D. Robertson[2],
Ken Duncan[2]
and Douglas B. Young[2]

Imperial College London, UK

[1]Centre for Integrative Systems Biology
at Imperial College (CISBIC),
Division of Molecular Biosciences,
Imperial College London,
South Kensington Campus,
London SW7 2AZ, UK

[2]Centre for Integrative Systems Biology
at Imperial College (CISBIC),
Department of Molecular Microbiology
and Infection,
Imperial College London,
South Kensington Campus,
London SW7 2AZ, UK
<d.young@imperial.ac.uk>

Abstract

Systems biology offers the potential for more effective selection of novel targets for anti-infective drugs. In contrast to conventional reductionist biology, a systems approach allows targets to be viewed in a wider context of the entire physiology of the cell, with the potential to identify key susceptible nodes and to predict synergistic effects of blocking multiple pathways. In addition to the holistic perspective provided by systems biology, the emphasis on quantitative analysis is likely to add further rigour to the process of target selection. Systems biology also offers the potential to incorporate different levels of information into the selection process. Consideration of data from microbial population biology may be important in the context of predicting future drug-resistance profiles associated with targeting a particular pathway, for example. This chapter provides an overview of major themes in the developing field of systems biology, summarising the core technologies and the strategies used to translate datasets into useful quantitative models capable of predicting complex biological behaviour.

Keywords: imaging, integrative systems biology, mathematical models, metabolic networks, protein interaction network, targets for anti-infective drugs, transciptional networks

1 Introduction

The current approach of target-driven drug discovery is underpinned by dramatic progress that has been achieved in molecular and structural biology within a framework provided by the revolution in genome sequencing. Sequences are available for most of the major pathogens and straightforward procedures are in place for the production of recombinant proteins required for drug discovery efforts based on high-throughput screens and structure-based compound optimisation. The challenge for the future of anti-infective drug development lies in target selection. Can we develop a rational approach to target identification that will allow us to produce new drugs and drug combinations that act faster than existing compounds, that are effective against the range of adaptive microbial phenotypes generated during infection, and that reduce the evolution of drug-resistant strains? To address this challenge we have to be able to evaluate potential targets within the context of the overall physiology of both pathogen and host with a level of predictive accuracy that matches the precision that we currently apply when working with the isolated targets (see Chapters 10 and 12). This will involve taking a step back from conventional reductionist approaches and entering the domain that is commonly referred to as systems biology, a conclusion also reached by the US Food and Drug Administration (FDA) in its report *Challenge and Opportunity on the Critical Path to New Medical Products* [1].

Investigation of intact biological systems is a relatively recent concept in the molecular biosciences. In ecology and epidemiology system-level descriptions of biological processes – often coupled with a rigorous quantitative framework – have a longer history, reaching back certainly to the first half of the 20th century. Advances in molecular biosciences have been achieved by a predominantly reductionist approach, based on isolation and analysis of individual components in preference to study of the system as a whole. As a result we now have rich and detailed data about the function of many genes and their protein products in an increasing number of species spanning all three kingdoms of life, and often a good understanding of how these are organised into local modules responsible for a range of cellular processes and signalling. The fledgling discipline of systems biology now aims to provide a global framework for the integrative, coherent and consistent analysis of all of the available data, moving beyond the purely descriptive towards a quantitative and predictive level of understanding.

From the perspective of infectious disease biology, an important goal of a systems-based approach will be to integrate information across a spectrum of biological complexity, with the 'system' ranging from an isolated microbe, to an individual infected host, and on to microbial and host populations. The evolution and spread of antibiotic resistance clearly involves a complex feedback between processes at the molecular and population levels for example, and an ability to link the molecular information emerging from functional genomics with the rich literature addressing host–pathogen (or host–vector–pathogen) systems from a population perspective will be essential for understanding and ultimately controlling infectious diseases.

Here we provide an outline of some of the experimental, theoretical and conceptual approaches that are involved in integrative systems biology and are considered in detail in subsequent chapters.

2 Data for systems biology: 'Omics, images and chemistry

A major impetus for the development of systems biology derives from technical advances associated with high-throughput sequencing [2] and chip-based systems [3, 4]. With the widespread availability of microarray formats for expression profiling, biologists whose primary focus was largely on the study of individual molecules or pathways were deluged with vast datasets comprising information on the simultaneous level of expression of every single gene in a cell or organism (the transcriptome) (see Chapter 2). While some simple clustering algorithms [5] provide an approach to analysing such datasets, it is clear that they contain a wealth of information that is not interpretable by conventional reductionist techniques. Analogous study of the total complement of proteins at a whole system level presents a greater technical challenge on account of the heterogeneity in their chemical and physical properties, but progress has been achieved by combining fractionation techniques such as two-dimensional gel electrophoresis with increasingly sophisticated mass spectrometry analysis [6, 7] (see Chapter 4). The ability to identify protein–protein interactions using yeast two-hybrid [8] and tandem affinity [9] purification systems has been particularly informative in mapping proteome networks (see Chapter 8). Analysis of protein-nucleic acid interactions [10, 11] at the level of transcriptional regulation generates an additional source of data that begins to link proteome and transcriptome information (see Chapter 4). Glycomic analysis based on mass spectrometry and nuclear magnetic resonance (NMR) techniques has provided insights into the further diversity generated by post-translational modification of proteins [12], and the same tools derived from physical chemistry allow quantitative analysis of the repertoire of small molecules that represent the cellular metabolome [13, 14] (see Chapter 5). At a higher level of complexity, metabonomic analysis provides an overview of metabolites in multicellular organisms, including the sharing of metabolite pools between host and microbe that is central both to commensal colonisation and to pathogen infection [14, 15] (see Chapter 10). Taken together, these 'omics datasets represent the starting material for the systems biologist, who faces the challenge of finding ways of maximising their integration and translation into usable information.

A second key source of data derives from imaging techniques. High-thoughput 'omics datasets are derived from analysis of biological systems at a population level, with differences between individual members of the population subsumed within an overall average. Technologies that derive data from single cells demonstrate that there is a significant underlying stochastic heterogeneity in the level of expression and in the spatial distribution of molecules within individual members of genetically clonal populations. In some cases these stochastic variations have been shown to be crucial in determining biological functions of the system [16], and an understanding at this level is a major component of systems biology.

Recent advances in fluorescent microscopy [17] have revealed an unprecedented degree of organisation and complexity in bacterial cells, despite their lack of membrane-bound cellular compartments. During the cell cycle many bacterial proteins localise to particular sites at specific times; understanding how such topological specificity is achieved is a fundamental question in cell biology. A recent example of proteins displaying previously unexplained dynamic protein localisation are the Spo0J/Soj proteins of *B. subtilis*, which are involved in chromosome segregation and transcriptional regulation. Using fluorescence microscopy Howard and colleagues [18] showed that Spo0J organises into compact foci associated with the nucleoid, while Soj undergoes irregular relocations from pole to pole or nucleoid to nucleoid. They propose that these irregularities are due in part to low copy number fluctuations: the relatively low numbers of the Spo0J/Soj proteins in a cell, together with the intrinsic probabilistic nature of their interactions, leading to large fluctuations in their dynamic behaviour. Stochasticity is vital for capturing the observed irregularity of the spatiotemporal protein dynamics for the Spo0J/Soj system.

The phenotypic tolerance to antimicrobial drugs associated with particular growth states of many microorganisms has also been shown to have a stochastic element [19, 20]. Integrating spatio-temporal information derived from single cell imaging with the type of information provided by high-throughput analysis of bulk populations is another central challenge for the systems biologist.

Biological systems are dynamic and observations recorded over time – particularly in response to some defined perturbation – provide critical information that is missing from a static analysis. Techniques for induction of relatively simple perturbations include changes to the cellular environment, induction or repression of selected genes, and addition of small molecule inhibitors (see also Chapter 3) [21, 22]. The use of chemical modulators is particularly informative in the context of anti-infectives. Changes in bacterial gene expression profiles induced by exposure to known drugs allows mapping of characteristic response networks [23], facilitating screening for compounds with novel mechanisms of action (see Chapter 2). Advances in genome re-sequencing technologies [24–26] present exciting opportunities for a chemical genomics approach to rapid target identification based on an initial chemical lead (see Chapter 3). Starting with a compound (of known or unknown structure) which has activity against a whole microbe, the target can be identified by isolating resistant mutants and identifying the corresponding genetic changes. This represents a very attractive approach to integration of chemistry, functional biology, and genetics.

3 Making models

When describing a biological system we have to determine first the level at which we wish to study the constituent processes and interactions. Often this will be determined by the nature and quality of the experimental data: if the data are plagued by high error levels it may not be possible or even desirable to formulate a detailed mathematical or conceptual model. In practice, most biological models are hybrids containing qualitative and quantitative elements.

3.1 Qualitative systems approach

Biologists have always relied on models to conceptualise how organisms work. Such models can be purely verbal models or descriptions of biological structures or processes. In a qualitative approach one uses only the most coarse-grained information about the constituents of a biological system. In the context of the Krebs cycle, for example, we do not care about the three dimensional structure of the enzymes or substrate molecules and their molecular interactions. In general no attempt is being made at predicting quantitative responses of a system or at quantifying results [27]. Qualitative (including verbal) models of the same system are very difficult to compare; if different researchers propose their own verbal models for a biological process it can be extremely difficult to decide to what extent these models are similar or not. Moreover they make almost exclusively linear assumptions: i.e., they make statements of the type "if A increases then B decreases". Incorporating feedback into a verbal model, for example, can become enormously cumbersome.

3.2 Quantitative systems approach

In a quantitative approach, as many details of a system are ignored as is possible (generally by trial and error). Again, for example, molecular structures may be ignored, but instead of a purely qualitative description of interactions and processes a mathematical description or function is now chosen to represent the entities making up the system and the interactions among them [28]. The mathematical model now requires us to specify our assumptions explicitly and from the outset and, once these have been determined, mathematical or computational analysis of the model will allow us to study its change over time (see Chapters 7 and 11). This is then compared to experimental data. Depending on the question at hand or the experimental data available the mathematical models can be very abstract and generic, or directly targeted at a particular biological problem. In the former case it may be possible, for example, to investigate systematically the expected behaviour of a certain type of theoretical model. This can then be compared qualitatively against experimental data. Especially when there is little data available such an approach has been very popular. This type of approach has also been used extensively in theoretical physics where, for example, highly simplified models of magnetic materials have been studied to qualitatively reproduce experimental results [29].

If more detailed data are available, and if a statistical approach can be devised which allows us to estimate the parameters of a mathematical model from such data, then more detailed predictive modelling approaches become possible. Such approaches have been highly successful, for example, in modelling the immune response to human immunodeficiency virus (HIV) [30], or in developing very detailed models of the human heart which can be used [31, 32], with some success, to model the effect of certain cardiovascular drugs (see Chapter 9).

Models of biological systems must, however, be understood not as realistic descriptions but as simplified representations of much more complicated entities. Almost all models will eventually be superseded by more sophisticated and more powerful models. In some areas – including for didactic purposes – even simple models retain their usefulness even if their limitations are known.

4 Networks

Molecular networks – in particular, metabolic, transcription regulation, and protein-interaction networks – offer the possibility of a coherent and consistent framework for the description of the whole complement of biological processes inside a cellular system [33] (see also Chapters 6 and 11). These networks have taken on a central role in computational systems biology. Statistical inference of networks [34–36], in particular co-expression networks estimated from microarray data, and the analysis of network structures have become important fields of research.

Networks can be described mathematically in terms of graphs (Fig. 1). Graphs occur in many different settings and as a result the theoretical description of graphs/networks has progressed independently in disciplines as varied as mathematics [37], computer science, statistical physics [38, 39], engineering and sociology. Integrating the different techniques developed in these disciplines and adapting them for the use in the modern life-sciences will allow us to analyse the increasing amount of network data currently being generated in systems biology [33].

One of the central features of natural networks is that they are highly heterogeneous: some nodes (whether genes, proteins or metabolites) have a large number of interaction partners, while most nodes interact with only a few other nodes in the network [38, 40]. This reflects some biologically intuitive relationships: we now know that some proteins are involved in many different processes and take an almost pivotal position in an organism's functional organisation (just like some highly promiscuous individuals – so-called super-spreaders – contribute to the spread of sexual

Protein interaction network data (just as the other network data discussed below) offer a highly idealised and partial representation of cellular processes. They will change over three different time-scales: changes will occur at the evolutionary (between species), developmental and physiological levels. At the moment the data will at most allow us to resolve differences between species. This, as well as the fact that present experimental techniques may only capture a subset of the interactions has to be kept in mind.

4.2 Transcriptional networks

Initiation and regulation of gene expression is currently best understood at the level of transcriptional gene regulation. Transcription factors bind to regulatory elements upstream of the genes they regulate and these relationships can be depicted using directed graphs [58]. In addition to experimental and labour-intensive validation of transcription factors and their binding sites in genomes a growing number of *in silico* approaches are being developed and applied across all domains of life [59]. These use either co-expression patterns of genes to identify those that are presumably regulated by the same (or a similar) transcription-factor; or they employ linguistic/evolutionary arguments to find regulatory elements in sequenced genomes [60]. At present our data on transcriptional networks is also incomplete and suffers probably from ascertainment problems (i.e., researchers have focussed on their 'favourite' genes and mapped them with great care without gaining a global overview). For other processes of gene regulation there is even more rudimentary understanding of the involved mechanisms/molecules and the structure of the underlying networks. Transcriptional networks include both qualitative descriptions and quantitative data in terms of fold changes in gene expression, as well as information about direction of the interaction: e.g., there is a difference between gene *A* coding for a transcription factor which initiates transcription on gene *B* or gene *B* controlling expression of *A*. It is still frequently overlooked that transcriptional regulation encompasses only a tiny fraction of gene expression regulation. Incorporation of post-transcriptional and post-translational processes is only starting to be considered.

4.3 Metabolic networks

The whole complement of enzymes and substrates inside cellular systems (or whole organisms) are increasingly described in terms of metabolic networks [61, 62] (see Chapter 5). These are a straightforward conceptual development from the notion of individual biochemical pathways (such as the Krebs cycle) towards a more integrative perspective (see Chapter 7). To a certain extent the integrative analysis of metabolic networks has progressed furthest as biochemical pathways are relatively straightforwardly described quantitatively using the familiar Michaelis-Menten theory of enzyme kinetics [27, 28]. Metabolic networks contain both qualitative and quantitative information.

In metabolic networks we can choose whether we want the enzymes or the substrates to be the nodes in the network. Over the past few years the view to denote enzymes as nodes of the metabolic network has prevailed.

Considerable work has gone into characterising the structure, evolution and functional organisation of these networks (see Chapters 6 and 11). Very simple mathematical models of network growth give rise to networks with structural properties similar to those observed in molecular networks [38, 63–65]. These networks offer an attractive perspective on biological systems but it is important to keep in mind their present limitations: (i) present network data are incomplete [66] and it is difficult to extrapolate from incomplete network data to the true network; (ii) experimental – in particular high-throughput – methodologies are notoriously noisy and data may be unreliable; (iii) some interactions may be too short-lived or weak to be observed experimentally but nevertheless have profound physiological importance; (iv) molecular networks are generally described in terms of (necessarily) simplified mathematical models, such as static graphs. In reality, however, they are highly dynamic and responsive objects. Simple models are slowly but steadily becoming too simplistic to capture the complexity of biological processes [67].

5 Integrative systems biology

While networks generated by different techniques are currently viewed independently, linking these together in integrated models is a central goal of systems biology (see Chapters 10 and 11). Clearly protein interactions depend in the first instance on genes being transcribed and translated; initiation of transcription in turn requires transcription factors which are themselves proteins. Enzymes, of course, are also proteins and are required for the metabolism inside a cell just as metabolic products are necessary to keep the protein synthesis going. By integrating the different forms of data, it should ultimately be possible, for example, to predict the proteome from knowledge of the genome, and to use knowledge of the transcriptome to derive insights into the metabolome.

Two examples serve to illustrate some of the challenges that need to be addressed in moving towards these ambitious goals. One hypothesis put forward in the context of linking genome to proteome, is that proteins involved in interactions with multiple other proteins (highly connected 'nodes') will be subject to increased pressure in favour of evolutionary conservation. While this is intuitively attractive, statistical analysis of data on protein interaction networks and genome conservation in *S. cerevisiae* and *C. elegans* showed that it was not the case [45]. An association was identified, however, between the degree of evolutionary conservation of a protein and its level of expression within the cell. A second example concerns the relationship between transcriptomic data and essential function. The adaptive responses that pathogens undergo during infection are most readily studied in terms of changes in gene expression (see Chapter 12). It would seem reasonable to infer that the induction of a gene in response to a particular environment will relate in some way to its required function but a simple comparison of list of genes that are upregulated – for example, in the case of a mycobacterial pathogen entering a host phagocyte [68] – displays little or no overlap with a list of genes identified as essential for survival. In a recent study of the factors underlying fungal virulence (using *S. cerevisae* as a model system), we have found that inclusion of protein interaction data does allow us to begin to link expression and essentiality datasets (M. Stumpf, unpublished observations). The usefulness of molecular network data has now been demonstrated for a number of different phenotypes, especially in *S. cerevisiae*; in light of such successes it seems natural to further explore whether it is possible to detect associations between network structures – rather than individual genes – and complex phenotypes. This would mean that rather than looking at individual genes or their protein products we would shift focus to the interactions directly. Given the lack of tangible success in mapping human genes underlying complex (disease) phenotypes, such a network centred approach ought to be worth considering.

6 New targets for anti-infective drug development

The initial impact of wide-scale pathogen genome sequencing has been to allow conventional charts of biochemical pathways to be annotated with gene names. Saturation mutagenesis tools have provided information on genes that are essential in particular growth media and, in some cases, under infection conditions. Systems biology aims to convert this static and informationally sparse framework into a dynamic network of nodes and fluxes. Quantitative models will highlight bottlenecks and nodes that are crucial for microbial viability and will distinguish between those at which a small or a large reduction in activity would be required for significant biological impact (see Chapter 7). The ability to input different types of data will allow models to be customised using information from genotypic data and from *in vivo* expression profiling to optimise for selection of targets that are appropriate in the context of existing drug resistance or in the context of phenotypic drug tolerance associated with latent tuberculosis and treatment of biofilm infections, for example. It can be anticipated that a systems biology framework will allow a rational approach to identification of synergistic drug combinations that will result in more rapid action and perhaps reduction in the evolution of resistance. Genetic experiments have shown that combining mutations which independently have no detectable impact on survival can result in 'synthetic lethality' [69, 70]. Similarly, it may be possible to identify drug combinations which result in a novel enhanced lethality by hitting two or more independent targets.

Systems biology may also help us in understanding infection processes in more detail. An illustrative outlook on what may be to come in the future is provided by a recent study by Uetz et al. [71] who studied interactions among human proteins and herpes-virus proteins. If or when the enormous experimental problems can be overcome – there is as yet no reliable experimental technique which allows us to test for transient or weak interactions – then such studies give much more detailed insights into infection biology at the molecular level with a distinct focus on the physical interaction *per se*. If we are willing to speculate for a moment then such approaches harbour a host of exciting possibilities waiting to be explored: we may for example be able to study why different species have different susceptibilities to different infectious agents – Simian Immunodeficiency Virus (SIV) and HIV are good examples for the subtle impact of cross-species effects – or we may study whether the molecular interactions between *P. falciparum* and their human hosts and fly vectors, respectively, can be exploited for clinical purposes.

As models evolve, they will integrate increasingly diverse sources of data. This could include information from structural biology and functional biochemistry that relate to the 'drugability' of targets. Pathogen–host systems biology comes with an additional component as infectious disease biology can only really be understood in an ecological and evolutionary framework: pathogens compete for a potentially limited host population, while hosts in turn mount an immune response against pathogens and may even develop suitable strategies against pathogens. There are a host of beautiful examples of apparent host–pathogen co-evolutionary dynamics (for example between lizards and some species of *Plasmodium*) [72]. In addition we must consider the interaction between the host and the drug (see Chapter 9); host metabolism or modification of the drug will also influence the way it interacts with its target and the system as a whole. Every effect we study at the molecular or cellular levels may lead to complicated (and long-term) feedback processes at the population level. Thus host–pathogen systems biology has to be even more immodest than other branches of the fledgling discipline of systems biology: it encompasses all levels from molecules all the way up to epidemiological dynamics at the eco-system level.

References

1 FDA (2004) The Critical Path to New Medical Products. http://www.fda.gov/oc/initiatives/criticalpath/
2 Kan CW, Fredlake CP, Doherty EA, Barron AE (2004) DNA sequencing and genotyping in miniaturized electrophoresis systems. *Electrophoresis* 25: 3564–3588
3 McGall GH, Christians FC (2002) High-density genechip oligonucleotide probe arrays. *Adv Biochem Eng Biotechnol* 77: 21–42
4 van Steensel B (2005) Mapping of genetic and epigenetic regulatory networks using microarrays. *Nat Genet* 37 Suppl: S18–24
5 Allison DB, Cui X, Page GP, Sabripour M (2006) Microarray data analysis: from disarray to consolidation and consensus. *Nat Rev Genet* 7: 55–65
6 Hernandez P, Muller M, Appel RD (2006) Automated protein identification by tandem mass spectrometry: Issues and strategies. *Mass Spectrom Rev* 25: 235–254
7 Liebler DC (2004) Shotgun mass spec goes independent. *Nat Methods* 1: 16–17
8 Fields S (2005) High-throughput two-hybrid analysis. The promise and the peril. *Febs J* 272: 5391–5399
9 Puig O, Caspary F, Rigaut G, Rutz B, Bouveret E, Bragado-Nilsson E, Wilm M, Seraphin B (2001) The tandem affinity purification (TAP) method: a general procedure of protein complex purification. *Methods* 24: 218–229
10 Ren B, Dynlacht BD (2004) Use of chromatin immunoprecipitation assays in genome-wide location analysis of mammalian transcription factors. *Methods Enzymol* 376: 304–315
11 Ren B, Robert F, Wyrick JJ, Aparicio O, Jennings EG, Simon I, Zeitlinger J, Schreiber J, Hannett N, Kanin E et al (2000) Genome-wide location and function of DNA binding proteins. *Science* 290: 2306–2309
12 Haslam SM, Gems D, Morris HR, Dell A (2002) The glycomes of *Caenorhabditis elegans* and other model organisms. *Biochem Soc Symp*: 117–134
13 Doherty MK, Beynon RJ (2006) Protein turnover on the scale of the proteome. *Expert Rev Proteomics* 3: 97–110
14 Nicholson JK, Holmes E, Wilson ID (2005) Gut microorganisms, mammalian metabolism and personalized health care. *Nat Rev Microbiol* 3: 431–438
15 Kitano H, Oda K (2006) Robustness trade-offs and host-microbial symbiosis in the immune system. *Mol Syst Biol* 2 doi: 10.1038/msb4100039
16 Howard M, Kruse K (2005) Cellular organization by self-organization: mechanisms and models for Min protein dynamics. *J Cell Biol* 168: 533–536
17 Yuste R (2005) Fluorescence microscopy today. *Nat Methods* 2: 902–904
18 Doubrovinski K, Howard M (2005) Stochastic model for Soj relocation dynamics in *Bacillus subtilis*. *Proc Natl Acad Sci USA* 102: 9808–9813
19 Balaban NQ, Merrin J, Chait R, Kowalik L, Leibler S (2004) Bacterial persistence as a phenotypic switch. *Science* 305: 1622–1625
20 Kussell E, Kishony R, Balaban NQ, Leibler S (2005) Bacterial persistence: a model of survival in changing environments. *Genetics* 169: 1807–1814

21 Andries K, Verhasselt P, Guillemont J, Gohlmann HW, Neefs JM, Winkler H, Van Gestel J, Timmerman P, Zhu M, Lee E et al (2005) A diarylquinoline drug active on the ATP synthase of *Mycobacterium tuberculosis*. *Science* 307: 223–227

22 Manjunatha UH, Boshoff H, Dowd CS, Zhang L, Albert TJ, Norton JE, Daniels L, Dick T, Pang SS, Barry CE 3rd (2006) Identification of a nitroimidazo-oxazine-specific protein involved in PA-824 resistance in *Mycobacterium tuberculosis*. *Proc Natl Acad Sci USA* 103: 431–436

23 Boshoff HI, Myers TG, Copp BR, McNeil MR, Wilson MA, Barry CE 3rd (2004) The transcriptional responses of *Mycobacterium tuberculosis* to inhibitors of metabolism: novel insights into drug mechanisms of action. *J Biol Chem* 279: 40174–40184

24 Albert TJ, Dailidiene D, Dailide G, Norton JE, Kalia A, Richmond TA, Molla M, Singh J, Green RD, Berg DE (2005) Mutation discovery in bacterial genomes: metronidazole resistance in *Helicobacter pylori*. *Nat Methods* 2: 951–953

25 Margulies M, Egholm M, Altman WE, Attiya S, Bader JS, Bemben LA, Berka J, Braverman MS, Chen YJ, Chen Z et al (2005) Genome sequencing in microfabricated high-density picolitre reactors. *Nature* 437: 376–380

26 Nuwaysir EF, Huang W, Albert TJ, Singh J, Nuwaysir K, Pitas A, Richmond T, Gorski T, Berg JP, Ballin J et al (2002) Gene expression analysis using oligonucleotide arrays produced by maskless photolithography. *Genome Res* 12: 1749–1755

27 Fell D (1996) *Understanding the Control of Metabolism*. Portland Press Ltd, UK

28 Murray JD (2001) *Mathematical Biology: An Introduction: Pts. 1 & 2*. Springer-Verlag New York Inc, USA

29 Fulde P (1995) *Electron Correlations in Molecules and Solids*. Springer-Verlag Berlin and Heidelberg GmbH & Co, Germany

30 Nowak M, May R (2000) *Virus Dynamics: Mathematical Principles of Immunology and Virology*. Oxford University Press, UK

31 Crampin EJ, Halstead M, Hunter P, Nielsen P, Noble D, Smith N, Tawhai M (2004) Computational physiology and the Physiome Project. *Exp Physiol* 89: 1–26

32 Noble D (2006) Systems biology and the heart. *Biosystems* 83: 75–80

33 de Silva E, Stumpf MPH (2005) Complex networks and simple models in biology. *J Royal Soc Interface* 2: 419–430

34 Dobra A, Hans C, Jones B, Nevins JR, West M (2004) Sparse graphical models for exploring gene expression data. *J Multiv Analysis* 90: 196–212

35 Schafer J, Strimmer K (2005) An empirical Bayes approach to inferring large-scale gene association networks. *Bioinformatics* 21: 754–764

36 Schäfer J, Strimmer K (2005) Learning large-scale graphical Gaussian models from genomic data. In: JF Mendes (ed.): *Science of Complex Networks: from Biology to the Internet and WWW (CNET 2004)*, The American Institute of Physics, USA

37 Bollobas B (1985) *Random Graphs*. Academic Press Inc (London) Ltd, UK

38 Dorogovtsev SN, Mendes JFF (2003) *Evolution of Networks: From Biological Nets to the Internet and WWW*. Oxford University Press, UK

39 Newman MEJ (2003) The structure and function of complex networks. *SIAM Review* 45: 167–256
40 Alm E, Arkin AP (2003) Biological networks. *Curr Opin Struct Biol* 13: 193–202
41 May RM, Lloyd AL (2001) Infection dynamics on scale-free networks. *Phys Rev E Stat Nonlin Soft Matter Phys* 64: 066112
42 Gagneur J, Krause R, Bouwmeester T, Casari G (2004) Modular decomposition of protein–protein interaction networks. *Genome Biol* 5: R57
43 Hallinan J (2004) Gene duplication and hierarchical modularity in intracellular interaction networks. *Biosystems* 74: 51–62
44 Pereira-Leal JB, Enright AJ, Ouzounis CA (2004) Detection of functional modules from protein interaction networks. *Proteins* 54: 49–57
45 Agrafioti I, Swire J, Abbott J, Huntley D, Butcher S, Stumpf MP (2005) Comparative analysis of the *Saccharomyces cerevisiae* and *Caenorhabditis elegans* protein interaction networks. *BMC Evol Biol* 5: 23
46 Mazurie A, Bottani S, Vergassola M (2005) An evolutionary and functional assessment of regulatory network motifs. *Genome Biol* 6: R35
47 Gavin AC, Bosche M, Krause R, Grandi P, Marzioch M, Bauer A, Schultz J, Rick JM, Michon AM, Cruciat CM et al (2002) Functional organization of the yeast proteome by systematic analysis of protein complexes. *Nature* 415: 141–147
48 Ho Y, Gruhler A, Heilbut A, Bader GD, Moore L, Adams SL, Millar A, Taylor P, Bennett K, Boutilier K et al (2002) Systematic identification of protein complexes in *Saccharomyces cerevisiae* by mass spectrometry. *Nature* 415: 180–183
49 Ito T, Chiba T, Ozawa R, Yoshida M, Hattori M, Sakaki Y (2001) A comprehensive two-hybrid analysis to explore the yeast protein interactome. *Proc Natl Acad Sci USA* 98: 4569–4574
50 Giot L, Bader JS, Brouwer C, Chaudhuri A, Kuang B, Li Y, Hao YL, Ooi CE, Godwin B, Vitols E et al (2003) A protein interaction map of *Drosophila melanogaster*. *Science* 302: 1727–1736
51 Li S, Armstrong CM, Bertin N, Ge H, Milstein S, Boxem M, Vidalain PO, Han JD, Chesneau A, Hao T et al (2004) A map of the interactome network of the metazoan *C. elegans*. *Science* 303: 540–543
52 Rual JF, Venkatesan K, Hao T, Hirozane-Kishikawa T, Dricot A, Li N, Berriz GF, Gibbons FD, Dreze M, Ayivi-Guedehoussou N et al (2005) Towards a proteome-scale map of the human protein–protein interaction network. *Nature* 437: 1173–1178
53 Stelzl U, Worm U, Lalowski M, Haenig C, Brembeck FH, Goehler H, Stroedicke M, Zenkner M, Schoenherr A, Koeppen S et al (2005) A human protein–protein interaction network: a resource for annotating the proteome. *Cell* 122: 957–968
54 Fribourg S, Romier C, Werten S, Gangloff YG, Poterszman A, Moras D (2001) Dissecting the interaction network of multiprotein complexes by pairwise coexpression of subunits in *E. coli*. *J Mol Biol* 306: 363–373
55 LaCount DJ, Vignali M, Chettier R, Phansalkar A, Bell R, Hesselberth JR, Schoenfeld LW, Ota I, Sahasrabudhe S, Kurschner C et al (2005) A protein interaction network of the malaria parasite *Plasmodium falciparum*. *Nature* 438: 103–107

56 Bader JS, Chaudhuri A, Rothberg JM, Chant J (2004) Gaining confidence in high-throughput protein interaction networks. *Nat Biotechnol* 22: 78–85
57 von Mering C, Krause R, Snel B, Cornell M, Oliver SG, Fields S, Bork P (2002) Comparative assessment of large-scale data sets of protein–protein interactions. *Nature* 417: 399–403
58 Shen-Orr SS, Milo R, Mangan S, Alon U (2002) Network motifs in the transcriptional regulation network of *Escherichia coli. Nat Genet* 31: 64–68
59 Qiu P (2003) Recent advances in computational promoter analysis in understanding the transcriptional regulatory network. *Biochem Biophys Res Commun* 309: 495–501
60 Boffelli D, Nobrega MA, Rubin EM (2004) Comparative genomics at the vertebrate extremes. *Nat Rev Genet* 5: 456–465
61 Almaas E, Kovacs B, Vicsek T, Oltvai ZN, Barabasi AL (2004) Global organization of metabolic fluxes in the bacterium *Escherichia coli. Nature* 427: 839–843
62 Fell DA, Wagner A (2000) The small world of metabolism. *Nat Biotechnol* 18: 1121–1122
63 Barabasi AL, Albert R (1999) Emergence of scaling in random networks. *Science* 286: 509–512
64 Berg J, Lassig M, Wagner A (2004) Structure and evolution of protein interaction networks: a statistical model for link dynamics and gene duplications. *BMC Evol Biol* 4: 51
65 Burda Z, Correia JD, Krzywicki A (2001) Statistical ensemble of scale-free random graphs. *Phys Rev E Stat Nonlin Soft Matter Phys* 64: 046118
66 Stumpf MP, Wiuf C, May RM (2005) Subnets of scale-free networks are not scale-free: sampling properties of networks. *Proc Natl Acad Sci USA* 102: 4221–4224
67 Stumpf MPH, Ingram PJ, Nouvel I, Wiuf C (2005) Statistical model selection methods applied to biological networks. *Proc Comp Systems Biol* 3
68 Stewart GR, Patel J, Robertson BD, Rae A, Young DB (2005) Mycobacterial mutants with defective control of phagosomal acidification. *PLoS Pathog* 1: 269–278
69 Tong AH, Drees B, Nardelli G, Bader GD, Brannetti B, Castagnoli L, Evangelista M, Ferracuti S, Nelson B, Paoluzi S et al (2002) A combined experimental and computational strategy to define protein interaction networks for peptide recognition modules. *Science* 295: 321–324
70 Tong AH, Evangelista M, Parsons AB, Xu H, Bader GD, Page N, Robinson M, Raghibizadeh S, Hogue CW, Bussey H et al (2001) Systematic genetic analysis with ordered arrays of yeast deletion mutants. *Science* 294: 2364–2368
71 Uetz P, Dong YA, Zeretzke C, Atzler C, Baiker A, Berger B, Rajagopala SV, Roupelieva M, Rose D, Fossum E et al (2006) Herpesviral protein networks and their interaction with the human proteome. *Science* 311: 239–242
72 Perkins SL (2001) Phylogeography of Caribbean lizard malaria: tracing the history of vector-borne parasites. *J Evol Biol* 14: 34–45

Progress in Drug Research, Vol. 64
(Helena I. Boshoff and Clifton E. Barry III, Eds)

Applications of transcriptional profiling in antibiotics discovery and development

By Hans Peter Fischer[1]
and Christoph Freiberg[2]

[1]Genedata AG,
Postfach 254,
4016 Basel, Switzerland
<Hans-Peter.Fischer@genedata.com>

[2]Bayer HealthCare AG,
Pharma Research & Development
(current address:)
Niederrhein University of Applied Sciences,
Department of Chemistry,
Adlerstraße 32,
47798 Krefeld, Germany
<Christoph.Freiberg@hs-niederrhein.de>

Abstract

This chapter will review specific applications of microarray technology and related data analysis strategies in antibacterial research and development. We present examples of microarray applications spanning the entire antibiotics research and development pipeline, from target discovery, assay development, pharmacological evaluation, to compound safety studies. This review emphasizes the utility of microarrays for a systematic evaluation of novel chemistry as antibiotic agents. Transcriptional profiling has revolutionized the process of target elucidation and has the potential to offer substantial guidance in the identification of new targets. Microarrays will continue to be a workhorse of anti-infectives discovery programs ranging from efficacy assessments of antibiotics ('forward pharmacology') to drug safety evaluations ('toxicogenomics').

1 Introduction

Since Fleming's discovery of the antibacterial activity of penicillin in 1928, discovery efforts in antibiotic research were mainly based on random cell-based screening and on the modification of already established chemical structures with antibacterial activity. However, the traditional approaches to antibiotic discovery are increasingly challenged by bacterial pathogens that rapidly develop resistance to established drugs. Although classical approaches to anti-infective drug discovery are still being used, new technologies show promise to significantly accelerate the discovery and development of novel drugs that are required to keep up with the increasing incidence of drug resistance [1]. In this context, molecular profiling technologies that enable the highly parallel quantification of mRNA, proteins or metabolites in a bacterial cell have attracted significant attention. In this review, we focus on applications of mRNA profiling technologies, sometimes referred to as microarray or DNA chip technologies.

Microarray technologies have greatly benefited from the availability of whole genome sequence data. In 1995, the genomic DNA sequence of the bacterium *Haemophilus influenzae* was deciphered as the first genome of a cellular organism [2]. In the decade since then, the complete genomic information of the majority of medically relevant bacterial species has been made available. Today, hundreds of microbial genomes are publicly available and can be used for developing specialized expression profiling technologies. In parallel, microarray technology has advanced tremendously for the investigation of whole-genome transcription profiles. Miniaturized arrays carrying DNA probes immobilized on solid surfaces enable the simultaneous measurement of the abundance of each transcript within a cell. Such a highly-parallel quantification of the transcriptional activity of each cellular gene has been shown to be an extremely valuable indicator for the physiological status of a cell and can provide in-depth information into regulatory networks of gene expression [3, 4].

Transcriptional profiling has been shown to be capable of supporting infectious disease research in various ways. The many diagnostic, prophylactic and therapeutic approaches, which are currently followed, comprise vaccine design [5], probiotic strategies [6, 7], resistance monitoring [8, 9] and discovery of novel natural product-derived or chemically synthesized drugs. In this review, we focus on the discovery and development of novel antibacterial agents. Transcriptional profiling has proven to be a key technology with many applications along the drug discovery and development pipeline, including (1) target identification and validation, (2) efficacy mechanism-of-action (MOA) characterization of drug candidates, sometimes referred to as 'forward pharmacology', (3) development of novel types of whole-cell assays, including pathway-specific reporter assays and biomarker assays, and (4) prospective drug safety and toxicology studies (see Fig. 1). Lastly, we will conclude by discussing systems biology concepts that aim at relating transcription profiling and quantitative pathway simulations, and the impact of these new strategies on antibacterial research and development.

2 Transcriptional profiling – highly parallel measurement of gene expression

Microarrays enable the simultaneous measurement of the expression of virtually all genes in a bacterial cell. Thus, a microarray experiment provides in-depth information about the transcriptional activity of all pathways and functional systems in a cell. In technical terms, different microarray types can be used. Depending on array size and spot density, microarrays or chips (usually glass slides) and so-called 'macroarrays' (nylon membranes) can be distinguished. While polymerase chain reaction (PCR)-products

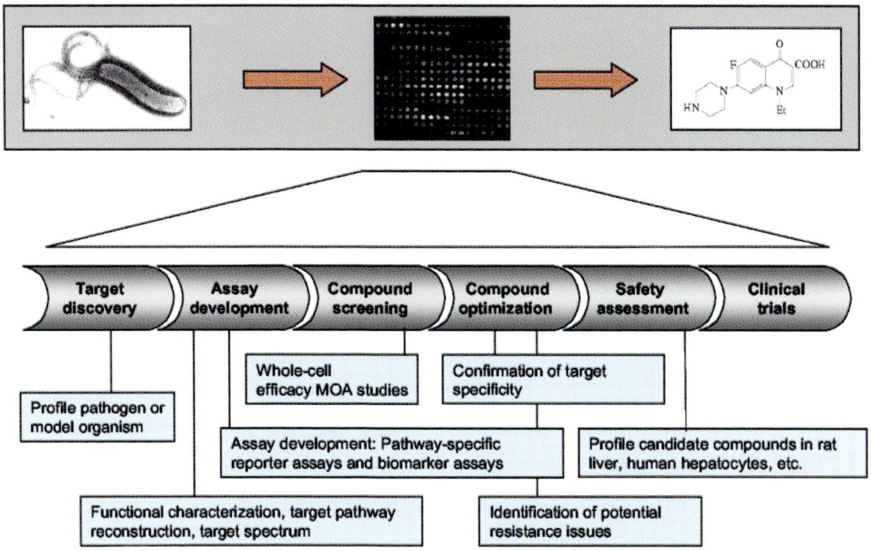

Figure 1.
Transcriptional profiling supports key steps of the antibiotics discovery and development pipeline. A schematic overview of the processes in which transcription profiling technologies are being used successfully or for which the potential utility of microarrays has been demonstrated. This includes (1) target identification and validation, (2) efficacy mechanism-of-action (MOA) characterization of drug candidates, (3) development of novel types of drug screening assays, and (4) prospective drug safety and toxicology studies (see text).

can be spotted on both types of arrays, oligonucleotides are generally immobilized on glass slides. For analysis of bacterial gene expression, PCR-products have the practical advantage that probes can be amplified directly from genomic DNA with each PCR-product representing one open reading frame (ORF) or gene. In fact, many of the currently available commercial microarrays are based on PCR products. However, the variable lengths of the PCR-products (especially for sequences shorter than 300 bp) and cross-hybridization of different transcripts to paralogous genes (typically for sequences showing >70% nucleotide identity over >200 bp sequence) may affect the specificity of the signals [10]. As a consequence, the PCR-based approach allows only the determination of the relative abundance of single transcripts when comparing two different samples. The PCR-based approach is not suitable for measuring the absolute amounts of different mRNA species, but is sensitive only to the fold changes of mRNA concentrations (which is why it is sometimes referred to as a 'two-channel technology'). By contrast, microarrays with gene-specific oligonucleotides of 50–100 bp are preferrable for measuring absolute mRNA concentrations [11]. Currently, the most commonly used oligonucleotide arrays are Affymetrix chips (http://www.affymetrix.com), which represent each gene by several pairs of perfectly matching oligonucleotides ('features') as well as mismatched controls. The feature signals can be used to estimate the absolute mRNA concentrations, using so-called 'condensing' algorithms. Remarkably, this oligonucleotide technology also allows for the experimental localization of the transcription start and termination sites as well as the determination of promoter sites and strand-specificity of bacterial mRNA [12].

About a decade ago, pre-made whole-genome microarrays were relatively pricey and only available for a few bacterial model organisms such as *Escherichia coli, Helicobacter pylori* and *Bacillus subtilis*. In addition, array suppliers often offered so-called 'custom-design' arrays, i.e., microarrays individually tailored to a customer's specific needs. However, the considerable set-up fees rendered this approach only viable for large-scale industrial research laboratories aiming at hundreds to thousands of microarray hybridization experiments per year. Apart from commercial suppliers, some laboratories have chosen to produce their own microarrays, as for instance successfully demonstrated at Stanford University (http://cmgm.stanford.edu/pbrown/mguide/index.html). Today, commercial off-the-shelf microarrays dominate the field. Commercial microarrays are now available for more and more bacterial species [13]. In the early days of microarray technologies, prokaryote-specific technical challenges of sample preparation including poor mRNA stability and the fact that bacterial transcripts lack polyadenlyation tails hindered the establishment of standardized experimental protocols for bacteria. In the meantime, optimized experimental protocols tailored to bacterial mRNA have been developed and are widely used within the microbiology research community. The recent drop in cost of commercial microarrays will certainly make transcriptional profiling more accessible for the various antimicrobial research applications in industrial as well as academic environments.

3 Comparison of the capabilities of transcriptomics and proteomics

RNA polymerase produces mRNA molecules, which represent the templates for protein synthesis. The transcriptome of a bacterial cell is therefore only an indirect indicator of a bacterium's physiological state, as it does not provide information about the proteins and metabolites, which determine the biochemical processes in the cell. Also, besides transcriptional control mechanisms, additional post-transcriptional processes can alter the amounts of active proteins, such as various translational control mechanisms as well as post-translational processes such as proteolysis and the processing and modification of proteins. However, several studies aimed at the comparison of the data derived from both mRNA and protein profiling technologies suggest that the majority of regulatory trends on the protein level are reflected by similar changes in the mRNA profiles [14–20]. Currently, proteomic technologies are not as well established as microarray technologies, especially with respect to reproducibility of data and ability to profile most of the protein species expressed at any one time, and protein analysis techniques are typically more labour-intensive due to their lower degree of automation. Also, some proteomic technologies such as the widely used 2-D gel electrophoresis technology focus only on the cytoplasmic subset of the cellular proteome, or are for technical reasons restricted to only a limited range of molecular weights and isoelectric values. Thus, microarray technology is advantageous for many drug discovery applications due to its comprehensive monitoring of all bacterial genes, its inherent high level of standardization and its ease-of-use. Nevertheless, protein profiling technologies are indispensable for studying processes on the post-transcriptional or post-translational level, such as for instance the effects caused by actinonin treatment [21, 22] (see Chapter 4).

4 The importance of experimental design and integrated data analysis systems

Any individual microarray experiment harbors a wealth of information, and many studies based on the biological interpretation of individual experiments have been published. However, the comparison of expression profiles across many different experimental conditions (e.g., different drug-induced stress responses) is of particular interest for understanding a bacterium's regulatory network. Incorporating larger numbers of microarray experiments enables comparisons based on statistical analyses, a critical requirement for well-educated decision making in pharmaceutical research. For instance, the comparison of a pathogen's transcriptional response to structurally different growth inhibitors is critical for deducing the regulatory networks underlying a pathogen's drug defense mechanisms or to predict mechanisms-of-actions (MOAs) of novel antibiotic structures. When dealing with such data sets, two major challenges arise.

Firstly, consistent and standardized conditions for drug treatment such as concentrations and exposure times have to be carefully chosen to enable comparison of profiles triggered by different compounds. Typically, compound concentrations are measured in units of the minimal inhibitory concentration (MIC), while treatment times are normally measured in units of the average bacterial replication time. For instance, previous studies report as optimal treatment times for *B. subtilis* a range of a few minutes after compound exposure up to more than one generation time (e.g., >40 minutes for *B. subtilis* in minimal medium [23]). The recent *B. subtilis* reference compendia approaches suggest that the optimal concentration window for compound MOA studies lies in the order of magnitude of the MIC, although generally concentrations are required that do not result in more than 15–25 % reduction of growth rate [24, 25].

Secondly, the typically large datasets comprising hundreds to thousands of experiments require standardized and statistically well-founded approaches. While standard clustering algorithms work well with relatively small data sets as has been successfully applied to the mRNA profiles induced by three anti-tuberculosis agents [26], the results of such methods are difficult to interpret when comparing dozens or more of stress-induced mRNA profiles. Also, most unsupervised clustering methods do not provide objective decision rules for characterizing the MOA of novel compounds. As known from studies with eukaryotic systems, more elaborate statistical methods are needed to optimally compare, cluster, categorize and annotate experiments and expression-relevant genes. For instance, algorithms that have been suggested for MOA classification purposes include support vector machines (SVMs), K-Nearest Neighbor Analysis, and Sparse Linear Discriminant Analysis [27–31]. Typically, in pharmaceutical research, whole data analysis workflow systems are required to systematically analyze drug-induced expression profiles in a standardized manner. Interactive, highly integrated visualization tools are required to discover trends in large and complex data sets (see Fig. 2). These systems can be set up and configured to combine sample and experiment data management systems with various normalization, filtering and statistical algorithms.

5 Discovering therapeutic targets

Despite the availability of so many complete genome sequences, the functions of many genes remain unclear, in particular if they share little sequence similarity with genes of known function. Expression profiling can be an efficient way to functionally characterize such genes. Co-expression of functionally uncharacterized genes across many experiments with others, of which the functional roles are known, indicates that the corresponding gene products are likely to be involved in the same pathway or protein complex. For instance, genes involved in motility and chemotaxis are controlled by an alternative sigma factor in many bacteria, which is part of the RNA polymerase complex. In the model bacterium *B. subtilis* the corresponding regulatory network could be comprehensively mapped by the identification of genes that are co-expressed with this sigma factor [13]. Using this approach, genes of unknown function could be functionally characterized. Similarly, expression profiles of bacteria growing under conditions thought to mimic the relevant environment of the organism during parasitism of the host, can lead to a more profound understanding of a pathogen's cellular processes during infection. For instance, transcriptional profiling of the lyme disease causing agent *Borrelia burgdorferi* under conditions simulating parasitism of the tick vector or during adaption to its mammalian host revealed a set of 150 genes that were differentially regulated in these environments [32]. This information enables the formulation of new testable hypotheses regarding the life cycle and virulence mechanisms of *B. burgdorferi*.

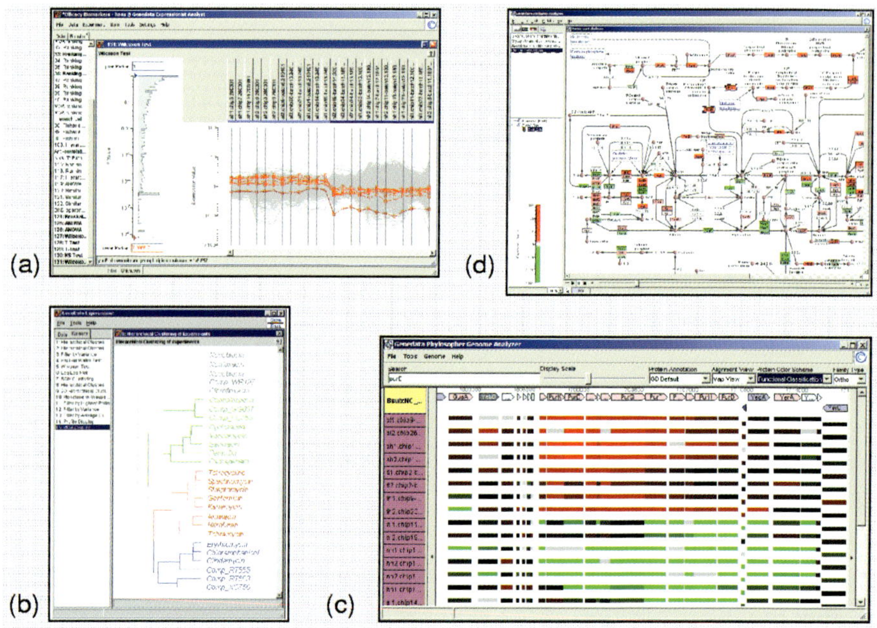

Figure 2.
Interpreting bacterial expression profiles requires integrated computational systems for a comprehensive statistical analysis and biological context analysis. (a) P-value distribution of *B. subtilis* genes expression profiles (left) when comparing the effect of treatment with trimethoprim (blue horizontal bar) and a quinolone (violet horizontal bar), both representing DNA replication inhibitors. The gene expression profiles discriminating best between the two compounds are colored in red. (b) Hierarchical clustering of antibiotics-induced gene expression profiles, based on the transcriptional activity of only a limited number of MOA-biomarkers. The visualized tree reflects the major categories of antibiotic mechanisms-of-action: inhibition of DNA replication (grey), cell wall biosynthesis (green), and protein biosynthesis (red and blue). (c) Integrating expression data and genome structure data to identify antibiotics-responsive operons. Tailored algorithms have been developed that consider whole genome organizations and microarray data across many different antibiotic stress experiments. The top row shows a subsection of the *B. subtilis* genome sequence with arrows corresponding to individual genes, while the rows underneath represent individual experiments, with the expression induction levels represented as red rectangles (= upregulated) and green rectangles (= downregulated). (d) Pathway context analysis. By overlaying expression data onto metabolic-, regulatory- or signaling pathway maps, new functional relationships can be discovered. Here, the characteristic response of the *B. subtilis* nucleotide biosynthesis pathway to treatment with the antibiotic novobiocin is demonstrated. Pathway context analyses are also very helpful for understanding a pathogen's resistance and defense mechanisms (screenshots from Genedata Expressionist® and Genedata Phylosopher®).

Expression profiling was also instrumental in identifying novel therapeutic targets in innovative approaches aimed at reduction of drug resistance or virulence of pathogens. For instance, studies with *Pseudomonas aeruginosa*, a medically relevant pathogen that infects especially immunocompromised individuals such as cystic fibrosis patients, have been utilized in approaches to develop drugs that target its virulence factors. *Pseudomonas* infections are extremely difficult to treat due to limited drug permeability through the cell envelope, very efficient drug efflux systems, and the capacity of the organism to form drug-resistant biofilms. *Pseudomonas* cells are known to communicate with each other via signaling molecules such as acyl-homoserine lactones which trigger expression of genes belonging to the so-called quorum-sensing regulon. Quorum-sensing is suspected to play an important role in chronic bacterial colonization leading to drug resistant biofilms. Hentzer et al. isolated a furanone derivative that was reported to block quorum-sensing [33]. Microarrays were used to obtain a transcriptional 'fingerprint' of the compound, showing that its underlying MOA is quorum-sensing inhibition. Rasmussen et al. found additional inhibitors of quorum-sensing in extracts of *Penicillium* strains [34]. In this study, microarrays were also used to determine the target specificity of those compounds. Such studies are pioneering the identification of novel targets of chemical entities that interfere with virulence or resistance mechanisms of bacteria.

In contrast to the previous examples, it should be noted that the targets currently preferred in the pharmaceutical industry are *in vitro* and *in vivo* essential targets, which are expressed under all growth conditions in a bacterium. In fact, the targets inhibited by the anti-infectives established in medicinal practice are largely represented by such 'essential' gene products. In the last decade, a number of genomics technologies such as parallel gene knock-out and conditional silencing methods have allowed the identification of most of the *in vitro* essential gene products of major bacterial pathogens (for a review, see [35, 36]). Although systematic knock-outs potentially reveal all essential genes by virtue of the inability to disrupt all ORFs, they do not provide any direct hints about their function; however, functional information is critical for developing target-based screening assays [37]. Expression profiling may be considered a complementary technology for elucidating the molecular and cellular function of uncharacterized essential genes. Thus, expression profiling has become a key component in the early stages of the antibacterial target discovery and validation process, supporting classical discovery strategies, but also guiding the way to innovative targets intended to interfere with the pathogen's resistance or virulence mechanisms.

6 Forward pharmacology

The systematic screening and characterization of compound libraries using microarrays is increasingly attracting attention. Natural product libraries as well as synthetic compound banks have great potential for harboring novel anti-infective lead structures; however, the systematic evaluation of their mechanisms is hampered by conceptual and technical hurdles. The measurement of changes in cellular mRNA levels triggered by compound treatment can help in elucidating the inhibitory mechanism of poorly understood drug candidates. Such compound-centric strategies aiming at deducing a chemical entity's cellular MOA are sometimes referred to as 'chemogenomics' [38] or 'forward pharmacology' [39]. In the context of the pharmaceutical drug discovery process, 'forward pharmacology' seems the most appropriate term, since the MOA identification represents an essential step in order to pharmacologically characterize a drug candidate. Indeed, microarrays were key in demonstrating that effects on the transcriptional level can be related to the physiological functions targeted by the respective compounds [14, 26, 40–43]. However, drugs generally also change the expression of a wide range of genes not directly linked to the target's function, which can obscure the primary antibiotic effect [44]. For instance, Brazas and Hancock discovered that the fluoroquinolone ciprofloxacin induces toxic gene products (so-called pyocins derived from latently integrated bacteriophages in the genome) making certain *Pseudomonas* strains more susceptible than the corresponding mutants with inactivated pyocin genes. Such induced pyocin genes are not the molecular target of ciprofloxacin or other fluoroquinolones, but obviously mediate antibiotic susceptibility [45].

To systematically deduce characteristic transcriptional 'fingerprints' that can be associated with specific drug mechanisms, the use of a comprehensive collection of diverse expression profiles that represent different cellular stress states (a so-called 'reference compendium approach') has been suggested. In an early pioneering study, Hughes et al. measured the levels of 6,000 yeast transcripts of knock-out mutants as well as compound-stressed cells, leading to expression profiles corresponding to 300 different physiological cell states [46]. Solely by a basic comparison and clustering of mRNA profiles, the topical anesthetic dyclonine, a drug with an as yet unknown MOA, could be predicted to interfere with ergosterol biosynthesis. This early yeast-based study pointed the way to how comparative expression analyses can be used for systematically classifying MOAs of anti-infectives with previously unknown targets. Since industrial antibacterial research has been primarily focused on combating multi-resistant Gram-positive bacteria, the phylogenetically related but non-pathogenic species *B. subtilis* has been chosen to become the first model bacterium for functional genomics-based antibacterial drug discovery. Freiberg et al. and Hutter et al. investigated the genome-wide transcriptional response of *B. subtilis* to a variety of drugs [24, 25]. These studies demonstrated the feasibility of microarray-based MOA classifications for antibacterial agents. For instance, the mechanism of inhibition by a novel antibacterial class of phenyl-thiazolylurea-sulfonamides originating from a lead optimization program on a screening hit from a biochemical target assay could be correctly characterized, just using the characteristic whole-genome expression response of *B. subtilis* to this compound. A comparison with a comprehensive expression profile compendium revealed that these compounds triggered the increased expression of the direct target phenylalanyl-tRNA synthetase as well as the stringent response, a regulatory event that was shown to be typical for aminoacyl-tRNA synthetase inhibition [24]. Similarly, a study using the pathogen *Mycobacterium tuberculosis* successfully demonstrated how a database of transcriptional profiles for diverse sets of drugs and growth-inhibitory conditions enabled to predict MOAs of agents lacking any mechanistic information [31]. For instance, the pyridoacridine alkaloid ascididemin, known to show anti-tumor, antiparasitic and anti-mycobacterial activity, was predicted to interfere with iron acquisition processes in *Mycobacterium tuberculosis,* a hypothesis that was subsequently independently validated. In addition, the upregulation of respiratory genes during treatment of *Mycobacterium tuberculosis* with phenothiazines led to the hypothesis that this class of drugs interfered with dehydrogenase function in the respiratory chain which was subsequently biochemically confirmed.

As the prediction of MOAs of uncharacterized substances is typically done by comparing the compound-induced mRNA profile with the ones triggered by reference compounds, it is important that the reference database includes compound-triggered mRNA profiles representing a broad variety of MOAs. However, for completely novel mechanisms the absence of reference compounds in the reference compendium means that MOA can not be elucidated based on simple comparison and/or clustering of transcriptional profiles. It has been proposed that this conceptual difficulty can be overcome by including mRNA profiles derived from mutants in which expression of genes representing potentially novel antimicrobial targets is controlled by regulatable promoters or by temperature sensitive mutations. The genetic downregulation of the target was proposed to mimic chemical inhibition of the gene product, resulting in similar mRNA profiles as would be expected during treatment with an inhibitor targeting the gene product under investigation. Again, studies using yeast were used to pioneer this strategy by including transcriptional profiles of promoter 'shut-off' strains for essential genes in the reference compendium [47]. Di Bernardo et al. used an expression profile compendium including the mRNA profiles of 215 strains carrying down-regulatable promoters upstream of essential genes as well as 300 additional profiles [38, 46]. The validity of their approach was proven by predicting the thioredoxin–thioredoxin reductase system as the target of the mechanistically uncharacterized anti-cancer compound (1-phenyl-1H-tetrazol-5-ylsulfonyl-butanenitrile; PTSB) which was subsequently independently confirmed.

In contrast to yeast, however, the experimental handling of conditional mutants under-expressing essential genes is non-trivial for many bacteria. In bacteria essential genes often need to be repressed by more than 99% in order to have an impact on the growth curves. Bacterial promoter systems are often too leaky to result in a transcriptional profile that clearly represents the cellular response that attempts to counteract the simulated effects of a chemical inhibitor of the gene under investigation. Thus, large-scale bacterial applications as required for reference compendium strategies are hampered for technical reasons. Nevertheless, in a recent proof-of-concept study, it could be shown that the approach of supplementing chemical reference compendia with conditional mutant profiles can be utilized successfully in bacteria. Expression profiles of *B. subtilis* conditional mutants enabled a characterization of the MOA of the natural product moiramide B, a compound known to possess antibacterial activity [24]. As a result of these studies, moiramide B was predicted to be the first antibiotic targeting the bacterial acetyl-CoA carboxylase. Moiramide B triggered a characteristic transcriptional response strongly resembling the profiles of mutants downregulating the enzyme's corresponding subunits. This example demonstrates that transcriptional profiling can lead to testable hypotheses, providing insights into drug-pathway or even drug-target interactions that were not previously anticipated. Indeed, the inhibition of the acetyl-CoA carboxylase by moiramide B could be independently confirmed by biochemical and genetic tests [48], validating the general applicability of reference compendium strategies for the elucidation of completely novel antibacterial mechanisms.

7 Developing reporter assays for pathway-specific compound screens

Reporter strains using gene promoters showing a transcriptional activation that is a signature for a specific MOA have been recognized as an efficient way to detect bioactive compounds interfering with specific pathways [13]. Such assays combine the advantages of the traditional whole-cell screening approaches and the directed, rational strategies of target-based assays. For the MOA-reporter assay approach, drug stress-specific promoters are fused to reporter genes such as the firefly luciferase gene. The resulting reporter strains are then used for assaying pathway-specific antibacterial compounds, and are typically applied in high-throughput compound library screening. Currently, the major bottleneck for following this approach is the identification of appropriately responding MOA-specific promoters. Microarray data have been shown to be key in the systematic discovery of suitable promoters for reporter assay development [49–51]. Microarrays are used to elucidate the regulatory architecture of the bacterial stress response to identify and characterize drug-responsive regulatory

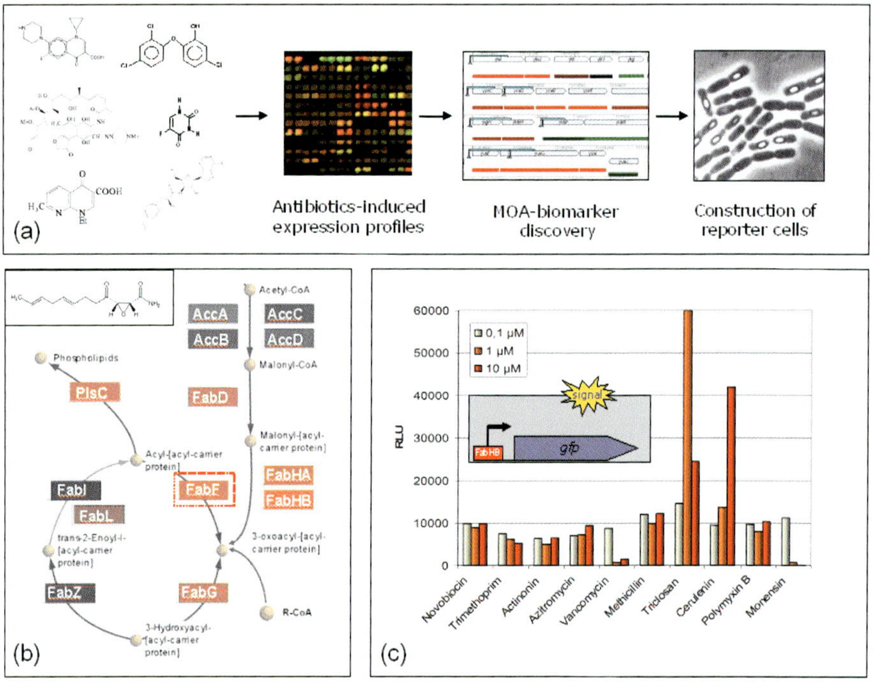

Figure 3.
A microarray-guided approach to drug screening assay development and high-throughput compound screening. To develop cell-based reporter assays, promoters are needed that respond in a highly mechanism-specific manner to compound exposure. An application from antibacterial drug discovery is exemplified in (a–c). A series of mRNA profiles representing the stress response of *B. subtilis* to various antibiotics has been analyzed to pinpoint stress-specific promoters (MOA biomarkers) in the context of the intended target pathway. The promoters are fused to a reporter gene resulting in reporter cells appropriate for high-throughput drug screening (a). In this example, fatty acid biosynthesis represents the target pathway of interest. The color-coded pathway activation pattern displayed in (b) reflects the pathways' reaction to exposure with cerulenin, a compound known to inhibit the gene product FabF (red dotted frame). Red rectangles indicate an upregulation of the respective genes, while the black rectangles correspond to non-responsive genes. This information is critical for identifying optimal promoters for reporter assay development (modified after [49], Phylosopher®, Genedata, Basel). Subsequently, a fatty acid pathway-specific reporter assay was developed, based on a new stress-inducible promoter (FabHB). The experimental validation of this data-driven approach is shown in (c). Luminescent light signals of the reporter assay were measured in response to ten antibiotics of different mechanisms-of-action. Significant signals are only detected for cerulenin and triclosan, the two fatty acid biosynthesis inhibitors among the tested antibiotics.

networks. Co-expressed genes and operons are generally controlled by the same transcriptional regulators, so that it is likely that they share common regulatory elements, such as transcription factor binding sites. The combination of DNA sequence-motif detection algorithms and expression-based correlation analyses allows a prediction of promoters controlling specific bacterial stress regulons. A genome-wide, systematic approach based on microarray data has been proposed by Fischer et al. [49]. In this study, microarray data was used to reconstruct the *B. subtilis* FapR-dependent regulon and to identify promoters whose activation is indicative of fatty acid biosynthesis stress (see Fig. 3). Indeed, Fischer et al. were able to construct assays based on the *in-silico* predictions and applied them successfully in a high-throughput screening setting. From the 900,000 screened compounds, more than 500 hits were identified, including at least four chemically novel types of structural hit clusters. These novel compounds were independently shown to efficiently inhibit the fatty acid biosynthesis pathway.

Systematic MOA-biomarker discovery strategies based on transcriptional profiling technologies produce significantly more suitable promoters than the traditional approaches based on classical low-throughput technologies [52–56]. Today, microarray-supported reporter assay development is instrumental in the systematic application of this elegant approach to detect bioactive compounds interfering with specific pathways.

8 Improving the compound selection and optimization process

The examples outlined above for mRNA profiling-based MOA predictions demonstrate the major contributions of transcriptional profiling to the early phases of the drug discovery process. However, microarray experiments are of great value even further downstream in the drug development pipeline, namely in the lead finding and chemical development process. Compounds identified in library screening campaigns of target-based assays might be profiled in order to confirm that their MOA against whole cells recapitulates the *in vitro* predictions. Transcriptional profiling is also used to prioritize compounds based on indications of undesirable side effects, such as transcriptional induction of detoxification or drug efflux systems. For instance, studies investigating the effect of triclosan on *M. tuberculosis* exhibit a striking upregulation of such bacterial defense systems [31]. Similarly, various antibacterial agents with aromatic character induce mycobacterial genes most likely involved in drug efflux and in detoxification such as monooxygenase, dioxygenase and methylase genes. Thus, expression profiling can aid in a systematic prioritization of screening hit compounds by focusing on the molecules showing no or little indications of drug resistance in their transcriptional response.

Chemical derivatisation programs following target-based screening campaigns typically result in large lead compound series. Important downstream profiling challenges such as cell penetration, pharmacokinetic stability, physicochemical profile and others cannot directly be addressed by expression profiling. However, there are valuable applications of transcriptional profiling for assessing and evaluating chemistry. For instance, it is well known that agents from natural product sources represent an attractive pool for finding novel antibiotic lead structures. Therefore, starting with a purified or *de novo* synthesized natural product and applying a forward pharmacology approach is extremely helpful to accelerate discovery programs such as described for the above-mentioned moiramide B [24]. Boshoff et al. report that crude extracts containing mixtures of different natural products can in some instances be successfully screened in transcriptional profiling experiments, since key metabolic responses can be observed within the expression patterns induced by the extracts [31]. Using this approach, the labor-intensive process of isolation of the active principle can be guided by microarray experiments, enabling an early prioritization of extracts with respect to novel or preferred MOAs.

Further downstream in the process of antibacterial drug development, expression profiling compendia are used to predict the target selectivity of compounds derived from chemical derivatization programs. For instance, in the case of acivicin, an antibacterial inhibitor reported to block histidine biosynthesis, the complex transcriptional response pattern of this compound led to the conclusion that additional off-target effects could contribute to bacterial growth inhibition [57]. The validation or rejection of such hypotheses can be optimally addressed by profile comparisons with a 'training set' of mRNA profiles derived from diverse nonspecifically acting compounds. Using this approach, expression profiling has promise of becoming an established tool for directing chemical derivatisation programs and for prioritising compounds with respect to target selectivity.

9 Assessing drug safety and toxicology

Microarray-based strategies are increasingly used not only to predict drug efficacy, but also to assess a compound's toxicity potential. The underlying hypothesis of this so-called 'toxicogenomics' approach (see also Chapter 9) is that toxicant-specific expression patterns in animals or cell lines can help in an early identification of antibiotics candidates that will exhibit adverse side effects. Previous studies showed that mRNA profiles generally agree with what is known from complementary methods, for both expression in tissues from animals treated *in vivo* and for cell cultures treated *in vitro* [58–62]. For instance, it has been reported that a compendium of expression patterns representing the transcriptional response of rats to liver toxins, enables prospective classification of potential hepatoxic mechanisms for development compounds [63]. Probably the most relevant applications of toxicogenomics lies in the detection of toxic effects that cannot be detected during preclinical or early phases of clinical trials [64, 65]. Idiosyncratic toxicity represents such a type of effect, which is known among others to be host dependent, i.e., the toxic effect cannot be detected in animals, but only in some human patients. For instance, the antibiotic trovafloxacin inhibiting the bacterial DNA gyrase and topoisomerase IV belongs to a generally well tolerated class of quinolones. Before the regulatory approval of trovafloxacin in 1997 there were no cases of hepatic failure in more than 7,000 patients. Since then, more than 2 million people have received this drug, resulting in 150 cases of reported liver toxicity [66]; however, the exact mechanism underlying this rare adverse effect has not yet been determined. Recently, it has been reported that comparative transcriptional profiling of trovafloxacin and other quinolones using isolated human hepatocytes revealed unique changes in mRNA levels triggered in the cells treated with trovafloxacin. Apparently, trovafloxacin causes mitochondrial damage and severely affects cellular functions which might cause hepatotoxicity [66]. It remains to be shown whether these studies will help in identifying distinct genes or gene groups that could serve as biomarkers for predicting a patient's risk for idiosyncratic hepatotoxicity.

10 Conclusion

Today, expression profiling analyses are firmly established in the pharmaceutical industry, in both the early drug discovery phases, as well as during later chemical development stages. Biomarker discovery strategies relying on transcriptional profiling are an emerging, highly useful, tool derived from microarray technology. Biomarker-based assays are already used to screen for novel chemotypes inhibiting specific targets or target pathways on a high-throughput scale.

Although driven by anti-infectives development, microarray technology has had many spin-off benefits. Microarrays are, for example, utilized for the development of pathogen diagnostic kits. These kits are employed in measuring strain-specific mRNA profiles. Related technologies are increasingly used for the identification of the genotype of bacterial strains by hybridizing genomic DNA on microarrays carrying oligonucleotides that cover the full genome sequence of the reference strain of the pathogen. This technique was performed for *Helicobacter pylori* [67], a bacterium that was discovered in 1982 by Marshall and Warren (for which they were awarded the Nobel Prize in 2005) as the infectious agent responsible for gastric ulcer disease [68]. *Helicobacter pylori* is distributed in at least half of the world's population with the many genomic variants of this bacterium determining pathogenesis and drug susceptibility [69]. The identification of bacterial polymorphisms allows a prediction of the resistance patterns that may be encountered when treating a patient. Hybridizing genomic DNA derived from a clinical isolate on microarrays containing oligonucleotides representing the sequenced reference strain can be used to identify deletions and mismatches hereby characterizing the exact nature of the infection in the patient which, in turn, would support tailored treatment strategies. Improving the currently existing diagnostic tools is an essential prerequisite for more focused therapies, because only a rapid detection of the causative agent and the properties of the expressed genes of the isolate allows for treatments based on narrow-spectrum antimicrobials

[70]. In addition, diagnostic microarrays are expected to provide the basis for a rational design of molecularly defined vaccines to replace poorly defined vaccines based on killed or attenuated pathogens, extracts thereof or on toxins inactivated by chemical treatment [5, 71, 72].

At the same time, with prices of microarrays decreasing to levels that are in reach of the majority of research institutions, a substantial increase in experimental throughput can be expected, so that high-content screening by entirely microarray-based approaches may become routine practice in the future. Microarrays would then allow for a direct evaluation of large compound libraries by probing the compound's effect on the whole bacterial cell. In this way, standardized, highly automated screens for the most efficacious compounds will significantly facilitate the search for novel antimicrobial lead structures. Transcriptional profiling information derived from microarray analyses is providing the groundwork for applications in systems biology. In the context of this review, the most noteworthy systems biology applications are dynamic pathway models that enable a numeric simulation of the temporal and spatial behavior of signaling and metabolic pathways. In fact, such comprehensive, predictive models of the cell will significantly facilitate the target selection process, and will undoubtedly lead to a better understanding of a pathogen's defence and resistance mechanisms. For some prokaryotic and eukaryotic model organisms, first proof-of-concept studies have been published (for example [73–76]). These studies indicate that the development of mathematical models that capture the essential features of metabolic or signaling pathways in a cell are indeed possible. For bacteria, initial studies have been published that aim at reverse-engineering the network of regulatory interactions between genes to determine the pathways and genes targeted by a compound [38]. As most systems biology studies address the investigation of large-scale properties of pathway networks, whole-genome transcription profiling will add important experimental proof for supporting specific mathematical models. Microarray data will also help in formulating hypotheses for expanding and refining existing models, for instance by fitting kinetic parameters to determine critical reaction constants.

Functional genomics technologies beyond transcription profiling can supplement the data that is required for gaining a better understanding of the integrated cellular system. Newly developed proteomics technologies (see for example [77] and Chapter 4) as well as innovative technologies for the parallel quantification of all cellular metabolites ('metabolic profiling' or metabolomics [78], Chapter 5) and metabolic flux patterns [79] represent essential building blocks in getting a holistic view of the bacterial cell. Together with integrative computational systems biology approaches these data will lay the foundation for successfully modeling the dynamics of biochemical pathways and complex physiological processes. Undoubtedly, such studies will have a major impact on our current understanding of the physiology of microbial pathogens, the human host's immune response to infection, as well as the effect of chemotherapy on the infectious agent and the host. This, in turn, will become a solid basis for discovering and developing innovative antimicrobials for combating infectious disease. Transcriptional profiling will undoubtedly continue to play an indispensable role in this process.

Acknowledgements

We are grateful to N. Brunner, L. Macko, and J. Cox for stimulating discussions and to O. Pfannes for critically reading the manuscript.

References

1 Spellberg B, Powers J, Brass E, Miller L, Edwards J Jr. (2004) Trends in antimicrobial drug development: implications for the future. *Clin Infect Dis* 38: 1279–1286

2 Fleischmann R, Adams M, White O, Clayton R, Kirkness E, Kerlavage A, Bult C, Tomb J, Dougherty B, Merrick J et al (1995) Whole-genome random sequencing and assembly of *Haemophilus influenzae* Rd. *Science* 269: 496–512

3 Goodman AL, Lory S (2004) Analysis of regulatory networks in *Pseudomonas aeruginosa* by genomewide transcriptional profiling. *Curr Opin Microbiol* 7: 39–44

4 Conway T, Schoolnik G (2003) Microarray expression profiling: capturing a genome-wide portrait of the transcriptome. *Mol Microbiol* 47: 879–889

5 Grandi G (2003) Rational antibacterial vaccine design through genomic technologies. *Int J Parasitol* 33: 615–620

6 Isolauri E, Salminen S, Ouwehand AC (2004) Probiotics. *Best Pract Res Clin Gastroenterol* 18: 299–313

7 Reid G, Gan BS, She YM, Ens W, Weinberger S, Howard JC (2002) Rapid identification of probiotic lactobacillus biosurfactant proteins by ProteinChip tandem mass spectrometry tryptic peptide sequencing. *Appl Environ Microbiol* 68: 977–980

8 Cui L, Lian JQ, Neoh HM, Reyes E, Hiramatsu K (2005) DNA microarray-based identification of genes associated with glycopeptide resistance in *Staphylococcus aureus*. *Antimicrob Agents Chemother* 49: 3404–3413

9 Morris RP, Nguyen L, Gatfield J, Visconti K, Nguyen K, Schnappinger D, Ehrt S, Liu Y, Heifets L, Pieters J et al (2005) Ancestral antibiotic resistance in *Mycobacterium tuberculosis*. *Proc Natl Acad Sci USA* 102: 12200–12205

10 Richmond C, Glasner J, Mau R, Jin H, Blattner F (1999) Genome-wide expression profiling in *Escherichia coli* K-12. *Nucleic Acids Res* 27: 3821–3835

11 Kane MD, Jatkoe TA, Stumpf CR, Lu J, Thomas JD, Madore SJ (2000) Assessment of the sensitivity and specificity of oligonucleotide (50mer) microarrays. *Nucleic Acids Res* 28: 4552–4557

12 Selinger DW, Saxena RM, Cheung KJ, Church GM, Rosenow C (2003) Global RNA half-life analysis in *Escherichia coli* reveals positional patterns of transcript degradation. *Genome Res* 13: 216–223

13 Freiberg C, Brunner NA (2002) Genome-wide mRNA profiling: impact on compound evaluation and target identification in anti-bacterial research. *Targets* 1: 20–29

14 Gmuender H, Kuratli K, Di Padova K, Gray CP, Keck W, Evers S (2001) Gene expression changes triggered by exposure of *Haemophilus influenzae* to novobiocin or ciprofloxacin: combined transcription and translation analysis. *Genome Res* 11: 28–42

15 Evers S, Di Padova K, Meyer M, Langen H, Fountoulakis M, Keck W, Gray CP (2001) Mechanism-related changes in the gene transcription and protein synthesis patterns of *Haemophilus influenzae* after treatment with transcriptional and translational inhibitors. *Proteomics* 1: 522–544

16 Betts J, Lukey P, Robb L, McAdam R, Duncan K (2002) Evaluation of a nutrient starvation model of *Mycobacterium tuberculosis* persistence by gene and protein expression profiling. *Mol Microbiol* 43: 717–731

17 Arfin SM, Long AD, Ito ET, Tolleri L, Riehle MM, Paegle ES, Hatfield GW (2000) Global gene expression profiling in *Escherichia coli* K12 – The effects of integration host factor. *J Biol Chem* 275: 29672–29684

18 Eymann C, Homuth G, Scharf C, Hecker M (2002) *Bacillus subtilis* functional genomics: global characterization of the stringent response by proteome and transcriptome analysis. *J Bacteriol* 184: 2500–2520

19 Khodursky AB, Peter BJ, Cozzarelli NR, Botstein D, Brown PO, Yanofsky C (2000) DNA microarray analysis of gene expression in response to physiological and genetic changes that affect tryptophan metabolism in *Escherichia coli*. *Proc Natl Acad Sci USA* 97: 12170–12175

20 Yoshida K, Kobayashi K, Miwa Y, Kang C, Matsunaga M, Yamaguchi H, Tojo S, Yamamoto M, Nishi R, Ogasawara N et al (2001) Combined transcriptome and proteome analysis as a powerful approach to study genes under glucose repression in *Bacillus subtilis*. *Nucleic Acids Res* 29: 683–692

21 Bandow JE, Becher D, Buttner K, Hochgrafe F, Freiberg C, Brotz H, Hecker M (2003) The role of peptide deformylase in protein biosynthesis: A proteomic study. *Proteomics* 3: 299–306

22 Bandow JE, Brötz H, Leichert LI, Labischinski H, Hecker M (2003) Proteomic approach to understanding antibiotic action. *Antimicrob Agents Chemother* 47: 948–955
23 Stulke J, Hanschke R, Hecker M (1993) Temporal activation of beta-glucanase synthesis in *Bacillus subtilis* is mediated by the GTP pool. *J Gen Microbiol* 139 (Pt 9): 2041–2045
24 Freiberg C, Fischer HP, Brunner NA (2005) Discovering the mechanism of action of novel antibacterial agents through transcriptional profiling of conditional mutants. *Antimicrob Agents Chemother* 49: 749–759
25 Hutter B, Schaab C, Albrecht S, Borgmann M, Brunner NA, Freiberg C, Ziegelbauer K, Rock CO, Ivanov I, Loferer H (2004) Prediction of mechanisms of action of antibacterial compounds by gene expression profiling. *Antimicrob Agents Chemother* 48: 2838–2844
26 Betts JC, McLaren A, Lennon MG, Kelly FM, Lukey PT, Blakemore SJ, Duncan K (2003) Signature gene expression profiles discriminate between isoniazid-, thiolactomycin-, and triclosan-treated *Mycobacterium tuberculosis*. *Antimicrob Agents Chemother* 47: 2903–2913
27 Gunther EC, Stone DJ, Gerwien RW, Bento P, Heyes MP, Staunton JE, Slonim DK, Coller HA, Tamayo P, Angelo MJ et al (2003) Prediction of clinical drug efficacy by classification of drug-induced genomic expression profiles *in vitro*. *Proc Natl Acad Sci USA* 100: 9608–9613
28 Bhattacharjee A, Richards WG, Staunton J, Li C, Monti S, Vasa P, Ladd C, Beheshti J, Bueno R, Gillette M et al (2001) Classification of human lung carcinomas by mRNA expression profiling reveals distinct adenocarcinoma subclasses. *Proc Natl Acad Sci USA* 98: 13790–13795
29 Staunton JE, Slonim DK, Coller HA, Tamayo P, Angelo MJ, Park J, Scherf U, Lee JK, Reinhold WO, Weinstein JN et al (2001) Chemosensitivity prediction by transcriptional profiling. *Proc Natl Acad Sci USA* 98: 10787–10792
30 Ramaswamy S, Tamayo P, Rifkin R, Mukherjee S, Yeang CH, Angelo M, Ladd C, Reich M, Latulippe E, Mesirov JP et al (2001) Multiclass cancer diagnosis using tumor gene expression signatures. *Proc Natl Acad Sci USA* 98: 15149–15154
31 Boshoff HI, Myers TG, Copp BR, McNeil MR, Wilson MA, Barry CE 3rd (2004) The transcriptional responses of *Mycobacterium tuberculosis* to inhibitors of metabolism: novel insights into drug mechanisms of action. *J Biol Chem* 279: 40174–40184
32 Revel A, Talaat A, Norgard M (2002) DNA microarray analysis of differential gene expression in *Borrelia burgdorferi*, the Lyme disease spirochete. *Proc Natl Acad Sci USA* 99: 1562–1567
33 Hentzer M, Wu H, Andersen JB, Riedel K, Rasmussen TB, Bagge N, Kumar N, Schembri MA, Song Z, Kristoffersen P et al (2003) Attenuation of *Pseudomonas aeruginosa* virulence by quorum sensing inhibitors. *Embo J* 22: 3803–3815
34 Rasmussen TB, Skindersoe ME, Bjarnsholt T, Phipps RK, Christensen KB, Jensen PO, Andersen JB, Koch B, Larsen TO, Hentzer M et al (2005) Identity and effects of quorum-sensing inhibitors produced by *Penicillium* species. *Microbiology* 151: 1325–1340

35 Freiberg C, Brotz-Oesterhelt H (2005) Functional genomics in antibacterial drug discovery. *Drug Discov Today* 10: 927–935
36 Miesel L, Greene J, Black TA (2003) Genetic strategies for antibacterial drug discovery. *Nat Rev Genet* 4: 442–456
37 Moir DT, Shaw KJ, Hare RS, Vovis GF (1999) Genomics and antimicrobial drug discovery. *Antimicrob Agents Chemother* 43: 439–446
38 di Bernardo D, Thompson MJ, Gardner TS, Chobot SE, Eastwood EL, Wojtovich AP, Elliott SJ, Schaus SE, Collins JJ (2005) Chemogenomic profiling on a genome-wide scale using reverse-engineered gene networks. *Nat Biotechnol* 23: 377–383
39 Gerhold DL, Jensen RV, Gullans SR (2002) Better therapeutics through microarrays. *Nat Genet* 32 Suppl: 547–551
40 Shaw KJ, Miller N, Liu X, Lerner D, Wan J, Bittner A, Morrow BJ (2003) Comparison of the changes in global gene expression of *Escherichia coli* induced by four bactericidal agents. *J Mol Microbiol Biotechnol* 5: 105–122
41 Wilson M, DeRisi J, Kristensen HH, Imboden P, Rane S, Brown PO, Schoolnik GK (1999) Exploring drug-induced alterations in gene expression in *Mycobacterium tuberculosis* by microarray hybridization. *Proc Natl Acad Sci USA* 96: 12833–12838
42 Sabina J, Dover N, Templeton LJ, Smulski DR, Soll D, LaRossa RA (2003) Interfering with different steps of protein synthesis explored by transcriptional profiling of *Escherichia coli* K-12. *J Bacteriol* 185: 6158–6170
43 Ng WL, Kazmierczak KM, Robertson GT, Gilmour R, Winkler ME (2003) Transcriptional regulation and signature patterns revealed by microarray analyses of *Streptococcus pneumoniae* R6 challenged with sublethal concentrations of translation inhibitors. *J Bacteriol* 185: 359–370
44 Brazas MD, Hancock RE (2005) Using microarray gene signatures to elucidate mechanisms of antibiotic action and resistance. *Drug Discov Today* 10: 1245–1252
45 Brazas MD, Hancock RE (2005) Ciprofloxacin induction of a susceptibility determinant in *Pseudomonas aeruginosa*. *Antimicrob Agents Chemother* 49: 3222–3227
46 Hughes TR, Marton MJ, Jones AR, Roberts CJ, Stoughton R, Armour CD, Bennett HA, Coffey E, Dai H, He YD et al (2000) Functional discovery via a compendium of expression profiles. *Cell* 102: 109–126
47 Mnaimneh S, Davierwala AP, Haynes J, Moffat J, Peng WT, Zhang W, Yang X, Pootoolal J, Chua G, Lopez A et al (2004) Exploration of essential gene functions via titratable promoter alleles. *Cell* 118: 31–44
48 Freiberg C, Schiffer G, Brunner N, Lampe T, Pohlmann J, Brands M, Haebich D, Ziegelbauer K (2004) Identification and characterization of the first class of potent bacterial acetyl-CoA carboxylase inhibitors with antibacterial activity. *J Biol Chem* 279: 26066–26073
49 Fischer HP, Brunner NA, Wieland B, Paquette J, Macko L, Ziegelbauer K, Freiberg C (2004) Identification of antibiotic stress-inducible promoters: a systematic approach to novel pathway-specific reporter assays for antibacterial drug discovery. *Genome Res* 14: 90–98

50 Hutter B, Fischer C, Jacobi A, Schaab C, Loferer H (2004) Panel of *Bacillus subtilis* reporter strains indicative of various modes of action. *Antimicrob Agents Chemother* 48: 2588–2594

51 Mascher T, Zimmer SL, Smith TA, Helmann JD (2004) Antibiotic-inducible promoter regulated by the cell envelope stress-sensing two-component system LiaRS of *Bacillus subtilis*. *Antimicrob Agents Chemother* 48: 2888–2896

52 Alksne LE, Burgio P, Hu W, Feld B, Singh MP, Tuckman M, Petersen PJ, Labthavikul P, McGlynn M, Barbieri L et al (2000) Identification and analysis of bacterial protein secretion inhibitors utilizing a SecA-LacZ reporter fusion system. *Antimicrob Agents Chemother* 44: 1418–1427

53 Bianchi AA, Baneyx F (1999) Stress responses as a tool to detect and characterize the mode of action of antibacterial agents. *Appl Environ Microbiol* 65: 5023–5027

54 Cao M, Salzberg L, Tsai CS, Mascher T, Bonilla C, Wang T, Ye RW, Marquez-Magana L, Helmann JD (2003) Regulation of the *Bacillus subtilis* extracytoplasmic function protein sigma(Y) and its target promoters. *J Bacteriol* 185: 4883–4890

55 Shapiro E, Baneyx F (2002) Stress-based identification and classification of antibacterial agents: Second-generation *Escherichia coli* reporter strains and optimization of detection. *Antimicrob Agents Chemother* 46: 2490–2497

56 Sun D, Cohen S, Mani N, Murphy C, Rothstein DM (2002) A pathway-specific cell based screening system to detect bacterial cell wall inhibitors. *J Antibiot (Tokyo)* 55: 279–287

57 Smulski DR, Huang LL, McCluskey MP, Reeve MJG, Vollmer AC, Van Dyk TK, LaRossa RA (2001) Combined, functional genomic-biochemical approach to intermediary metabolism: Interaction of acivicin, a glutamine amidotransferase inhibitor, with *Escherichia coli* K-12. *J Bacteriology* 183: 3353–3364

58 Ulrich RG, Rockett JC, Gibson GG, Pettit SD (2004) Overview of an interlaboratory collaboration on evaluating the effects of model hepatotoxicants on hepatic gene expression. *Environ Health Perspect* 112: 423–427

59 Waring JF, Halbert DN (2002) The promise of toxicogenomics. *Curr Opin Mol Ther* 4: 229–235

60 Kramer JA, Pettit SD, Amin RP, Bertram TA, Car B, Cunningham M, Curtiss SW, Davis JW, Kind C, Lawton M et al (2004) Overview on the application of transcription profiling using selected nephrotoxicants for toxicology assessment. *Environ Health Perspect* 112: 460–464

61 Hamadeh HK, Bushel PR, Jayadev S, Martin K, DiSorbo O, Sieber S, Bennett L, Tennant R, Stoll R, Barrett JC et al (2002) Gene expression analysis reveals chemical-specific profiles. *Toxicol Sci* 67: 219–231

62 Amin RP, Vickers AE, Sistare F, Thompson KL, Roman RJ, Lawton M, Kramer J, Hamadeh HK, Collins J, Grissom S et al (2004) Identification of putative gene based markers of renal toxicity. *Environ Health Perspect* 112: 465–479

63 Waring JF, Jolly RA, Ciurlionis R, Lum PY, Praestgaard JT, Morfitt DC, Buratto B, Roberts C, Schadt E, Ulrich RG (2001) Clustering of hepatotoxins based on mechanism of toxicity using gene expression profiles. *Toxicol Appl Pharmacol* 175: 28–42

64 Ellinger-Ziegelbauer H, Stuart B, Wahle B, Bomann W, Ahr HJ (2004) Characteristic expression profiles induced by genotoxic carcinogens in rat liver. *Toxicol Sci* 77: 19–34

65 Ellinger-Ziegelbauer H, Stuart B, Wahle B, Bomann W, Ahr HJ (2005) Comparison of the expression profiles induced by genotoxic and nongenotoxic carcinogens in rat liver. *Mutat Res* 575: 61–84

66 Liguori MJ, Anderson LM, Bukofzer S, McKim J, Pregenzer JF, Retief J, Spear BB, Waring JF (2005) Microarray analysis in human hepatocytes suggests a mechanism for hepatotoxicity induced by trovafloxacin. *Hepatology* 41: 177–186

67 Salama N, Guillemin K, McDaniel TK, Sherlock G, Tompkins L, Falkow S (2000) A whole-genome microarray reveals genetic diversity among *Helicobacter pylori* strains. *Proc Natl Acad Sci USA* 97: 14668–14673

68 Marshall BJ, Warren JR (1984) Unidentified curved bacilli in the stomach of patients with gastritis and peptic ulceration. *Lancet* 1: 1311–1315

69 Go MF (2002) Review article: natural history and epidemiology of *Helicobacter pylori* infection. *Aliment Pharmacol Ther* 16 Suppl 1: 3–15

70 Cordwell S, Nouwens A, Walsh B (2001) Comparative proteomics of bacterial pathogens. *Proteomics* 1: 461–472

71 Klade CS (2002) Proteomics approaches towards antigen discovery and vaccine development. *Curr Opin Mol Ther* 4: 216–223

72 Serruto D, Adu-Bobie J, Capecchi B, Rappuoli R, Pizza M, Masignani V (2004) Biotechnology and vaccines: application of functional genomics to *Neisseria meningitidis* and other bacterial pathogens. *J Biotechnol* 113: 15–32

73 Schmid JW, Mauch K, Reuss M, Gilles ED, Kremling A (2004) Metabolic design based on a coupled gene expression-metabolic network model of tryptophan production in *Escherichia coli. Metab Eng* 6: 364–377

74 Swameye I, Muller TG, Timmer J, Sandra O, Klingmuller U (2003) Identification of nucleocytoplasmic cycling as a remote sensor in cellular signaling by databased modeling. *Proc Natl Acad Sci USA* 100: 1028–1033

75 Reed JL, Vo TD, Schilling CH, Palsson BO (2003) An expanded genome-scale model of *Escherichia coli* K-12 (iJR904 GSM/GPR). *Genome Biol* 4: R54

76 Koffas M, Stephanopoulos G (2005) Strain improvement by metabolic engineering: lysine production as a case study for systems biology. *Curr Opin Biotechnol* 16: 361–366

77 Lee WC, Lee KH (2004) Applications of affinity chromatography in proteomics. *Anal Biochem* 324: 1–10

78 Jonsson P, Johansson AI, Gullberg J, Trygg J, AJ, Grung B, Marklund S, Sjostrom M, Antti H, Moritz T (2005) High-throughput data analysis for detecting and identifying differences between samples in GC/MS-based metabolomic analyses. *Anal Chem* 77: 5635–5642

79 Shimizu K (2004) Metabolic flux analysis based on 13C-labeling experiments and integration of the information with gene and protein expression patterns. *Adv Biochem Eng Biotechnol* 91: 1–49

Progress in Drug Research, Vol. 64
(Helena I. Boshoff and Clifton E. Barry III, Eds)

Chemical genetics: An evolving toolbox for target identification and lead optimization

By Helena I. Boshoff
and Cynthia S. Dowd

National Institutes of Health,
Rockville, MD 20852, USA
<hboshoff@niaid.nih.gov>

Abstract

Chemical genetics combines chemistry with biology as a means of exploring the function of unknown proteins or identifying the proteins responsible for a particular phenotype. Chemical genetics is thus a valuable tool in the identification of novel drug targets. This chapter describes the application of chemical genetics in traditional and systems-based approaches to drug target discovery and the tools/approaches that appear most promising for guiding future pharmaceutical development.

1 Genomic approaches to identifying drug targets

The availability of complete genome sequences from simple organisms such as *Mycoplasma* to complex vertebrates such as humans has accelerated the development of systems biology as a field. The value of genome sequences does not lie in knowing the number of genes of a particular organism (approximately 30,000 in humans versus 470 in *Mycoplasma*, for example) [1, 2] but in the information gained from exploring the network of interactions between the protein products. Understanding these networks would greatly benefit drug discovery since the networks provide information about pathway essentiality as well as redundancy. Successful drugs ideally target non-redundant, essential pathways of the organism.

Protein interaction networks based on protein–protein interactions have partially extended our understanding of the network maps, although in many cases the function of the protein remains elusive. Partial protein interaction networks have been reported for several pathogens such as *Mycobacterium tuberculosis* [3], *Helicobacter pylori* [4], *Plasmodium falciparum* [5] and *Rickettsia sibirica* [6]. These have been investigated with the hope of finding interactions that point to the function of unknown proteins through 'guilt-by-association' as well as pinpointing promising drug targets.

Essentiality screens are another way that investigators have used genomic information to glean information about processes required for survival of different organisms. Essentiality screens in *Mycoplasma* indicated that approximately 73 % of the genes were required for viability [7] whereas 53 % of *Haemophilus influenzae* genes appear to be important for growth [8]. In *M. tuberculosis* a similar screen indicated that at least 614 of the 4,000 encoded genes were essential for growth *in vitro* [9]. Of the genes that were not essential for growth *in vitro*, 194 were essential for growth *in vivo* in infected mouse tissues with many of these being genes unique to mycobacteria [10]. Genes that are essential for growth could be potential drug targets. However, many genes deemed essential have no known function, and target function is often a prerequisite for drug development.

2 The genomic interface of chemistry and biology: Chemical genetics

Chemical genetics is a multidisciplinary research field that combines chemistry with genetics as a means of probing gene function in cells. It allows exploration of the genes responsible for specific phenotypes as well as providing a means for the identification of function of unknown genes. Two approaches to chemical genetics have been pursued: forward chemical genetics and reverse chemical genetics (Fig. 1).

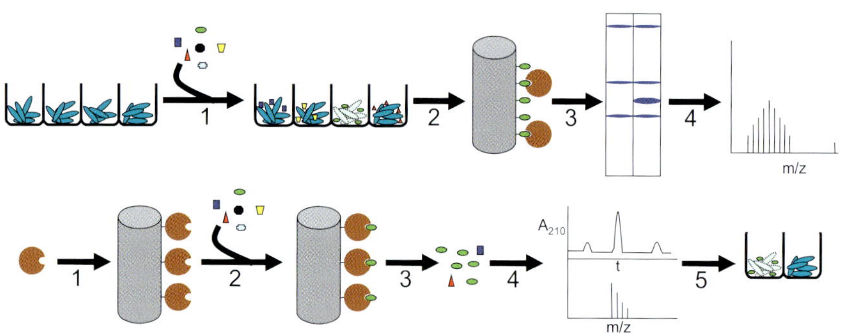

Figure 1.
Comparison of forward and reverse chemical genetics. In forward chemical genetics (top), small molecule libraries are used to find a compound that results in a phenotype of interest. In this example small molecules are identified that result in cell lysis (1). The protein target of the compound can subsequently be identified by affinity chromatography using the molecule linked to a solid support (2). Bound proteins are subsequently identified by SDS-PAGE (3) where specifically bound protein appears as a unique band (second lane) as compared to the non-specific control sample (first lane). The protein can be characterized by mass spectrometric methods (4). In reverse chemical genetics (bottom), the protein of interest is bound to an affinity column (1) and used to find small molecule ligands (2). The small molecule is eluted (3) and identified by mass spectrometry (4). The phenotype of the small molecule is then characterized (5).

In classical forward genetics, the underlying basis of a cellular phenotype is sought by identifying the causative gene. This is usually done by creating libraries of mutants and screening the mutants for the loss or gain of a particular phenotype. Mutations can be generated by saturating transposon mutagenesis, chemical mutagenesis, or by irradiation. Alternatively, the gene responsible for a phenotype can be identified through large-scale gene function screening using expression libraries or libraries of antisense expression constructs. The drawback of forward genetics is that generation of random mutations is not possible at the level of genome saturation since essential genes cannot be functionally deleted. In addition, overexpression of genes is often not associated with a phenotype that explains gene function whereas the time required for the functional consequences of downregulation of gene expression allows buffering by compensatory systems. These obstacles can be overcome using forward chemical genetics. In this approach, a small molecule library is used to perturb protein function and the small molecule that results in the phenotype of interest is then isolated. This approach has the advantage that small molecules rapidly perturb function, are able to interact with a single aspect of a protein's function, can be used to disrupt protein–protein interactions, and can cause both gain as well as loss of function.

In classical reverse genetics, the function of an uncharacterized gene can be investigated by the creation of mutants by site-directed mutagenesis, overexpression of the corresponding protein product, or by creation of an allelic knockout. The expression of a gene can also be downregulated or aborted through titratable promoters, antisense RNA or short-interfering RNAs. The disadvantage of classical reverse genetics is that knockouts cannot be created of essential genes and that cellular networks can adapt to genetic perturbations within a timeframe required for generation of mutant cell lines which can mask the phenotypic effects of functional knockouts. More recent approaches using regulatable systems to downregulate gene expression can overcome such drawbacks [11, 12]. In reverse chemical genetics, the function of uncharacterized proteins is studied through the use of membrane-permeable small molecule inhibitors of the protein under investigation to probe the effect of perturbation of function on cellular physiology. In this way, a small molecule, known to interact with a particular *in vitro* target, yields information about how inhibition of that target affects cellular processes.

2.1 Chemical genetics as a tool in systems biology

The advantage of a small molecule chemical genetics approach is that the phenotypic effect of the perturbation is obtained with cells having little time to adapt to the small molecule through altering expression and function of compensatory pathways which directly mimics pharmacological interventions. In forward chemical genetic screens, one particular phenotype such as mitotic spindle arrest, protein acetylation, or secretion of a protein, can be the result of inhibition of one (or under non-ideal conditions, more) of a series of proteins in a sub-network of cellular metabolism. Thus, deciphering the mechanism of action of a small molecule inhibitor can be used in mapping components of the perturbed network. Small molecule ligands may inhibit one aspect of a protein's function while not affecting another aspect of its activity, and some small molecule inhibitors can augment or diminish the effect of another small molecule. Establishing the network of chemical genetic interactions using small molecules can shed further light on the protein and genetic network maps.

An example of the use of small molecules to map a protein network was reported by Huang et al. [13] where a map of the target-of-rapamycin (TOR) signaling network in yeast was compiled. A library of 16,320 small molecules was screened to find compounds that modulated the growth inhibitory effect of rapamycin on yeast cells using an assay based on visual inspection of growth phenotype during compound exposure in rapamycin-containing medium. From this screen, six compounds were identified that abrogated the antiproliferative effect of rapamycin, while 57 compounds were identified that were synthetically lethal in combination with rapamycin. To unravel the effects of these small molecules on the TOR signaling network, transcriptional profiling experiments of yeast exposed to various concentrations of these molecules and/or rapamycin, were performed. To identify the targets of two of the small molecules, a biotin-capture approach was employed. The two compounds were labeled with biotin in a position which did not affect their *in vivo* phenotype. These biotinylated ligands were used to probe protein chips containing nearly the entire yeast proteome. Fluorescently labeled streptavidin was used to identify spots that contained bound biotin-conjugates. In this way, new members of the TOR sub-network were identified.

Koeller et al. [14] used small molecule inhibitors of histone and/or tubulin acetylases as molecular probes to partially elucidate cellular networks affected by acetylation of these proteins. To identify the relationship between pharmacophores and the resulting biological phenotypes, Haggarty et al. [15] mapped phenotypes of protein deacetylase inhibitors onto the chemical space computed by principle component analysis of the molecular descriptors of their 1,3-dioxane-based library of 7,200 compounds. In this way regions in chemical space could be correlated with phenotypic effects. Systematic mapping of chemical space using biological phenotypes would accelerate interpretation of chemical genetic networks.

Much of the data that has been generated from chemical genetics has been collected in several databases, many of which are publicly available. The KEGG resource contains information on small molecule ligands, their interacting proteins, and the metabolic networks that are associated with the pathways containing these proteins (http://www.genome.jp/kegg/). Public databases of small molecules such as ChemDB (http://cdb.ics.uci.edu) provide information on properties such as predicted solubility, three-dimensional structure and availability of more than 4 million compounds with more than 8 million isomers [16]. ChemBank (http://chembank.broad.harvard.edu/) and PubChem (http://pubchem.ncbi.nlm.nih.gov/) are two databases of small molecules and their associated biological activities.

2.2 Phenotypic screens in forward chemical genetics

Screening of large compound libraries efficiently requires the use of high-throughput screens (HTS). In reverse chemical genetics where a single or a few proteins are used to find small molecule binders, assay development is often straightforward, requiring an assay based on a property of the library or the protein's known function. In forward chemical genetic screens, however, a particular phenotype on a whole cell or whole organism level is sought. This makes high-throughput screening more difficult, often involving sophisticated components. Recently, several screens have been developed to detect agents with antiproliferative properties in an effort to map cellular mechanisms in cancer. Some of these screens have relied on microscopic detection of changes in cellular proliferation using automated microscopes linked to analysis software that can process data generated from 96-, 384- and 1536-well plates with cells and reagents dispensed by automated liquid handling systems [17, 18]. Screens based on microscopic analyses can detect complex phenotypic characteristics including cell morphology, changes in fluorescence in one or more channels, changes in parameters such as nuclear size, cytoplasmic area, cell perimeter, shape and biogenesis of the mitotic spindle, and changes in fluorescence intensity [19]. Wilson et al. [20] identified a quinazolinone inhibitor of tubulin polymerization using incorporation of a fluorescent DNA stain as a microscopic readout of change in DNA polymerization state to screen a library of 13,399 compounds.

Simpler cellular assays have been used where expression of reporter constructs, such as green fluorescent protein or firefly luciferase under control of the promoter of a gene associated with a particular phenotype, are monitored after compound exposure [18, 19]. Other screens depend on changes in expression of surface markers that can be detected by surface labeling with antibodies [21].

Large-scale screening is not only possible with cell cultures, but can also be performed on whole organisms such as zebrafish embryos [22–24]. Zebrafish are amenable to HTS because they are easy to culture in 96-well plates, develop outside the mother, are a good example of vertebrate development, are transparent, and are a good model for certain aspects of human disease. In recent years, a wealth of genetic information on zebrafish has become available. This includes large-scale mutagenesis screens and gene inactivation studies by short interfering RNAs and antisense morpholinos [24]. This information facilitates interpretation of data gathered from such chemical genetics endeavors. Peterson et al. [22] applied forward chemical genetics by screening a library of 1,100 small molecules for morphological defects on 1-, 2-, and 3-day old embryos. Several molecules were found that affected various aspects of development. Khersonsky et al. [23] screened a tagged triazine library of 1,536 small molecules against zebrafish embryos with the tags allowing subsequent affinity purification of proteins that bound to the triazine hit. Zebrafish have also been used in high-throughput screening of drugs to detect changes in heart rate by use of continuous video monitoring [25], a study that showed that molecules that caused QT prolongation in humans resulted in bradycardia in fish.

Small molecule microarrays have also been used in screens. In one study [26] a poly-lactide/glycolide copolymer impregnated with small libraries of molecules was used as the small molecule microarray. This circumvented the requirement for attachment of the compounds to the array surface. Monolayers of cells were then grown on top of the microarray, and phenotypic effects due to slow release of embedded small molecules were screened by microscopic analysis. The drawbacks to this approach include the fact that compounds are released to the cells from the onset of the experiment, only cells that grow as monolayers can be screened, and the size of the microarray is dictated by the distance required between spots in order to prevent cross-contamination.

2.3 Target identification strategies

The targets of hits obtained in phenotypic screens must subsequently be identified using affinity matrices, affinity linkers, or other methods. In some cases the targets of inhibitors can be deduced from their known biological activities in combination with information gained from the use of genetic mutants. The mode of action of Taxol, a natural product with potent antiproliferative activity, was deduced from the existing knowledge of other poisons, many targeting microtubules, which similarly caused cells to arrest in mitosis. *In vitro* studies with purified tubulin were used to demonstrate that Taxol promoted microtubule assembly and stabilized polymerized tubulin in contrast to several other microtubule poisons that destabilized microtubules [27]. The target of the antibiotic rifampicin was found through the use of rifampicin-resistant bacteria which were found to harbor mutations in the genes encoding RNA polymerase [28].

2.3.1 Target identification: Affinity-based methods

In affinity chromatography, the small molecule is derivatized with a chemical group that allows attachment to a solid support (Fig. 1). Derivatization of the small molecule carries the risk of losing affinity to its original target due to steric hindrance or alteration of attractive properties of the molecule. Attachment of a linker, such as triethyleneglycol, to the small molecule has been successfully used in affinity chromatography [29]. A good example of target identification through the use of affinity chromatography is the identification of the target of FK506 [30]. Structure-activity relationships had previously revealed important structural features required for FK506 activity which facilitated the placement of an amino-tag. This derivatized analog of FK506 was linked to a solid support. A protein from the cell lysate was identified that specifically bound to the FK506-affinity matrix. This was called FKBP for FK506 binding protein. It was later demonstrated that FK506 bound to a family of proteins (FKBPs) with the original protein target designated FKBP12.

The protein target of a small molecule can also be found by direct affinity labeling. Small molecule libraries can be designed so that the library members contain specific electrophilic or chemical crosslinking groups. These groups will form a covalent attachment to one or more amino acid residues on the target involved in ligand binding. Alternatively, the small molecule can be modified with a reactive moiety after its initial identification, but ideally this requires knowledge of structure-activity relationships (SAR) so that the modification does not affect the desired phenotypic change. Modified proteins can subsequently be identified based on intrinsic properties of the small molecule binder such as fluorescence or radioactivity. The target of L-583916 [31] was found by direct labeling of the protein. This compound inhibits leukotriene production by macrophages, neutrophils, and mast cells by a mechanism that did not involve any enzymes known to be involved in leukotriene production. Based on structure-activity relationships of similar compounds that modulated or were inactive in inhibition of leukotriene production, an analog of L-583916 was produced that contained an aromatic azide. The azide could be used for affinity labeling of the target. The small molecule was further labeled with ^{125}I. After incubation with cell lysates and photoactivation of the compound, the target protein was identified by SDS-PAGE and autoradiography. Competition experiments using unlabeled L-583916 revealed that an 18 kDa protein was specifically labeled. Interestingly, this protein was detected using affinity chromatography with an analog of L-583916, but would not have been identified as the specific target of the small molecule inhibitor since several proteins in addition to the 18 kDa target bound weakly to the column.

2.3.2 Target identification: Proteomic approaches

The target of a specific small molecule has also been found using a more global approach: looking at changes in the organism's proteome in response to treatment by the small molecule. The target of FK506 was found using a global proteomics approach. In this report, a tritiated FK506 analog was incubated with cell lysate from a T cell line and subsequently fractionated by protein chromatographic procedures. SDS-PAGE analysis led to the identification of a 12 kDa FKBP [32, 33]. The target of bengamides, a group of natural products with antiproliferative activities isolated from marine sponges, were found by analyzing 2D gels of treated *versus* untreated cells. This analysis revealed that a few proteins from the treated cells had altered isoelectric points due to retention of the methionine initiator. This led to the demonstration that the bengamides inhibited methionine aminopeptidase [34].

2.3.3 Target identification: Target titration

An approach utilized by Lum et al. [35] to identify protein targets of small molecule inhibitors used a library of 3,503 yeast strains, each containing a unique molecular barcode in one allele of a specific gene. The heterozygous strains were combined and grown in the presence of an inhibitor. The barcode tags of the cultures before and after exposure to the inhibitor were amplified, labeled with different fluorescent dyes, and used to probe DNA microarrays of yeast genes. Changes in relative abundance of a barcode due to altered susceptibility of a mutant strain to the inhibitor were detected by measuring changes in fluorescence intensities of the two fluorophores between DNA amplified before and after treatment. In this way, strains that were hypersusceptible to a particular inhibitor due to deletion of one gene in a heterozygous mutant were useful in identifying the targets of known and unknown inhibitors.

Multicopy suppression of a phenotype can be used to identify a target. Li et al. [36] screened a library of 8,640 compounds in an *E. coli* growth inhibitory assay. The protein targets of the hits were subsequently sought by screening for restoration of growth in clones expressing a genomic library. Restoration of growth was in most cases due to overexpression of multi-drug efflux systems although the target of two leads was identified and confirmed to be dihydrofolate reductase.

2.3.4 Target identification: Expression cloning

McPherson and co-workers [37] utilized an expression cloning approach to identify the target of a small molecule. In this approach, cDNAs are generated by polymerase chain reaction (PCR) with primers that allow transcription, ligation to a puromycin DNA linker, and *in vitro* translation to generate a protein–nucleic acid conjugate. This complex is incubated with the small molecule under investigation which has been immobilized to a solid support. Unbound protein–nucleic acid complexes are subsequently washed off and bound complexes are eluted with excess free ligand or with sodium hydroxide. The resulting DNA can now be amplified by PCR and subjected to further rounds of selection followed by cloning and identification of the protein.

The validity of this approach was demonstrated by the use of an immobilized FK506-biotin conjugate using protein–nucleic acid fusions generated from human kidney, liver and bone marrow transcripts to pull out FKBP12 , a known FK506 binding protein [37]. This approach would be especially useful for target proteins that are present in low abundance since these targets would easily be disregarded by methods that depend on direct detection of bound protein from complex extracts. The disadvantage of this approach, in addition to the requirement for an active immobilized ligand as previously discussed and the lengthy procedure, is that success depends on the size of the protein required for binding to the small molecule since full-length long cDNAs are not easily obtained. Thus, the method selects against large proteins. This is demonstrated by the fact that the known larger FK506 targets were not pulled out by this method.

2.3.5 Target identification: Transcriptional approaches

Databases of transcriptional profiles elicited by small molecule inhibitors can aid in identification of both the protein targets and the cellular subnetworks that are affected by these agents [38, 39]. Kung et al. [40] used transcriptional profiles generated from analog-sensitive mutants of specific kinases to identify the targets of uncharacterized kinase inhibitors. Their strategy used yeast kinase mutants with functionally silent mutations in the highly conserved ATP-binding site which are sensitive to inhibition by specific small molecule inhibitors. Transcriptional profiles of the kinase mutants during exposure to characterized inhibitors could be compared to transcriptional profiles generated by the uncharacterized kinase inhibitors. This analysis aided in the identification of the targets of these molecules. Gene clusters were also identified that were predictive of inhibition of each kinase. The combination of gene clusters that were affected by the agents under investigation pinpointed the kinase targets of the drugs. This is an especially useful approach for kinases since the highly conserved nature of the ATP binding pocket of these proteins results in several kinase inhibitors inhibiting more than one kinase so that the signaling sub-networks perturbed by such small molecules can be difficult to map.

2.4 Hurdles in target identification

While the above discussion depicts a variety of methods for target identification, it should be understood that such processes have obstacles that must be overcome. Firstly, identification of a protein target depends on a reasonable affinity between the small molecule and its target protein. As is often the case, concentrations required to detect a phenotypic change can be on the order of 1 μM which is far from the ideal of nM range potencies [41]. As a result, the true target proteins of hits found in many phenotypic screens remain unidentified. Secondly, many compounds in small molecule libraries are quite hydrophobic which leads to significant non-specific binding to cellular components. Thus, target identification through affinity selection requires stringent wash conditions to dissociate non-specific hydrophobic interactions. Compounds with low binding affinities are inevitably dissociated in such washes. Thirdly, the abundance of the target protein affects the success of its identification. Highly abundant proteins that bind to the small molecule in an affinity-based method are easily enriched and subsequently detected. However, proteins expressed in low-copy numbers are not easily detected above the non-specific background. The success of detection of FKBP as the FK506 target was in part due to the highly abundant nature of this cytosolic protein [30, 41]. In general, the molar ratio between compound and target is far from ideal. Specific binding of a protein would be improved if the target protein is present in excess of its ligand since this would allow the target to effectively compete with proteins of lower specificity. However, during most affinity selection methods, the amount of small molecule ligand vastly out numbers its target, leaving excess binding sites available to non-target proteins.

There are several solutions to overcome these practical hurdles. To discern target from non-target protein hits, one can increase the amount of protein loaded on the affinity matrix by, for example, including cell lysate from *Escherichia coli*. Alternately, two affinity matrix purifications can be run in parallel. One affinity matrix should contain the small molecules of interest, and the other should contain a structurally similar but inactive molecule. In this way, proteins that bind to the two matrices can be compared, and the true target can be found [41]. Finally, comparison of differentially bound proteins can be done by labeling each set differently. For example, one set could be labeled with a light label and the other with an isotopically heavy label (e.g., ICAT reagents [42]) or by two different fluorophores.

Identification of the target can further be complicated by the presence of more than one target in the cell and non-specific interactions. The potency of compounds that give positive hits in phenotypic screens can subsequently be improved by medicinal chemistry efforts even before the target has been identified, but the maturation of libraries into molecules of high affinity depends on the success of finding initial hits and being able to distinguish apparent hits from non-specific effects. Fantin et al. [43] developed a parallel screening assay where an immortalized cell line was transformed with the *neu* oncogene whereas the negative control screen consisted of non-transformed cells. Compounds that affected membrane potential in a *neu*-dependent manner could thus be distinguished from compounds with non-specific effects. Co-screening of control cell lines and cells transformed with a variety of reporter constructs have been used in other studies to find drugs that kill cells in a gene-specific manner [44, 45].

2.5 Library design

One of the most important components of a chemical genetics approach using small molecules, forward or reverse, is the design of the chemical library to be used. Chemical libraries can be broadly classified as arising from diversity-oriented synthesis (DOS) or focused library synthesis (FLS). DOS libraries, most useful in forward chemical genetics, examine a variety of scaffolds and structural classes of compounds. The goal of the library is to examine as much structural space as possible. The result can be the identification of multiple new targets. FLS libraries, by contrast, center around one or a small number of closely related scaffolds. The molecules in an FLS library are closely related and can be used in either forward or reverse chemical genetics approaches.

When designing a library, several points are to be considered. These points have been described by YT Chang in a series of reviews on the topic [29, 46, 47]. Briefly, the ideal scaffold should contain three elements: 1) several diversity points; 2) undemanding chemical synthesis; and 3) rigidity to minimize nonspecific protein binding. The reasons for these elements are two-fold: to increase the number of compounds with maximal diversity and purity and to decrease the rate of false positives.

Over the past few years, there have been several examples of chemical library synthesis that has resulted in biologically active molecules (see reviews [29, 46–48]). The choice of scaffold in these examples can be seen as coming from natural product origin or compounds with known biological activity. Natural products have been very important for the discovery of novel biologically-active structural classes as well as new targets. Because of this, using a structural moiety that arose from a natural substance can be a fruitful starting point for a chemical library. Libraries have been built around shikimic acid and dimethylbenzopyran, both moieties found in several natural products [49–52]. Alternatively, chemical libraries can be built upon scaffolds with known biological activity. In a forward chemical genetics approach, Schultz's group prepared a combinatorial library using purine as a scaffold with variation at three positions. The library was initially made and examined to identify novel inhibitors of kinase family members [53]. In addition to kinase inhibitors, compounds were identified with a variety of other activities including sulfotransferase inhibitors

[54, 55], osteogenesis induction [56], and microtubule assembly inhibitors [57, 58]. Libraries based on ceramides [59] and sulfonamides [60–62] have been produced as well.

More recently, libraries have been designed to facilitate identification of the target. In classical forward chemical genetics, the target of an active compound would be elucidated by some means of labeling, purification, and identification. Practically, this often involves modifying the active compound with a new structural motif that will covalently bind to the target. This type of modification can often be deleterious to the activity of the compound so an extensive synthetic effort must be made in order to put the 'tag' in the most appropriate place. Recent work by YT Chang and others has produced tagged libraries where the compounds to be screened already contain the motif required for target labeling. Therefore, no additional SAR or synthetic work is necessary before identifying the target. An example of a tagged library was reported by the Chang group. In this report, a series of triazines were prepared with a triethyleneglycol linker attached [23]. Upon identifying an active molecule, the linker was attached to an agarose bead. This combination was used to identify the target molecule.

2.6 Fishing for small molecule ligands in reverse chemical genetics

In reverse chemical genetics, small molecules that bind to a protein of interest are selected from a compound library. These small molecules are subsequently used in whole cell/organism assays to explore the function of the protein under investigation. Traditional methods of identifying small molecule ligands are affinity chromatography, affinity labeling of the target protein (as previously discussed), and screening libraries of small molecules for enzyme inhibition.

Recently, several strategies to discover novel lead compounds against specific targets have been reported. Many of these approaches are fragment-based, relying on an improved entropic gain after tethering two low-affinity ligands (Fig. 2). Several of these approaches also take advantage of recent advances in synthetic and analytical techniques such as combi-

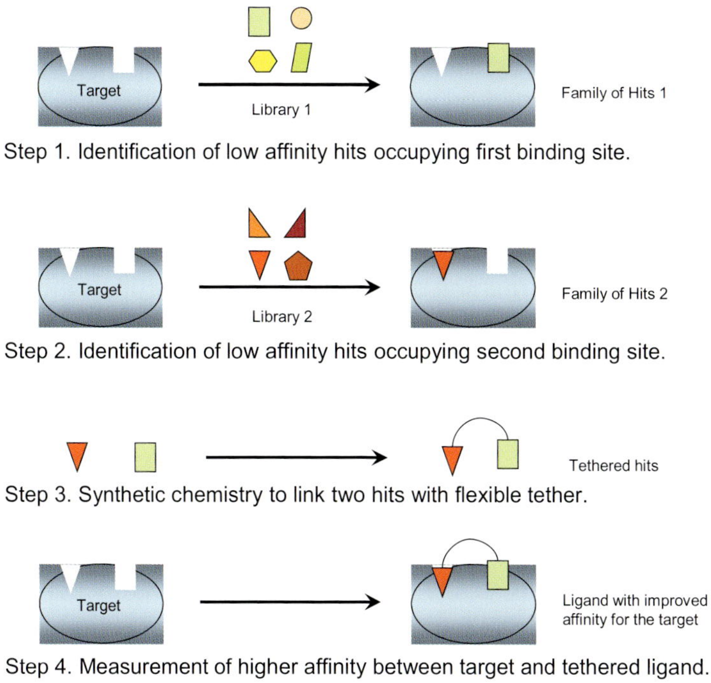

Figure 2.
General scheme for NMR-based screening strategies. This approach to ligand discovery uses two rounds of small molecule screening to identify two low-affinity ligands which bind to separate sites on the protein of interest. Linking the two low-affinity small molecules with a flexible tether results in a single molecule with increased affinity to the protein. This process is facilitated by using the protein's structural information to guide tether design and location on the small molecules.

natorial chemistry, 2D nuclear magnetic resonance (NMR), or orthogonal reactions.

2.6.1 NMR-based approaches

In pioneering work, Steve Fesik's group at Abbott Laboratories developed 'SAR by NMR' [63]. In this approach, binding of a series of small molecules to the target protein is examined by 2D NMR. From these experiments, the relative binding locations of small molecules can be mapped onto a target. The small molecules may have weak (mM–μM) binding affinities. Two small molecules that bind to proximal sites on the protein are then synthetically linked (Fig. 2). The resulting tethered ligand displays stronger affinity (μM-nM) to the target due to the entropic gain from the tether. This fragment-based method was used to identify ligands for FKBP [63], stromelysin [64, 65], and the antiapoptotic protein Bcl-x_L [66] among many other targets.

In a second NMR-based approach termed SAR by interligand nuclear Overhauser effect (SAR by ILOEs), Becattini et al. measured interactions between ligands to gain information about small molecules that bind in proximal binding sites on the target [67]. They then used molecular modeling and synthesis to generate a small number of compounds to be evaluated. Their work resulted in the identification of a series of bidentate small molecule inhibitors of Bid, a protein important in apoptosis.

A third NMR-based approach is called SHAPES [68]. This approach uses NMR to screen a small library of compounds. The compounds in the library are chosen based on common structural shapes and drug-like qualities found in biologically active molecules. NMR experiments are conducted using mixtures of the target and sets of compounds from the SHAPES library. Either 1D 1H NMR or 2D NOESY NMR can be used in the screening process, the latter giving clear binding results for mixtures of compounds. The hits, many of which are weak (μM–mM) binders, are used to refine larger collections of compounds for additional rounds of screening. The SHAPES approach has distinct advantages in that ^{15}N-labeled protein is not required and it is amenable to targets of variable size. For example, the authors screened their SHAPES library against several enzyme targets including p38 MAP kinase (42 kDa) and inosine-5′-monophosphate dehydrogenase (224 kDa).

2.6.2 Systems-based ligand design

In a novel approach, Sem et al. focused on structurally-related targets and the development of bivalent ligands for these related targets [69]. Their method relied on the hypothesis that members of the same 'pharmacofamily' will have similar binding sites for ligands. In their pharmacofamily, the oxidoreductases, a co-factor binding site was common to all members of the pharmacofamily. All members of the family also had an adjacent binding site that bound substrate. The authors created bivalent ligands comprised of a co-factor moiety (common binding element) and a variable element that gave target specificity to the ligand. NMR SOLVE was used to determine the placement of a linker between the common binding element and the specificity ligand. Specific inhibitors for the related enzymes lactate dehydrogenase, DOXPR (1-deoxy-D-xylulose-5-phosphate reductoisomerase), and DHPR (dihydrodipicolinate reductase) were found by this approach.

2.6.3 Site-directed ligand discovery

In this approach, a protein target with a free cysteine is exposed to a library of disulfide-containing small molecules [70]. The experiment is conducted in partially reducing conditions such that disulfide exchange occurs between the small molecules and the target. Adducts formed between the target and compounds with weak binding affinity are then detected by mass spectrometry. The hits were then optimized with the aid of X-ray crystallography to generate nM inhibitors of thymidylate synthase.

2.6.4 Combinatorial small molecule libraries

Maly et al. used an approach that combined identification of weak binding fragments, combinatorial chemistry, and facilitated tether synthesis [71]. They screened a small molecule library where each molecule contained a common chemical linkage group. Pairs of hit molecules are linked together combinatorially using a flexible linker. The combinatorial library is screened to ascertain the tightest binding ligands. An inhibitor of c-Src with an IC_{50} of 64 nM was identified by this approach. This method does not require 3D knowledge of the target and incorporates tether synthesis early in the strategy hereby decreasing required synthesis.

2.6.5 *In situ* click chemistry

Several years ago, a novel approach to identifying small molecule ligands was reported which took advantage of a unique chemical reaction between an azide and an alkyne (Fig. 3). This reaction, to yield a triazole, occurs in aqueous solution and in the presence of most other functional groups. It is referred to as the 'click' reaction [72]. The application to chemical genetics came when the click reaction was used with a biological target to assemble complementary small molecule ligands [73, 74]. Using a small

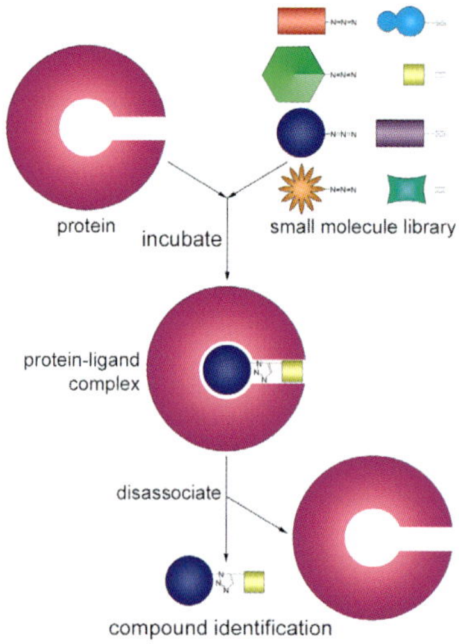

Figure 3.
The use of click chemistry to find novel inhibitors. Small molecule building blocks are incubated with a protein of interest. The building blocks consist of two small molecule libraries containing either an azide or terminal alkyne group. Binding of the building blocks in adjacent sites on the protein may position the alkyne and azide substituents in close proximity to one another, leading to the formation of a triazole. The triazole product is identified by mass spectrometry. When tested in a subsequent experiment, the triazole hit is expected to have higher affinity for the protein than the individual building blocks.

library of tacrine and phenylphenanthridinium azides and acetylenes, a series of fM inhibitors for acetylcholinesterase were identified.

2.6.6 Small molecule microarrays

Identification of small molecules that bind to a protein of interest can be facilitated by the use of small molecule microarrays (reviewed in [75]). In small molecule arrays, surface-attached compounds are spatially separated on a solid surface such as a glass slide. The protein of interest is labeled, for example by a fluorophore or radioisotope, incubated with the array, washed, and the spots with bound protein are identified by fluorimetry or autoradiography. Koehler et al. [76] used a library of 12,396 members attached to a glass slide to find ligands that bound to a glutathione S-transferase-transcription factor fusion protein. Bound protein was detected using an antibody recognizing glutathione S-transferase.

2.6.7 Barcode tags

Another approach utilizes polyamide nucleic acid (PNA) tags on library members. The sequence-specific PNA tag encodes the identity of the small molecule based on its synthetic history. The protein of interest is incubated with the fluorescently labeled PNA-tagged library, the complexes are separated from unbound library members by size exclusion chromatography,

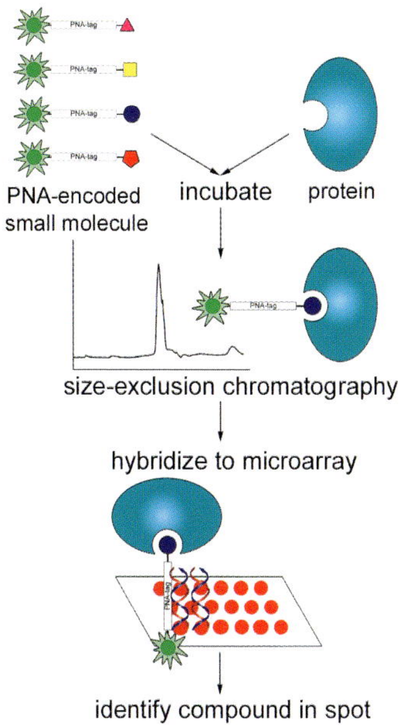

Figure 4.
Reverse chemical genetic screen using a polyamide nucleic acid (PNA) tagged chemical library. The PNA-tagged library is incubated with the protein of interest. Unbound library members are subsequently removed by size exclusion chromatography. The purified PNA-tagged protein is hybridized to an array carrying oligonucleotides complementary to the original PNA library. Positive identification of the small molecule hit is achieved from the array as the PNA tags encode the synthetic history of the small molecule.

and the ligand is subsequently identified by a microarray containing complementary oligonucleotides (Fig. 4). The PNA-tagged approach was used to identify substrates of proteases [77, 78] using a library of 192 PNA-tagged potential protease substrates prepared by split and pool combinatorial synthesis.

2.6.8 Affinity selection – Mass spectrometry

Affinity selection of small molecule binders followed by identification of the compound by mass spectrometry (MS) is another convenient approach for finding small molecules that interact with unknown proteins (Fig. 5). This is performed by incubating the protein of interest with a library of small molecules. The protein–ligand complexes are subsequently separated from unbound molecules by standard chromatographic techniques such as gel filtration, the complexes are dissociated by, for example, reverse phase chromatography, and the small molecule in question is identified by MS or tandem MS. The advantage of this approach is that the protein under investigation does not need to be modified, thereby retaining its

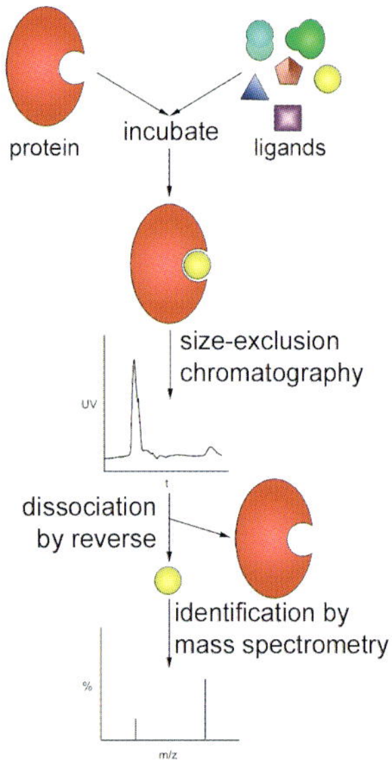

Figure 5.
Reverse chemical genetic screens through affinity selection of ligands followed by mass spectrometric identification. Novel ligands that bind to a protein of interest are identified by incubation of the protein with a small molecule library. The ligand–protein complexes are separated by size exclusion chromatography, then the small molecule is dissociated by reverse-phase chromatography. The small molecule ligand is then identified by mass spectrometry. Mass spectrometric identification is greatly facilitated through the use of mass-encoded libraries.

functionality. In addition, other non-specific effects such as binding of small molecules to the matrix in affinity chromatography are avoided.

Annis and co-workers [79] used an affinity selection – MS method to identify compounds that bound to the *E. coli* dihydrofolate reductase enzyme. In their approach, they utilized a 2,500-member combinatorial library of mass-encoded compounds. After solution-phase binding to the protein, complexes were separated from unbound molecules by rapid size exclusion chromatography performed at low temperature, to allow retrieval of low affinity complexes, followed by dissociation by reverse phase chromatography and drug identification by liquid chromatography (LC)–MS. The precise chemical identity of small molecule binders was performed using LC-MS/MS. In another approach, a library of 44,440 compounds distributed in multi-well plates in groups of four was incubated with fluorescently labeled *Staphylococcus aureus* YihA, a protein of unknown function that is essential in *E. coli* and *B. subtilis* [80]. The mixture was directly assayed by capillary electrophoresis and fluorimetric detection. Binding of ligand resulted in altered mobility of the protein. The identity of a hit was deduced by deconvolution of the compounds in the wells. From the 115 small molecule ligands detected in the capillary electrophoresis assay, 80 compounds inhibited the growth of at least one of five bacterial pathogens tested.

Compounds that are identified as small molecule ligands in reverse chemical genetic screens are subsequently assayed against whole cells in order to probe the function of the protein in question. The advantage of the chemical genetic screens is that potential binders can be found that potentially bind to a variety of surfaces of the protein. Thus, binders may inhibit enzymatic activity of a protein, modulate enzymatic activity of the protein, or affect protein–protein interactions.

2.7 Orthogonal chemical genetics

Chemical genetics is a term also used to describe the methodology in which proteins are engineered to alter their substrate selectivity. This allows modified chemical analogs to be employed that can distinguish the activity of the protein of interest from other enzymes/proteins in the cell. This approach has been widely used to investigate the function of kinases using chemically modified substrates or inhibitors that specifically interact with the genetically modified kinases. Juris and co-workers [81] identified otubain 1 as a substrate for the *Yersinia* protein kinase YpkA by genetically engineering YpkA to alter its ATP substrate selectivity. YpkA is a virulence factor in *Yersinia* spp. that is activated in the host cell resulting in disruption of the actin cytoskeleton. The only previously identified substrate of YpkA was actin. The 'gatekeeper' residue of YpkA, a conserved bulky hydrophobic amino acid, was mutated to the smaller amino acids alanine or glycine, thereby allowing binding of analogs of ATP with a bulky substituent at the N^6 position of ATP. Radiolabeled γ–^{32}P,N^6-phenylethyl ATP was preferentially utilized by the mutated YpkA, distinguishing its activity from other cellular kinases. Mutant YpkA phosphorylated actin as expected, as well as a 36 kDa protein which was identified as otubain 1 by a combination of MALDI-TOF (matrix-assisted laser desorption ionization time-of-flight) and MALDI-PSD (matrix-assisted laser desorption ionization post source decay) mass spectrometry. This result was further confirmed by *in vitro* demonstration of otubain phosphorylation by YpkA in the presence of actin as well as the interaction of these three proteins *in vivo*.

25 Milan DJ, Peterson TA, Ruskin JN, Peterson RT, MacRae CA (2003) Drugs that induce repolarization abnormalities cause bradycardia in zebrafish. *Circulation* 107: 1355–1358

26 Bailey SN, Sabatini DM, Stockwell BR (2004) Microarrays of small molecules embedded in biodegradable polymers for use in mammalian cell-based screens. *Proc Natl Acad Sci USA* 101: 16144–16149

27 Schiff PB, Fant J, Horwitz SB (1979) Promotion of microtubule assembly *in vitro* by taxol. *Nature* 277: 665–667

28 Yura T, Ishihama A (1979) Genetics of bacterial RNA polymerases. *Annu Rev Genet* 13: 59–97

29 Mitsopoulos G, Walsh DP, Chang YT (2004) Tagged library approach to chemical genomics and proteomics. *Curr Opin Chem Biol* 8: 26–32

30 Harding MW, Galat A, Uehling DE, Schreiber SL (1989) A receptor for the immunosuppressant FK506 is a cis-trans peptidyl-prolyl isomerase. *Nature* 341: 758–760

31 Miller DK, Gillard JW, Vickers PJ, Sadowski S, Leveille C, Mancini JA, Charleson P, Dixon RA, Ford-Hutchinson AW, Fortin R et al (1990) Identification and isolation of a membrane protein necessary for leukotriene production. *Nature* 343: 278–281

32 Siekierka JJ, Hung SH, Poe M, Lin CS, Sigal NH (1989) A cytosolic binding protein for the immunosuppressant FK506 has peptidyl-prolyl isomerase activity but is distinct from cyclophilin. *Nature* 341: 755–757

33 Siekierka JJ, Staruch MJ, Hung SH, Sigal NH (1989) FK-506, a potent novel immunosuppressive agent, binds to a cytosolic protein which is distinct from the cyclosporin A-binding protein, cyclophilin. *J Immunol* 143: 1580–1583

34 Towbin H, Bair KW, DeCaprio JA, Eck MJ, Kim S, Kinder FR, Morollo A, Mueller DR, Schindler P, Song HK et al (2003) Proteomics-based target identification: bengamides as a new class of methionine aminopeptidase inhibitors. *J Biol Chem* 278: 52964–52971

35 Lum PY, Armour CD, Stepaniants SB, Cavet G, Wolf MK, Butler JS, Hinshaw JC, Garnier P, Prestwich GD, Leonardson A et al (2004) Discovering modes of action for therapeutic compounds using a genome-wide screen of yeast heterozygotes. *Cell* 116: 121–137

36 Li X, Zolli-Juran M, Cechetto JD, Daigle DM, Wright GD, Brown ED (2004) Multicopy suppressors for novel antibacterial compounds reveal targets and drug efflux susceptibility. *Chem Biol* 11: 1423–1430

37 McPherson M, Yang Y, Hammond PW, Kreider BL (2002) Drug receptor identification from multiple tissues using cellular-derived mRNA display libraries. *Chem Biol* 9: 691–698

38 Boshoff HI, Myers TG, Copp BR, McNeil MR, Wilson MA, Barry CE 3rd (2004) The transcriptional responses of *Mycobacterium tuberculosis* to inhibitors of metabolism: novel insights into drug mechanisms of action. *J Biol Chem* 279: 40174–40184

39 Butcher RA, Schreiber SL (2005) Using genome-wide transcriptional profiling to elucidate small-molecule mechanism. *Curr Opin Chem Biol* 9: 25–30

40 Kung C, Shokat KM (2005) Small-molecule kinase-inhibitor target assessment. *Chembiochem* 6: 523–526
41 Burdine L, Kodadek T (2004) Target identification in chemical genetics: the (often) missing link. *Chem Biol* 11: 593–597
42 Ranish JA, Yi EC, Leslie DM, Purvine SO, Goodlett DR, Eng J, Aebersold R (2003) The study of macromolecular complexes by quantitative proteomics. *Nat Genet* 33: 349–355
43 Fantin VR, Berardi MJ, Scorrano L, Korsmeyer SJ, Leder P (2002) A novel mitochondriotoxic small molecule that selectively inhibits tumor cell growth. *Cancer Cell* 2: 29–42
44 Torrance CJ, Agrawal V, Vogelstein B, Kinzler KW (2001) Use of isogenic human cancer cells for high-throughput screening and drug discovery. *Nat Biotechnol* 19: 940–945
45 Simons A, Dafni N, Dotan I, Oron Y, Canaani D (2001) Establishment of a chemical synthetic lethality screen in cultured human cells. *Genome Res* 11: 266–273
46 Khersonsky SM, Chang YT (2004) Strategies for facilitated forward chemical genetics. *Chembiochem* 5: 903–908
47 Khersonsky SM, Chang YT (2004) Forward chemical genetics: library scaffold design. *Comb Chem High Throughput Screen* 7: 645–652
48 Stockwell BR (2004) Exploring biology with small organic molecules. *Nature* 432: 846–854
49 Nicolaou KC, Pfefferkorn JA, Barluenga S, Mitchell HJ, Roecker AJ, Cao G-Q (2000) Natural product-like combinatorial libraries based on privileged structures. 3. The "Libraries from Libraries" principle for diversity enhancement of benzopyran libraries. *J Am Chem Soc* 122: 9968–9976
50 Nicolaou KC, Pfefferkorn JA, Mitchell HJ, Roecker AJ, Barluenga S, Cao G-Q, Affleck RL, Lillig JE (2000) Natural product-like combinatorial libraries based on privileged structures. 2. Construction of a 10,000-membered benzopyran library by directed split-and-pool chemistry using nanokans and optical encoding. *J Am Chem Soc* 122: 9954–9967
51 Nicolaou KC, Pfefferkorn JA, Roecker AJ, Cao G-Q, Barluenga S, Mitchell HJ (2000) Natural product-like combinatorial libraries based on privileged structures. 1. General Principles and solid-phase synthesis of benzopyrans. *J Am Chem Soc* 122: 9939–9953
52 Tan DS, Foley MA, Stockwell BR, Shair MD, Shreiber SL (1999) Synthesis and preliminary evaluation of a library of polycyclic small molecules for use in chemical genetic assays. *J Am Chem Soc* 121: 9073–9087
53 Gray NS, Wodicka L, Thunnissen AM, Norman TC, Kwon S, Espinoza FH, Morgan DO, Barnes G, LeClerc S, Meijer L et al (1998) Exploiting chemical libraries, structure, and genomics in the search for kinase inhibitors. *Science* 281: 533–538
54 Armstrong JI, Portley AR, Chang YT, Nierengarten DM, Cook BN, Bowman KG, Bishop A, Gray NS, Shokat KM, Schultz PG et al (2000) Discovery of carbohydrate sulfotransferase inhibitors from a kinase-directed library. *Angew Chem Int Ed Engl* 39: 1303–1306

55 Verdugo DE, Cancilla MT, Ge X, Gray NS, Chang YT, Schultz PG, Negishi M, Leary JA, Bertozzi CR (2001) Discovery of estrogen sulfotransferase inhibitors from a purine library screen. *J Med Chem* 44: 2683–2686
56 Wu X, Ding S, Ding Q, Gray NS, Schultz PG (2002) A small molecule with osteogenesis-inducing activity in multipotent mesenchymal progenitor cells. *J Am Chem Soc* 124: 14520–14521
57 Chang YT, Wignall SM, Rosania GR, Gray NS, Hanson SR, Su AI, Merlie J Jr, Moon HS, Sangankar SB, Perez O et al (2001) Synthesis and biological evaluation of myoseverin derivatives: microtubule assembly inhibitors. *J Med Chem* 44: 4497–4500
58 Rosania GR, Chang YT, Perez O, Sutherlin D, Dong H, Lockhart DJ, Schultz PG (2000) Myoseverin, a microtubule-binding molecule with novel cellular effects. *Nat Biotechnol* 18: 304–308
59 Chang Y-T, Choi J, Ding S, Prieschl EE, Baumruker T, Lee J-M, Chung S-K, Schultz PG (2002) The synthesis and biological characterization of a ceramide library. *J Am Chem Soc* 124: 1856–1857
60 Kim SW, Hong CY, Lee K, Lee EJ, Koh JS (1998) Solid phase synthesis of benzylamine-derived sulfonamide library. *Bioorg Med Chem Lett* 8: 735–738
61 Ryckebuscha A, Déprez-Poulaina R, Debreu-Fontainea M-A, Vandaelea R, Mourayb E, Grellierb P, Sergheraert C (2002) Parallel synthesis and anti-malarial activity of a sulfonamide library. *Bioorg Med Chem Lett* 12: 2595–2598
62 Yokoi A, Kuromitsu J, Kawai T, Nagasu T, Sugi NH, Yoshimatsu K, Yoshino H, Owa T (2002) Profiling novel sulfonamide antitumor agents with cell-based phenotypic screens and array-based gene expression analysis. *Mol Cancer Ther* 1: 275–286
63 Shuker SB, Hajduk PJ, Meadows RP, Fesik SW (1996) Discovering high-affinity ligands for proteins: SAR by NMR. *Science* 274: 1531–1534
64 Olejniczak ET, Hajduk PJ, Marcotte PA, Nettesheim DG, Meadows RP, Edalji R, Holzman TF, Fesik SW (1997) Stromelysin inhibitors designed from weakly bound fragments: effects of linking and cooperativity. *J Am Chem Soc* 119: 5828 –5832
65 Hajduk PJ, Sheppard G, Nettesheim DG, Olejniczak ET, Shuker SB, Meadows RP, Steinman DH, Carrera J, Marcotte PA, Severin J et al (1997) Discovery of Potent nonpeptide inhibitors of stromelysin using SAR by NMR. *J Am Chem Soc* 119: 5818 –5827
66 Petros AM, Dinges J, Augeri DJ, Baumeister SA, Betebenner DA, Bures MG, Elmore SW, Hajduk PJ, Joseph MK, Landis SK et al (2006) Discovery of a potent inhibitor of the antiapoptotic protein Bcl-xL from NMR and parallel synthesis. *J Med Chem* 49: 656–663
67 Becattini B, Sareth S, Zhai D, Crowell KJ, Leone M, Reed JC, Pellecchia M (2004) Targeting apoptosis via chemical design: inhibition of bid-induced cell death by small organic molecules. *Chem Biol* 11: 1107–1117
68 Fejzo J, Lepre CA, Peng JW, Bemis GW, Ajay, Murcko MA, Moore JM (1999) The SHAPES strategy: an NMR-based approach for lead generation in drug discovery. *Chem Biol* 6: 755–769

69 Sem DS, Bertolaet B, Baker B, Chang E, Costache AD, Coutts S, Dong Q, Hansen M, Hong V, Huang X et al (2004) Systems-based design of bi-ligand inhibitors of oxidoreductases: filling the chemical proteomic toolbox. *Chem Biol* 11: 185–194

70 Erlanson DA, Braisted AC, Raphael DR, Randal M, Stroud RM, Gordon EM, Wells JA (2000) Site-directed ligand discovery. *Proc Natl Acad Sci USA* 97: 9367–9372

71 Maly DJ, Choong IC, Ellman JA (2000) Combinatorial target-guided ligand assembly: identification of potent subtype-selective c-Src inhibitors. *Proc Natl Acad Sci USA* 97: 2419–2424

72 Kolb HC, Finn MG, Sharpless KB (2001) Click chemistry: Diverse chemical function from a few good reactions. *Angew Chem Int Ed Engl* 40: 2004–2021

73 Lewis WG, Green LG, Grynszpan F, Radic Z, Carlier PR, Taylor P, Finn MG, Sharpless KB (2002) Click chemistry *in situ*: acetylcholinesterase as a reaction vessel for the selective assembly of a femtomolar inhibitor from an array of building blocks. *Angew Chem Int Ed Engl* 41: 1053–1057

74 Manetsch R, Krasiski A, Radi Z, Raushel J, Taylor P, Sharpless KB, Kolb HC (2004) *In situ* click chemistry: Enzyme inhibitors made to their own specifications. *J Am Chem Soc* 126: 12809–12818

75 Walsh DP, Chang YT (2004) Recent advances in small molecule microarrays: applications and technology. *Comb Chem High Throughput Screen* 7: 557–564

76 Koehler AN, Shamji AF, Schreiber SL (2003) Discovery of an inhibitor of a transcription factor using small molecule microarrays and diversity-oriented synthesis. *J Am Chem Soc* 125: 8420–8421

77 Winssinger N, Damoiseaux R, Tully DC, Geierstanger BH, Burdick K, Harris JL (2004) PNA-encoded protease substrate microarrays. *Chem Biol* 11: 1351–1360

78 Winssinger N, Ficarro S, Schultz PG, Harris JL (2002) Profiling protein function with small molecule microarrays. *Proc Natl Acad Sci USA* 99: 11139–11144

79 Annis DA, Nazef N, Chuang CC, Scott MP, Nash HM (2004) A general technique to rank protein-ligand binding affinities and determine allosteric *versus* direct binding site competition in compound mixtures. *J Am Chem Soc* 126: 15495–15503

80 Lewis LM, Engle LJ, Pierceall WE, Hughes DE, Shaw KJ (2004) Affinity capillary electrophoresis for the screening of novel antimicrobial targets. *J Biomol Screen* 9: 303–308

81 Juris SJ, Shah K, Shokat K, Dixon JE, Vacratsis PO (2006) Identification of otubain 1 as a novel substrate for the *Yersinia* protein kinase using chemical genetics and mass spectrometry. *FEBS Lett* 580: 179–183

Progress in Drug Research, Vol. 64
(Helena I. Boshoff and Clifton E. Barry III, Eds)

Proteomic profiling of cellular stresses in *Bacillus subtilis* reveals cellular networks and assists in elucidating antibiotic mechanisms of action

By Julia E. Bandow[1]
and Michael Hecker[2]

[1] Pfizer Global Research and Development,
Pfizer Inc.,
Ann Arbor, Michigan, USA
<julia.bandow@pfizer.com>

[2] Institute for Microbiology,
Ernst-Moritz-Arndt Universität Greifswald,
Greifswald, Germany

Abstract

Proteomic profiling provides a global view of the protein composition of the cell. In contrast to the static nature of the genome sequence, which provides the blueprint for all protein-based cellular building blocks, the proteome is highly dynamic. The protein composition is constantly adjusting to facilitate survival, growth, and reproduction in an ever-changing environment. In a quest to understand the regulation of cellular networks in bacteria and the role of individual proteins in the adaptation process, the proteomic response to stress and starvation was analyzed in wild-type and mutant strains. The knowledge derived from these proteomic studies was applied to investigating the bacterial response to antibiotics. It was found that proteomics presents a powerful tool for hypothesis generation regarding antibiotic mechanism of action.

1 Introduction

Bacillus subtilis has long been the Gram-positive model organism for studies of bacterial physiology. Since it is a non-pathogenic bacterium that lives in the soil, one may wonder what attributes led *B. subtilis* to this modest fame. Besides being easily grown and handled under laboratory conditions two reasons stand out. First, physiologists were fascinated by the ability of *B. subtilis* to survive hostile environmental conditions by producing robust dormant endospores that germinate when conditions become more favorable. Sporulation and germination presented the opportunity to study cell differentiation in an organism of relatively low complexity (for recent review see [1]). Secondly, *B. subtilis* was a great organism for functional analyses because it was easily genetically modified due to natural competence – which enables the cells to take up intact DNA from the growth medium and incorporate DNA into their own genome via homologous recombination. Proteomic analyses have been part of physiological and functional investigations of *B. subtilis* since the early 1980s and have contributed to the understanding of the sequential expression of proteins during sporulation [2, 3]. At that time, two-dimensional gel electrophoresis, now considered the classic platform for proteomic profiling, had only recently been described by O'Farrell [4] and Klose [5]. It was capable of separating hundreds of proteins with great resolution but comparative analysis relied on visual inspection of gels or gel images and was therefore qualitative in nature and hardly comprehensive. Later, proteins were identified using

N-terminal sequencing or amino acid composition analysis, cumbersome processes that many times were in vain because no matching protein or DNA sequence could be found in the sparsely-populated databases.

A series of major developments have caused the landscape of proteomic profiling to look quite different today: (1) the availability of genomic sequences of entire organisms combined with (2) huge progress in the field of protein mass spectrometry (MS) have enabled the high throughput identification of proteins from 2D gels; (3) 2D gels can now be run with much higher reproducibility, and (4) the development of specialized image analysis software has facilitated the study of large numbers of samples, allowing statistical analysis of protein expression. 'Proteomic maps', annotated gel images on which identified proteins are labeled, are rapidly established with these methods and in the case of bacteria cover a high percentage of transcribed open reading frames. Together with the growing knowledge on protein function and the mapping of proteins to metabolic and regulatory pathways these proteome maps provide a good starting point for comparative analyses that lead to new hypotheses or biological insights.

Comprehensive proteome maps for *B. subtilis* have been published [6, 7] that cover about 40% of the open reading frames expressed under exponential growth conditions and about 20% of all encoded open reading frames. Importantly, the majority of proteins belonging to major metabolic pathways like citric acid cycle, amino acid or nucleotide metabolism, as well as transcription elongation and translational apparatus are identified on standard 2D gels and allow detailed monitoring of vital cellular functions. In this chapter, we will briefly discuss the relevant methods and then turn to the important contributions of proteomics to understanding the enormous capacity of bacteria to adapt to changes in their environment and growth conditions. Proteomic studies have also provided key insights into the make up of bacterial regulatory networks and functional units and resolved their interplay over time. We will further show how the study of bacterial survival strategies led to practical applications in antibacterial drug discovery, providing insights into compound mechanism of action, confidence in safety of compounds, as well as generating hypotheses around new targets.

2 The tools of proteomic profiling

The vast majority of proteomic studies in *B. subtilis* that aimed at answering physiological questions were performed utilizing pulse labeling with L-[^{35}S]-methionine to capture 'snapshots' of protein synthesis, followed by two-dimensional gel electrophoresis for protein separation, and mass spectrometry for protein identification. We will briefly summarize the principles of these technologies here.

2.1 Pulse labeling experiments

Pulse labeling experiments (Fig. 1) have played a key role in the analysis of bacterial stress responses. In particular, they enabled the study of physiological changes over time. Profiling of the total accumulated protein of

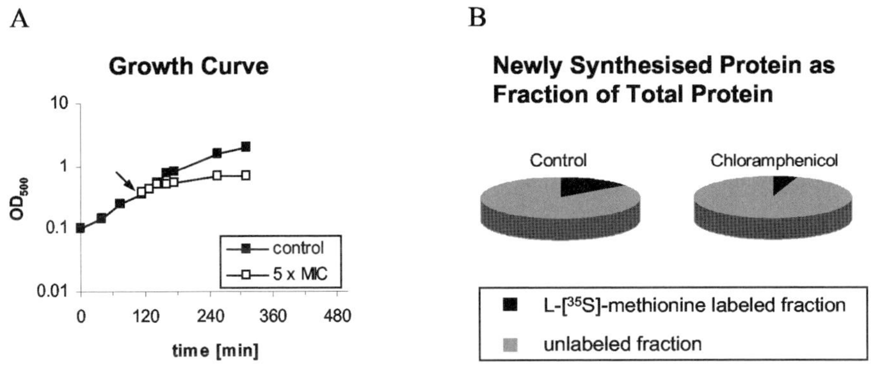

Figure 1a and b.
Pulse labeling experiments allow comparison of protein amount and protein synthesis. Exposure to chloramphenicol at a concentration of 15 µg/ml for 10 min is used here as an example for proteomic profiling of protein synthesis using pulse labeling with *L*-[^{35}S]-methionine and protein amounts using silver staining. (A) Growth curve of *B. subtilis*. The arrow indicates the addition of chloramphenicol to the medium. Aliquots of the control culture and chloramphenicol treated culture are labeled with *L*-[^{35}S]-methionine for 5 min beginning 10 min after addition of the antibiotic. Cells are then harvested and lyzed for proteomic profiling. (B) Total protein is measured by Bradford assay and radioactivity is measured using a scintillation counter. The addition of the protein synthesis inhibitor chloramphenicol leads to a decrease in protein synthesis rates, which is reflected by the smaller fraction of radio labeled protein in the antibiotic-treated sample.

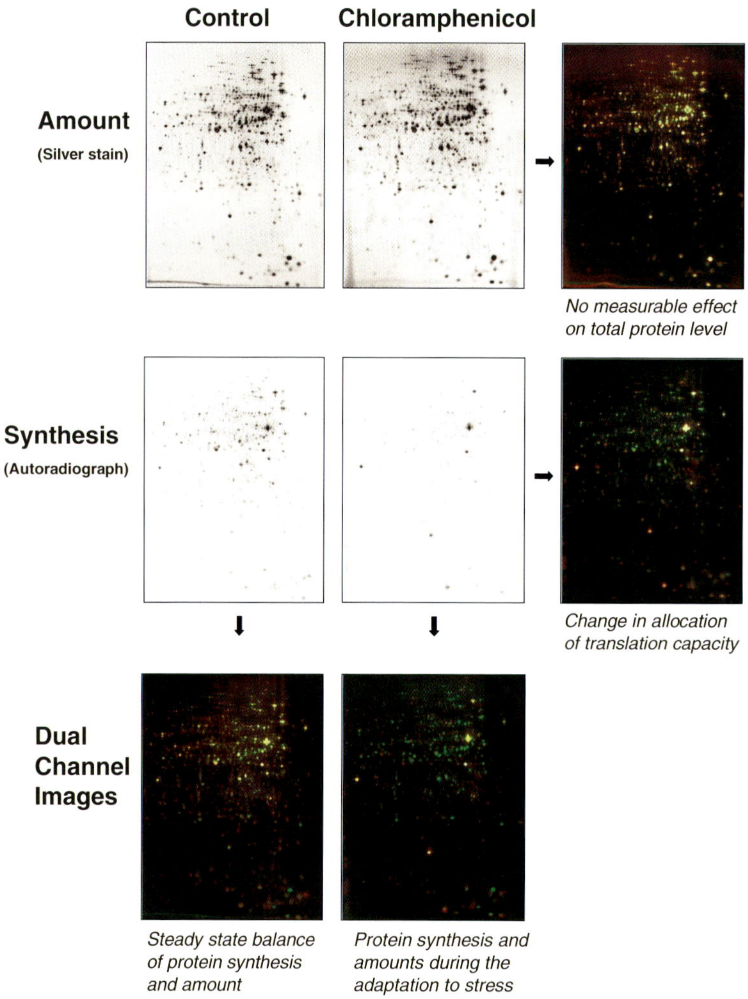

Figure 1c.
(C) Proteins are separated on 2D gels and stained with silver nitrate. Gels are then dried and exposed to phosphor screens, which are scanned to generate autoradiographic images. The overall pattern of the accumulated protein is not changed much between the control and the chloramphenicol treated cells (top row). When comparing the proteomic profile of the proteins newly synthesized during the pulse in the control and antibiotic treated samples (second row) the differences in translation capacity allocation become apparent. The dual channel images (third row) are overlays of the silver stained gel images (green) and the autoradiographs (red). These dual channel images allow comparing protein synthesis and amount. The control sample shows a balance of protein synthesis and amount which is evidenced by most proteins being yellow, whereas in the chloramphenicol treated sample most proteins appear green, which means that they are no longer synthesized but still present in stainable amounts (consistent with protein synthesis inhibition).

cell cultures under different conditions is not a sensitive enough tool to analyze the rapid changes occurring in bacterial responses because of the relatively long *in vivo* half-life of proteins. Rather than looking at the total cellular protein, a lot of which comes as a legacy of growth in 'good times' it is much more informative to examine changes taking place in the short transition period during which cells adapt to meet current challenges. This is achieved by metabolic labeling of newly synthesized proteins with radio-labeled amino acids for a short period of time (5 min) before cell harvest. The readout is not unlike that of RNA profiling studies in principle, however, the relatively long half-life of proteins is in contrast to the snapshot of RNA profiling that is often dominated by the relative instability of bacterial RNA (the half life of most mRNAs in *B. subtilis* is less than 5 min under exponential growth conditions). Dual channel imaging has been developed and applied in the context of studying the adaptation of *B. subtilis* to heat shock and oxidative stress [8]. This very intuitive graphical tool aligns the autoradiograph of a 2D gel depicting only newly synthesized proteins with the image of the stained gel showing the total accumulated protein, thereby directly visualizing changes in the relative rates of specific protein synthesis. The image of the autoradiograph is assigned the false-color red and the image of the stained gel is colored green. Proteins synthesized in higher amounts in response to an imposed change in growth conditions stand out in bright red while proteins whose synthesis is downregulated appear green. The magnitude of the change in synthesis rates can also be quantified using image analysis software. Where protein amount and synthesis are balanced, the protein spots appear yellow. Under exponential growth conditions this is the case for most protein spots. However, when the cells are adapting to changes in their environment they shift protein production predominantly to those proteins that are vital to the adaptive response to the stress imposed. At the same time cells often stop producing proteins that are not required any longer in non-growing cells to avoid wasting nutrients. The majority of the downregulated proteins remain abundant, and are often still present at levels sufficient to continue to fulfill their cellular function. This aspect of the stress response cannot be monitored on the mRNA level.

2.2 2D gel electrophoresis and mass spectrometry

Two-dimensional gel electrophoresis, first developed in 1975, is still the major workhorse in comparative proteomic profiling analysis. Complex protein mixtures like cell lysates are separated into individual protein components based on two physicochemical properties, the isoelectric point (first dimension) and molecular weight (second dimension). Isoelectric points are a function of the globular structure of proteins and are performed under mostly native conditions. The isoelectric focusing for the experiments described in this chapter was for the most part performed in immobilized pH gradient gel (IPG) strips [8]. After the isoelectric focusing protein disulfides are reduced and alkylated *in situ* in separate steps before the plastic-backed gel is placed onto a large denaturing SDS-PAGE gel for the second electrophoresis step. Unfortunately, these separation techniques do not extend well to membrane proteins, primarily because of the difficulties of maintaining native structure for the isoelectric focusing step (denatured proteins migrate primarily as a function of their amino acid composition) which is an important limitation of proteomic approaches. Over the years visualization methods have also evolved. Coomassie Brilliant Blue G-250 and silver stains have gradually been supplemented by the sensitive and more quantitative fluorescence-based Sypro Ruby stain. Likewise, different methods have been used for analysis. As image analysis software tools improved in accuracy and speed the visual inspection of hundreds of protein spots across many gel images was mostly replaced by automated quantitative analysis (although it is fair to say that a good amount of time is still spent on visual quality control). Protein spots of interest are excised from the 2D gel for mass spectrometric analysis. Peptide mass fingerprinting (PMF) provides high-throughput protein identification [9]. Peptide masses detected in a tryptic digest of an isolated protein spot are compared to a database containing peptide masses of all proteins predicted by *in silico* calculation based on the genome sequence. In cases where PMF is not conclusive peptides can be analyzed by tandem mass spectrometry [10], which provides partial amino acid sequence information and is similarly interpreted through searches against a database.

3 Proteomic contributions to understanding bacterial physiology

Proteomics has greatly contributed to our knowledge of physiological adaptive responses. The following sections will describe what we have learned about the major proteins and pathways in adaptation processes, how they are connected and how they are regulated.

3.1 Uncovering stimulons, regulons, and proteomic signatures

During exponential growth bacterial cells produce and turn over proteins maintaining a steady state that supports regular cell growth and division. Experiments that disturb this steady state force the cells to respond to the perturbation by adjusting their protein composition in order to overcome the challenge and survive. By exposing cells to a variety of metabolic insults, regulatory processes are exposed, revealing key protein components whose concentrations are adjusted to facilitate successful adaptation. Any particular factor chosen to disturb the system is referred to as stimulus.

Proteomic experiments first addressed those stimuli that *B. subtilis* is likely to routinely encounter in its natural environment such as heat shock, salt stress, oxidative stress, oxygen, amino acid, or glucose limitation [2, 8, 11–13]. Adaptation to glucose limitation [13] is a practical example of how the proteomic response can be monitored over time. Pulse labeling was performed as a function of time, beginning with a control time point reflecting the steady state of exponential growth phase and different time points along the course of adaptation. At each time point a fraction of the culture was labeled with L-[^{35}S]-methionine for 5 min providing insight into which proteins are synthesized at any given point in the process. These snapshots put together in sequence provide a 'time-lapse movie' showing which components of the proteome come into play at particular stages of adaptation. Any component that is either upregulated or downregulated in response to the disturbance of the steady state is part of the stimulon – the total of all changes induced by a stimulus.

Bacteria are extremely fast responders. Within minutes the protein expression pattern can change completely if the stimulus warrants dramatic changes, leaving no group of proteins untouched. In the case of heat

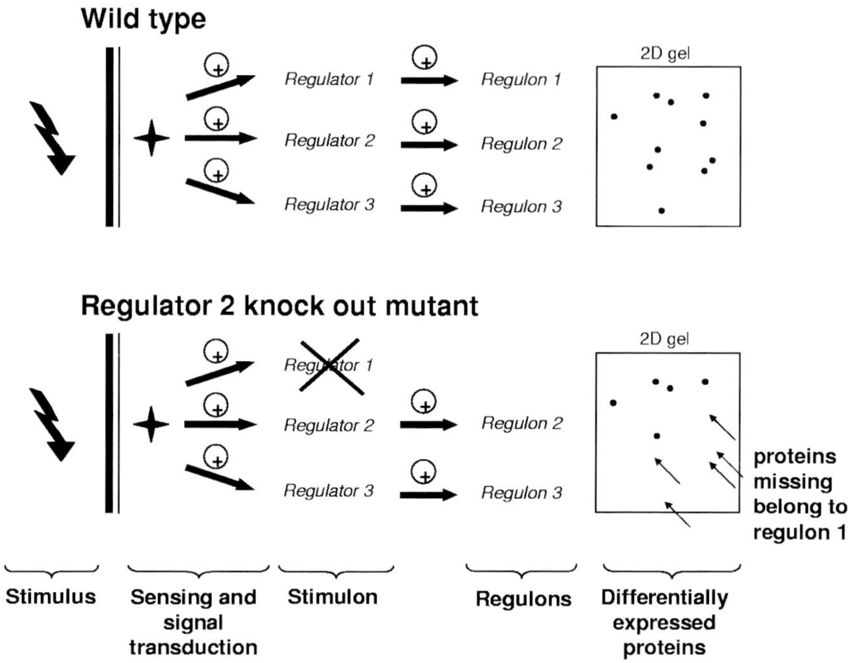

Figure 2.
Elucidation of stimulons and regulons using proteomics. All proteins that are differentially produced in response to a particular change in conditions (stimulus) form a stimulon. The upregulation and downregulation of proteins can be identified on 2D gels. Often times multiple regulators are involved in orchestrating the cellular response to a stimulus, each one controlling those proteins that belong to its regulon. The protein profile of knock out mutants lacking a critical regulator can be compared to the wild type to identify the members of the regulon.

shock and glucose limitation, expression rates of the majority of proteins are either upregulated or downregulated [8, 13]. Mutant analyses are a useful tool to analyze how these changes are orchestrated. Performing the same stress or nutrient limitation experiment with mutants that lack crucial regulators like transcription factors, repressors, or alternative sigma factors reveal which proteins are coordinated by a regulator under the conditions tested (Fig. 2). Heat shock experiments revealed that at least four different regulators are involved in coordinating a large number of heat shock responsive proteins in *B. subtilis*: for example, the repressor HrcA which binds to the controlling inverted repeat of chaperone expression (CIRCE) element [14], the alternative sigma factor SigB [15], the repressor CtsR [16, 17], and the two-component system CssR/S [18]. Each regulator controls a specific set of proteins referred to as a regulon. Interestingly, many regulators react in response to more than one stimulus and therefore the proteins controlled by them are part of more than one stimulon. Proteins can also be regulated by more than one regulator and therefore be part of more than one regulon. The *clpC* operon is a prototypical example of an operon under dual control. Upon heat shock it is transcribed from a SigB-dependent promoter, but a SigA-dependent promoter can compensate in a *sigB* mutant exposed to heat shock. This promoter, recognized by the house-keeping sigma factor SigA, is responsible for *clpC* induction upon hydrogen peroxide stress or puromycin treatment in the wild-type [19]. It is evident that the adaptational networks are of considerable complexity. In addition to different regulators acting in parallel there are also regulators that are activated in sequence. Glucose limitation is an excellent example of sequential regulation [13]. In the transient phase, at the onset of glucose limitation, the cells respond by inducing a set of proteins known as SigB-dependent general stress proteins, which are thought to protect the cell from future damage [20, 21]. Cells then activate the stringent response, shutting down many house-keeping proteins in order to conserve metabolites in nutrient-limited conditions. This response is initiated by the alarmone guanosine tetraphosphate (ppGpp) and leads to downregulation of the translational machinery, proteins involved in amino acid synthesis and other vegetative proteins [22]. At the same time, cells express proteins that help them access alternative carbon sources, which in the presence of glucose are repressed by CcpA. In parallel, at least some cells seem to initiate sporulation in a Spo0A-dependent fashion. This protein expression profiling experiment of glucose-starved cells was supplemented by mRNA profiling confirming most of the protein data [23]. This transcriptional analysis, however, did not reveal those proteins whose synthesis has been switched off in glucose-starved cells but that were still present and probably still active.

3.2 Revealing complex responses

In analyzing a variety of different stress factors and growth conditions it was recognized that regulons and subsets of regulons could be simultaneously part of the response to a variety of stimuli. In analyzing the response to cold and heat shock in *Escherichia coli* as well as treatment with antibiotics that inhibit translation, Van Bogelen and Neidhardt [24] found that there was overlap between the response to cold shock and the treatment with erythromycin and chloramphenicol, antibiotics that target the peptidyl-transferase step in translation, whereas the response to heat shock had many responder proteins in common with those inhibitors causing mistranslation. This led to the introduction of the term proteomic signatures, which consist of one or more proteins that are diagnostic of a physiological condition [25]. As we will see later, particularly the concept of proteomic signatures has greatly benefited the mechanism of action studies for novel drugs. Thus, certain antibiotics result in a proteomic signature identical to the cold shock-like response by virtue of their ability to upregulate proteins of the translation apparatus. This suggests that translational capacity is the limiting factor for cell growth at cold temperatures as well as when peptidyl-transferase is inhibited. On the other hand, the induction of chaperone systems like GroES/GroEL is an indication of an increase in the number of misfolded proteins in the cell which occurs upon heat shock and treatment with aminoglycosides. In addition to proteomic signatures that consist of upregulated or downregulated proteins, 2D gel-based proteomics can also reveal direct effects of stimuli if they modify or damage proteins. Oxidative stress is a good example: several regulons are induced in response to hydrogen peroxide, paraquat, and/or diamide (PerR, Fur, CtsR, OhrR) serving as indicators for oxidative damage [26, 27]. An additional change reveals direct evidence of alteration of several proteins particularly sensitive to oxidative damage, because protein migration patterns are altered if cysteines are oxidised to sulfonic acid resulting in migration at a more acidic pI. With different labeling strategies non-native disulfide bonds formed as a result of protein oxidation can also be visualized on 2D gels [28, 29]. Attempts have also been made at deciphering the S-nitrosoproteome of organisms. Nitrosylation of proteins can be rapid and reversible and often occurs by formation of S-nitrosothiols of cysteine residues. S-nitrosothiols decompose in the presence of thiols and reduced metal cations and determining the extent of S-nitrosylation can be difficult. One method for stabilizing these groups involves firstly blocking thiols with a rapidly acting thiol-reactive agent, reduction of S-nitrosothiols with subsequent labeling of the resulting thiol groups with a fluorescent or biotinylated methanethiosulfonate derivative [30]. The nitrosoproteome of *Mycobacterium tuberculosis* that results from exposure of the organism to nitric oxide was established as a way of identifying the vulnerable targets of this antimicrobial [31]. The nitrosoproteins identified were all enzymes, many of them essential, and could indicate their potential as drug targets. The phosphoproteome of *B. subtilis* has also been established as a means of probing dynamic metabolic processes in bacterial cells [32].

4 Proteomics in antibacterial drug discovery

The proteomic analysis of bacterial response to stress demonstrates that the expression pattern is exquisitely fine-tuned and provides a very sensitive monitor of environmental changes. Approaches in antibacterial drug discovery are changing. For decades the discovery of novel antibacterial agents began with the observation that bacterial growth was inhibited by a compound *in vivo* and/or in a host. Subsequent efforts to elucidate the mechanism of action often took many years, during which compounds were often already in use to treat patients. Since the mid 1990s, with the availability of entire bacterial genome sequences, this approach was mostly replaced by rational drug discovery. Drug targets were picked based on essentiality of a gene and evolutionary conservation of the target across species yet evolutionary divergence from potential host homologs [33, 34]. High throughput *in vitro* assays are designed to search for specific inhibitors of these 'golden targets'. Out of thousands of compounds screened, the few compounds that successfully inhibited the target were tested for antibacterial activity *in vivo*.

Proteomics can make contributions to both general approaches to antibacterial discovery programs. When antibacterial activity is observed but the mechanism of action is not known, proteomic profiles can reveal the mechanism of action by comparison to inhibitors with known mechanism of action. Even when no reference compound with matching profile is available, marker proteins and proteomic signatures can be used to interpret the physiological changes invoked by the compound. This may very well lead to testable hypotheses about the mechanism of action. If compounds found in an *in vitro* assay are tested for antibacterial activity, proteomic profiles can be used to confirm that this same target is affected during treatment of whole cells with the inhibitor. Protein profiles of conditional mutants of the target gene will generally resemble the protein profile of the inhibitor. Protein profiling can additionally identify compounds that have undesired effects by comparing compound profiles to profiles of agents that exhibit general toxicity. RNA profiling can contribute in a similar way to mechanism of action studies [34, 35].

The best time point for antibiotic proteomic profiling is typically early exponential growth phase. Cells have ample nutrients and are in a steady state of regular division where the protein pattern is quite stable. In this growth phase cells have the greatest ability to respond to stress imposed on them because neither energy nor nutrients limit their ability to respond.

4.1 Reference compendium

A reference compendium of protein profiles contains annotated protein profiles that visualize differences and provide quantitation of the changes in protein expression compared to control conditions [36, 37]. It is most helpful when these changes can be related to the knowledge about the physiological state of the cells. The power of a reference compendium depends on the diversity of conditions and treatments represented in the database. Ideally, the database will contain groups of protein profiles corresponding to a number of similar stimuli, for instance structurally different inhibitors of the same molecular target or inhibitors that target different steps in a metabolic pathway, so that protein signatures or marker proteins can be defined for particular physiological conditions. The largest and most diverse compendium to date has been published for *B. subtilis* [38]. It contains the protein profiles for 30 different agents with antimicrobial activity, some of which are antibiotics with established as well as unknown mechanisms of action, others are general cytotoxic agents such as detergents and DNA intercalators which in themselves have no value as drugs due to universal toxicity, but which serve to define the metabolic pathways that are activated after defined cellular insults. Furthermore, the reference compendium contains protein profiles of a conditional mutant that provide proof of concept for the regulation of particular proteins in response to certain stresses [39]. Profiles of compounds with unknown mechanism of action stemming from antibacterial research programs were compared to the reference profiles [38, 40, 41] and are now included. Large numbers of well-characterized physiological conditions in the reference compendium increase the chances of finding a match for compounds with unknown mechanism. A reference compendium that includes profiles for all essential gene products would be very helpful in assigning mechanisms of action to novel antimicrobial agents.

4.2 Stress response studies give insight into mechanisms of drug action

The extensive study of the responses of *B. subtilis* to different stress conditions provided important insights into the structures of bacterial adaptation networks and therefore was an invaluable prerequisite for the antibiotic studies. Beyond the general understanding of regulatory networks specific aspects discovered in these initial experiments benefited the interpretation of drug response analyses. Antibiotic exposure is not unlike exposure to other life threatening stress factors and the resulting adaptational responses evolved securing a competitive advantage in the environment. Protein signatures established for different physiological conditions can prove very useful in the interpretation of antibiotic protein profiles. Cells treated with a novel inhibitor of phenylalanyl-tRNA synthetase for example showed a proteomic signature known to be characteristic for the stringent response [41] – a mechanism triggered by uncharged tRNAs occupying the A-site of the ribosome. The stringent response is mediated by ppGpp synthesis that results in subsequent shut-down of protein synthesis and other growth-oriented activities like expression of ribosomal proteins and is therefore metabolically similar to aminoacyl-tRNA synthetase inhibition. Additionally, the protein profile was highly similar to that elicited by Mupirocin – a known inhibitor of isoleucyl-tRNA synthetase – with the important difference that the phenylalanyl-tRNA synthetase inhibitor induced the targeted phenylalanyl tRNA synthetase instead of the isoleucyl-tRNA synthetase.

4.3 Novel compound classes with unknown mechanisms of action

A novel pyrimidinone compound, BAY 50-2369, which was structurally related to a natural compound TAN 1057 A/B, was discovered to have antibacterial activity but the mechanism of action was unknown. The protein profile of *B. subtilis* after treatment with this compound was highly similar to that of erythromycin, chloramphenicol, tetracycline, and fusidic acid – all compounds known to directly or indirectly inhibit peptidyl-transferase activity. Protein synthesis inhibitors are strongly represented in the reference compendium. Based on their protein profiles and signatures in *B. subtilis* they can be sorted into three distinct groups: (1) those that interfere directly or indirectly with peptidyl-transferase activity (erythromycin, chloramphenicol, tetracycline, fusidic acid), (2) those that cause mis-translation and, as a result, incorrectly folded proteins (aminoglycosides), and (3) those that lead to abortive translation (puromycin). Based on the similarity of the proteomic profile of Bay 50-2369 to that of inhibitors of peptidyl-transferase activity, the mechanism of action could be narrowed down rapidly [38] (Fig. 3). In independent experiments peptidyl-transferase was confirmed as the target for TAN 1057 A/B [42].

4.4 Proteomic analysis of conditional mutants – a powerful tool for target validation

Essential genes hold valuable promise as targets for antibiotics since disruption of essential functions should inhibit bacterial growth. Several potential new targets have been identified based on essentiality and the absence of close homologs in humans, whose inhibition could potentially cause cessation of bacterial growth. To analyze cells that lack essential gene functions, conditional mutants have to be generated that are able to grow under permissive conditions, while providing the possibility to tightly downregulate the expression of the essential gene. While complicated to construct and often unstable, these mutants provide excellent

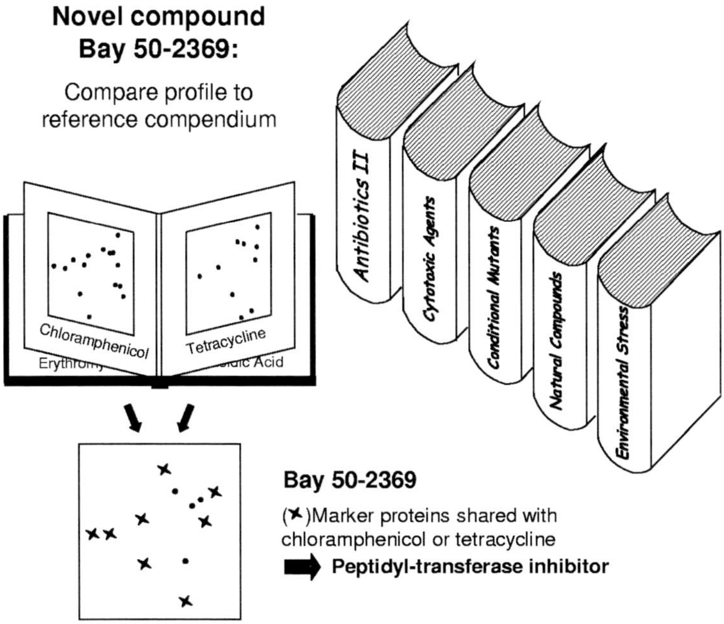

Figure 3.
Reference compendium. Comparing protein profiles of novel compounds to the reference compendium can generate hypotheses about the mechanism of action. The example shows how the mechanism of action of Bay 50-2369 was identified.

tools to study changes in the protein profile upon limitation of an essential gene function. The change in the protein profile is very similar to that of cells in which the same cellular function is inhibited by a small molecule inhibitor. This was shown in a proof of concept study, which compared protein profiles of a conditional *B. subtilis* deformylase mutant and the protein profiles of wild-type *B. subtilis* treated with the deformylase inhibitor actinonin [39]. Regardless of whether deformylase function was impaired genetically or by the inhibitor, the protein profiles revealed the same dramatic changes in the protein expression pattern. New protein spots with slightly more acidic pIs appeared next to existing protein spots. These pI shifts of newly synthesized proteins are caused by the uncleaved formyl-residue that masks the N-termini of proteins.

Conditional mutants have been used for proof of concept studies to verify that downregulation of the gene has the desired effect of ceasing bacterial growth [43]. Protein profiles of these conditional mutants greatly enhance the value of the reference compendium, as they provide a reference profile for inhibition of targets for which inhibitors have not yet been identified. Compounds that are identified in *in vitro* target inhibition screening and show inhibition of growth can be tested in proteomic profiling experiments to confirm the *in vivo* mechanism of action by comparison to the reference profile.

4.5 Identification of potential safety issues

In some cases proteomics can reveal potential issues that are related to safety profiles of compounds. For instance, the reference compendium contains chemicals that are known DNA-damaging agents. Marker proteins for DNA damage include RecA, a regulatory protein involved in the DNA repair process. In *B. subtilis* the expression of prophage PBSX is RecA-dependent and the prophage proteins are induced upon treatment with DNA-damaging reagents mitomycin C and 4-nitroquinoline-1-oxide [38]. If these proteins are induced they warrant scrutiny in investigating the potential of the tested compounds being DNA-damaging and thus their suitability as anti-infectives. However, agents that result in DNA damage are not necessarily poor drug candidates since inhibition of specific proteins involved in maintenance of DNA metabolism may also result in a profile indicative of DNA repair. This is seen in the upregulation of the RecA-dependent SOS regulon during treatment of bacteria with fluoroquinolones [44] as a result of double-stranded DNA breaks introduced in the chromosome by topoisomerase inhibition. Protein signatures containing proteins that serve as markers for interference with membrane integrity are currently being characterized. Compounds in this class of inhibitors span a range of mechanisms of action: agents such as gramicidin A that result in the formation of ion channel for monovalent cations, agents such as gramicidin S that cause membrane depolarization, molecules such as monensin that complex of Group IA and IIA metal cations and interfere with their transport across the membrane, valinomycin which creates potassium channels across the phospholipid bilayer and detergents such as Triton X-100. Interestingly, the profiles of the tested compounds are very dissimilar [38]. The variety of responses elicited by these various membrane function disruptive agents indicates that *B. subtilis* has evolved to respond specifically to mechanistically different challenges of membrane integrity. This suggests that different sensory and response mechanisms exist in *B. subtilis* to counteract the loss of critical functions of the cell membrane. To date, not enough membrane-targeting inhibitors have been tested to link specific proteomic signatures to the impairment of particular physiological membrane functions.

4.6 New targets – a rare proteomics contribution

When the genome sequencing projects were first launched, it was anticipated that global profiling methods would reveal new targets. The cross-species comparison of essential bacterial genes on the DNA level has led to the identification of potential antibacterial targets that were not yet exploited [33]. Proteomics has traditionally not been used in identifying new potential targets since protein expression profiles reveal the cellular response to a stimulus rather than the actual target. However, recently an example of proteomics aiding new target identification has been described [40]. The mechanism of action of a novel class of bactericidal compounds, the acyldepsipeptides, was investigated using two different approaches: proteomic profiling and the mapping of mutations in resistant mutants utilizing a genomic plasmid library. The proteomic profile did not match any of the previously obtained profiles. The protein expression profile elicited by the acyldepsipeptides was characterized by the accumulation of the degradation products of GroEL, DnaK, Tig, and EF-Tu in new protein spots on the gel as well as the induction of ClpP. The induction of these proteins is consistent with the presence of protein degradation products or misfolded proteins in the cell as has been observed during treatment with aminoglycosides. However, accumulation of specific protein fragments was not observed with aminoglycosides, indicating that this presented a new proteomic signature. The hypothesis generated from these profiling experiments was that the compound activates a protease that induced the degradation of the proteins of which the degradation products were observed and, in turn, that the protein fragments induced the production of the Clp protease and chaperones. This hypothesis was tested and confirmed by transforming the sensitive parental strain with a genomic library created from resistant mutants, which revealed that ClpP was the target of acyldepsipeptides. These studies were extended by subsequent binding studies between the protease and the acyldepsipeptides and protein activity measurements. Acyldepsipeptides initiate a catastrophic cycle in which newly synthesized proteins are vulnerable to degradation by the deregulated protease. This provides an example of how proteomics can shed light on the mode of action of unknown drugs leading to the generation of testable hypotheses. Interestingly, unlike most drugs which inhibit a specific target, the acyldepsipeptides perturb the balance of the cellular system by activating the ClpP protease, a function that is usually tightly controlled, and uncoupling ClpP activity from auxiliary proteins that normally function as regulatory safeguards. This highlights the value of proteomics in elucidating mechanistically and conceptually novel mechanisms of action of new anti-infectives.

References

1 Piggot PJ, Hilbert DW (2004) Sporulation of *Bacillus subtilis*. *Curr Opin Microbiol* 7: 579–586
2 Wachlin G, Hecker M (1984) Protein biosynthesis following heat shock in *Bacillus subtilis*. *Z Allg Mikrobiol* 24: 397–401 (German)
3 Richter A, Hecker M (1986) Heat-shock proteins in *Bacillus subtilis*: a two-dimensional electrophoresis study. *FEMS Microbiol Lett* 36: 69–71
4 O'Farrell PH (1975) High resolution two-dimensional electrophoresis of proteins. *J Biol Chem* 250: 4007–4021
5 Klose J (1975) Protein mapping by combined isoelectric focusing and electrophoresis of mouse tissues. *Humangenetik* 26: 231–243
6 Buttner K, Bernhardt J, Scharf C, Schmid R, Mader U, Eymann C, Antelmann H, Volker A, Volker U, Hecker M (2001) A comprehensive two-dimensional map of cytosolic proteins of *Bacillus subtilis*. *Electrophoresis* 22: 2908–2935
7 Eymann C, Dreisbach A, Albrecht D, Bernhardt J, Becher D, Gentner S, Tam le T, Buttner K, Buurman G, Scharf C et al (2004) A comprehensive proteome map of growing *Bacillus subtilis* cells. *Proteomics* 4: 2849–2876
8 Bernhardt J, Buttner K, Scharf C, Hecker M (1999) Dual channel imaging of two-dimensional electropherograms in *Bacillus subtilis*. *Electrophoresis* 20: 2225–2240
9 Henzel WJ, Billeci TM, Stults JT, Wong SC, Grimley C, Watanabe C (1993) Identifying proteins from two-dimensional gels by molecular mass searching of peptide fragments in protein sequence databases. *Proc Natl Acad Sci USA* 90: 5011–5015
10 Mann M, Hendrickson RC, Pandey A (2001) Analysis of proteins and proteomes by mass spectrometry. *Annu Rev Biochem* 70: 437–473

11 Volker U, Engelmann S, Maul B, Riethdorf S, Volker A, Schmid R, Mach H, Hecker M (1994) Analysis of the induction of general stress proteins of *Bacillus subtilis*. *Microbiology* 140: 741– 752

12 Antelmann H, Bernhardt J, Schmid R, Mach H, Volker U, Hecker M (1997) First steps from a two-dimensional protein index towards a response-regulation map of *Bacillus subtilis*. *Electrophoresis* 18: 1451–1463

13 Bernhardt J, Weibezahn J, Scharf C, Hecker M (2003) *Bacillus subtilis* during feast and famine: visualization of the overall regulation of protein synthesis during glucose starvation by proteome analysis. *Genome Res* 13: 224–237

14 Zuber U, Schuman W (1994) CIRCE, a novel heat shock element involved in regulation of heat shock operon *dnaK* of *Bacillus subtilis*. *J Bacteriol* 176: 1359–1363

15 Benson AK, Haldenwang WG (1993) The sigmaB-dependent promoter of the *Bacillus subtilis sigB* operon is induced by heat shock. *J Bacteriol* 175: 1929–1935

16 Kruger E, Hecker M (1998) The first gene of the *Bacillus subtilis clpC* operon, *ctsR*, encodes a negative regulator of its own operon and other class III heat shock genes. *J Bacteriol* 180: 6681–6688

17 Derre I, Rapoport G, Masdek T (2000) The CtsR regulator of stress is active as a dimer and specifically degraded *in vivo* at 37 degrees C. *Mol Microbiol* 38: 335–347

18 Darmon E, Noone D, Masson A, Bron S, Kuipers OP, Devine KM, van Dijl JM (2002) A novel class of heat and secretion stress-responsive genes is controlled by the autoregulated CssRS two-component system of *Bacillus subtilis*. *J Bacteriol* 184: 5661–5671

19 Kruger E, Msadek T, Hecker M (1996) Alternate promoters direct stress-induced transcription of the *Bacillus subtilis clpC* operon. *Mol Microbiol* 20: 713–723

20 Hecker M, Völker U (1998) Non-specific, general and multiple stress resistance of growth-restricted *Bacillus subtilis* cells by the expression of the σ^B regulon. *Mol Microbiol* 29: 1129–1136

21 Brody MS, Vijay K, Price CW (2001) Catalytic function of an alpha/beta hydrolase is required for energy stress activation of the sigma(B) transcription factor in *Bacillus subtilis*. *J Bacteriol* 183: 6422–6428

22 Eymann C, Homuth G, Scharf C, Hecker M (2002) *Bacillus subtilis* functional genomics: global characterization of the stringent response by proteome and transcriptome analysis. *J Bacteriol* 184: 2500–2520

23 Koburger T, Weibezahn J, Bernhardt J, Homuth G, Hecker M (2005) Genome-wide mRNA profiling in glucose starved *Bacillus subtilis* cells. *Mol Genet Genomics* 274: 1–12

24 VanBogelen RA, Neidhardt FC (1990) Ribosomes as sensors of heat and cold shock in *Escherichia coli*. *Proc Natl Acad Sci USA* 87: 5589–5593

25 VanBogelen RA, Schiller E, Thomas JD, Neidhardt FC (1999) Diagnosis of cellular states of microbial organisms using proteomics. *Electrophoresis* 20: 2149–2159

26 Mosterz J, Scharf C, Hecker M, Homuth (2004) Transcriptome and proteome analysis of *Bacillus subtilis* gene expression in response to superoxide and peroxide stress. *Microbiol* 150: 497–512

27 Leichert LI, Scharf C, Hecker M (2003) Global characterization of disulfide stress in *Bacillus subtilis*. *J Bacteriol* 185: 1967–1975
28 Leichert LI, Jakob U (2004) Protein thiol modifications visualized *in vivo*. *PloS Biol* 2: e333
29 Hochgraefe F, Mostertz J, Albrecht D, Hecker M (2005) Fluorescence thiol modification assay: oxidatively modified proteins in *Bacillus subtilis*. *Mol Microbiol* 58: 409–425
30 Yang Y, Loscalzo J (2005) S-nitrosoprotein formation and localization in endothelial cells. *Proc Natl Acad Sci USA* 102: 117–122
31 Rhee KY, Erdjument-Bromage H, Tempst P, Nathan CF (2005) S-nitroso proteome of *Mycobacterium tuberculosis*: Enzymes of intermediary metabolism and antioxidant defense. *Proc Natl Acad Sci USA* 102: 467–472
32 Levine A, Vannier F, Absalon C, Kuhn L, Jackson P, Scrivener E, Labas V, Vinh J, Courtney P, Garin J et al (2006) Analysis of the dynamic *Bacillus subtilis* Ser/Thr/Tyr phosphoproteome implicated in a wide variety of cellular processes. *Proteomics* 6: 2157–2173
33 Mills SD (2003) The role of genomics in antimicrobial discovery. *J Antimicrob Chemother* 51: 749–752
34 Freiberg C, Brotz-Oesterhelt H (2005b) Functional genomics in antibacterial drug discovery. *Drug Discovery Today* 1: 927–935
35 Freiberg C, Fisher HP, Brunner NA (2005a) Discovering the mechanism of action of novel antibacterial agents through transcriptional profiling of conditional mutants. *Antimicrob Agents Chemother* 49: 749–759
36 Brötz-Oesterhelt H, Bandow JE, Labischinski H (2005) Bacterial proteomics and its role in antibacterial drug discovery. *Mass Spectrom Rev* 24: 549–565
37 Freiberg C, Brotz-Oesterhelt H, Labischinski H (2004) The impact of transcriptome and proteome analyses on antibiotic drug discovery. *Curr Opin Microbiol* 7: 451–459
38 Bandow J, Brötz H, Leichert LIO, Labischinski H, Hecker M (2003) Proteomic approaches to understanding antibiotic action. *Antimicrob Agents Chemother* 47: 948–955
39 Bandow JE, Becher D, Buttner K, Hochgrafe F, Freiberg C, Brötz H, Hecker M (2003). The role of peptide deformylase in protein biosynthesis: a proteomic study. *Proteomics* 3: 299–306
40 Brötz-Oesterhelt H, Beyer D, Kroll HP, Schroeder W, Hinzen B, Raddatz S, Paulsen H, Bandow JE, Sahl HG, Labischinski H (2005) Dysregulation of bacterial proteolytic machinery by a new class of antibiotics. *Nat Med* 11: 1082–1087
41 Beyer D, Kroll HP, Endermann R, Schiffer G, Siegel S, Bauser M, Pohlmann J, Brands M, Ziegelbauer K, Haebich D et al (2004) New class of bacterial phenylalanyl-tRNA synthetase inhibitors with high potency and broad-spectrum activity. *Antimicrob Agents Chemother* 48: 525–532
42 Boddecker N, Bahador G, Gibbs C, Mabery E, Wolf J, Xu L, Watson J (2002) Characterization of a novel antibacterial agent that inhibits bacterial translation. *RNA* 8: 1120–1128

43 Apfel CM, Locher H, Evers S, Takacs B, Hubschwerlen C, Pirson W, Page MG, Keck W (2001) Peptide deformylase as an antibacterial drug target: target validation and resistance development. *Antimicrob Agents Chemother* 45: 1058–1064

44 Boshoff HI, Myers TG, Copp BR, McNeil MR, Wilson MA, Barry CE 3rd (2004) The transcriptional responses of *Mycobacterium tuberculosis* to inhibitors of metabolism: novel insights into drug mechanisms of action. *J Biol Chem* 279: 40174–40184

Progress in Drug Research, Vol. 64
(Helena I. Boshoff and Clifton E. Barry III, Eds)

Elucidating the mode-of-action of compounds from metabolite profiling studies

By Jesper Højer-Pedersen,
Jørn Smedsgaard
and Jens Nielsen

Center for Microbial Biotechnology,
BioCentrum-DTU,
Technical University of Denmark,
Kgs. Lyngby, Denmark
<jn@biocentrum.dtu.dk>

Abstract

Metabolite profiling has been carried out for decades and is as such not a new research area. However, the field has attracted increasing attention in the last couple of years, and the term metabolome is now often used to describe the complete pool of metabolites associated with an organism at any given time. Mass spectrometry (MS) and nuclear magnetic resonance (NMR) spectroscopy are the best candidates for comprehensive analysis of the metabolome and the application of these technologies is presented in this chapter. In this relation, the importance of efficient metabolite screening for discovery of novel drugs is discussed. Related to metabolite profiling, the principals underlying the application of labeled substrates to quantify *in vivo* metabolic fluxes are introduced, and the chapter is concluded by discussing the perspectives of metabolite measurements in systems biology.

Keywords: drug discovery, metabolite profiling, fingerprinting, MS, CE-MS GC-MS, LC-MS, flux analysis, systems biology, metabolite analysis

1 Introduction

Although metabolite profiling studies have been carried out for decades they have recently attracted increased attention as a tool in functional genomics and systems biology [1–6], and the term metabolome has been coined to described the complete pool of cellular metabolites. The metabolome is the concentration of all low molecular weight metabolites under specified conditions by analogy to the use of the terms genome, transcriptome and proteome, and was first mentioned in the literature in 1998 [7, 8]. A major component of the metabolome (the primary metabolites in central metabolism) is conserved across species which makes it possible to develop generic analytical techniques that can be applied uniformly, in contrast to the situation for genes, transcripts and proteins that are species-specific. The metabolome can be further divided into the endo- and the exo-metabolome that cover the metabolites inside and outside the cell, respectively, although obviously some metabolites are present in both the endo- and the exo-metabolome since they are transported across the cell membrane.

Metabolite profiles are the signature of physiological states. The central dogma in biology hierarchically links genes, transcripts and proteins, but metabolites cannot be simply characterized as a direct product of proteins.

However, proteins catalyze the conversion of metabolites and the catalytic activity of enzymes is a prerequisite for most metabolic reactions. Metabolites are therefore indirectly a downstream consequence of patterns of gene expression [9, 10]. Metabolites are also the intermediates of biochemical reactions that form metabolic pathways. These pathways are highly interconnected and constitute a metabolic network that serves many different functions in a living cell. Metabolite concentrations are determined by the kinetics of the different enzymes that produce and consume the metabolite, hence the metabolite concentrations are indirectly influenced by gene transcription, mRNA translation and stability, protein–DNA interactions, protein–protein interactions, post-translational modifications etc. Metabolite concentrations therefore provide dynamic and integrative information on the many different processes operating in a living cell, and are therefore very likely to be direct indicators of developmental, genetic and environmental changes, which to some degree is complementary to the genetic information [7, 11–13]. The mode-of-action of small molecule enzyme inhibitors is also theoretically directly reflected in the metabolite profiles [13, 14] and an analysis of extracellular metabolite profiles from biofluids or fermentation broths has the potential of providing reporters of mode-of-action [15, 16]. Adaptive changes in metabolism often are accumulated outside the cells and the effects will be amplified as a function of time.

In this chapter we will present some of the current analytical techniques for metabolite profiling and discuss the potential of metabolite profiling in the context of identification of novel anti-infectives and systems biology with a special emphasis on metabolite profiling of microorganisms. Metabolite analysis contributes to various research fields, but the type of data sought depends on the actual application. Table 1 lists examples of application of metabolite data.

2 Microbial metabolite profiling

In principle, metabolite profiling includes the chemical analysis of a broad range of molecules. A metabolite profiling strategy typically consists of an analytical method that – although it might be directed towards certain

Table 1.
Examples of application of metabolite data and the metabolite analysis strategy supporting this application

Application	Metabolite Analysis Strategy
Classification	Comprehensive (and qualitative) metabolite profiling
Drug discovery	Comprehensive and qualitative metabolite profiling
Pathogenicity	Specific and targeted analysis of a limited number of metabolites
Systems biology	Quantitative analysis of (primary) metabolites

chemical classes of molecules – covers detection of both known and unknown molecules. The ideal metabolite profiling method would cover the whole metabolome; but the distinct physical and chemical properties of metabolites make a joint analysis of all of them difficult (or perhaps even impossible). It is therefore most likely that an array of analytical techniques will be required to cover the whole metabolome, with the detection methods requiring a very wide dynamic range since specific metabolite concentrations typically cover nine orders of magnitude (mM – pM) [17].

Several different definitions of metabolite analysis strategies have been suggested in the literature [17–20] and to avoid misunderstandings we have outlined the definitions used in this chapter in Table 2. Whereas metabolite profiling typically includes qualitative and even quantitative identifi-

Table 2.
Overview of definitions used in relation to metabolite analysis

Term	Definition
Metabolite profiling	Chemical analysis of several metabolites aiming at identification and quantification
Metabolite fingerprinting	Metabolic signature of intracellular metabolites
Metabolite footprinting	Metabolic signature of extracellular metabolites
Metabolome	The metabolome is the comprehensive set of low-molecular-weight molecules (metabolites) associated with an organism at any given time. The metabolome comprises the endometabolome (intracellular metabolites) and the exometabolome (extracellular metabolites)
Metabolomics	Application and integration of metabolite data in a genomics context [20] e.g., functional genomics, metabolic engineering or systems biology

cation of metabolites, metabolic fingerprinting [11] and footprinting [12, 16] are metabolite analysis strategies that return a metabolic signature as a qualitative view of the intracellular or extracellular metabolites, respectively. As such, identification of the chemical structure of each metabolite is not required, and these techniques are typically fast and capable of being automated, which makes them well suited for screening.

Sample preparation is a critical issue whenever one is dealing with metabolite profiling, but beyond the scope of the chapter hence we refer to the literature for more details on this issue [21–24]. Our main focus will be on mass spectrometry (MS) and nuclear magnetic resonance (NMR) spectroscopy, since these are very likely to be the leading techniques for metabolite profiling in the future. Table 3 compares MS- and NMR-based methods and outlines the respective advantages and disadvantages for the

Table 3.
Comparison of specific metabolite profiling techniques

Technique	**(+) Advantages** **(–) Drawbacks**	**Reference**
Direct infusion MS	(+) Fast (+) High sensitivity (–) Matrix effects	Smedsgaard et al. (2004) [28] Castrillo et al. (2003) [92]
GC-MS	(+) High resolution (+) Spectral libraries available (–) Derivatization usually required	Strelkov et al. (2004) [42]
LC-MS	(+) Complement GC-MS (–) Matrix effects, but less than direct infusion MS	Wu et al. (2005) [54]
CE-MS	(+) High resolution (–) Complex setup	Soga et al. (2003) [59]
NMR	(+) Unbiased (–) Limited sensitivity (–) Limited resolution	Raamsdonk et al. (2001) [11]
LC-NMR-MS	(+) Combination of comprehensive and complementary techniques (–) Slow	—

References are selected from a microbial point of view

two techniques. A more detailed description of the technologies is presented in the following sections.

2.1 Mass spectrometry

MS has more or less been the driving force for development of metabolomics, especially because it allows high sensitivity and selectivity [19, 25]. Any technology related to MS relies on measuring the mass-to-charge ratio of ions and there are several mass analyzer technologies available for acquiring mass spectra. In Table 4 the four most common technologies are described. The quadrupole mass analyzer is the most popular mainly because it is robust and fairly cheap. The time-of-flight (TOF) instruments have been widely applied for protein analysis, but lately they have also been used for metabolite profiling. These instruments have become more and more popular due to the development of detection systems giving higher mass resolution and better mass accuracy.

2.1.1 Direct infusion MS

The introduction of atmospheric pressure ionization (API) techniques in the late 1980s revolutionized mass spectrometric analysis of biomolecules by enabling an easy coupling of MS to liquid chromatography. The most popular API technique is electrospray ionization (ESI) that allows analysis of polar molecules up to several thousand Daltons.

Direct infusion MS is carried out by injecting the sample directly into the ion source without any prior separation. This allows the determination of a signature of the masses of molecules present in the sample. Typically the analysis time is 2–3 min and direct infusion MS is well-suited for high-throughput screening. The data is compact and the acquisition is fast, but one should be aware of matrix effects that might reduce the signal for some compounds, as they loose the 'battle' for charges in the ESI process (see more about matrix effects in the section about liquid chromatography MS). Nevertheless, direct infusion MS is powerful for screening. For ESI molecular ionization is typically obtained by protonation $[M + H]^+$ or deprotonation $[M - H]^-$, but adduct formation with e.g., Na^+, NH_4^+ and Cl^- is also common. When more complex molecules are analyzed, solvent adducts also appear, e.g., $[M + H_2O + H]^+$ and $[M + CH_3OH + H]^+$, and more

Table 4.
Description of common mass spectrometry (MS) technologies in relation to metabolites profiling

MS Technology	Description
Quadrupole (Q)	The quadrupole functions as a mass filter that only allows passage to the detector of ions with a set mass-to-charge ratio. The quadrupole can be operated in single ion monitoring mode for a specific mass or scan mode to acquire a mass spectrum. The quadrupole is constructed by four metal rods on which an oscillating and a constant potential is applied to control the transmission of ions. The quadrupole is a low resolution detector and the accuracy of mass is within unit mass.
Ion-trap (TRAP)	The ion-trap operates by trapping the ions and sequentially ejecting them to the detector where they are counted. Additionally, the ion-trap enables fragmentation experiments that are useful for determining structures or for increased specificity. Theoretically there are no limitations on the number of fragmentations one can perform, thus MS^n is possible. Similarly to the quadrupole the ion-trap normally returns masses within unit mass.
Time-of-flight (TOF)	The ions are accelerated through an electrical field to obtain the same kinetic energy of $E = \frac{1}{2}(m/z)v^2$. The ions then pass through an evacuated flight tube of constant length (s) and the time of flight (t) is measured. From the flight time the mass-to-charge (m/z) is easily calculated, since $v = s/t$. The TOF technology returns high-resolution data and mass accuracies around 5 ppm can be obtained.
Fourier transform ion cyclotron resonance (FTICR)	FTICR is one of the more recent technologies for MS. The heart of a FTICR MS is a trapping cell located in a magnetic field. The ions are excited and will move in a circular orbit with a specific frequency that is determined by the mass, charge and velocity. The frequency signal is Fourier transformed and used to deduce the mass spectrum. FTICR is superior when it comes to resolution and accuracy, and masses can be determined with < 1 ppm error.
Hyphenated technologies	Combination of the above mentioned technologies expands the MS capabilities. Triple quadrupole detectors are suited for tandem MS and allow high sensitivity for trace analysis. The Q-TOF also enables tandem MS and accurate masses is obtained. These are just two examples of hyphenated technologies.

complex ions like $[2M + H]^+$ and $[M - H + 2Na]^+$ are frequently observed. For larger molecules like peptides and proteins multiply charged ions $[M + nH]^{n+}$ are also very common.

Direct infusion MS has been successfully used in several different classification studies. Smedsgaard and co-workers [26–29] have used direct infusion MS to profile secondary metabolites from filamentous fungi in relation to chemotaxonomy, allowing the classification of closely-related species of *Penicillium*. From the mass spectra several secondary metabolites could be identified based on their mass and isotope patterns. Similarly, direct infusion MS was used for identification of bacteria by analysis of crude cell extracts [30]. Here, five bacterial strains were studied and the predominant biomarkers from the analysis were found to be phospholipids, glycolipids and proteins. Application of high resolution mass spectrometers (Table 4), e.g., Time of Flight (TOF) or Fourier Transform Ion Cyclotron Resonance instruments, can further increase the chemical information from direct infusion MS, since they make it possible to determine the accurate mass of compounds. Here compositionally different compounds that have the same unit mass can be separated on the mass scale, e.g., lysine ($C_6H_{14}N_2O_2$; M = 146.1055 Da) and glutamine ($C_5H_{10}N_2O_3$; M = 146.0691 Da), and from the accurate mass measurement the elemental composition can be directly computed [29, 31, 32].

Figure 1 shows a mass spectrum resulting from direct infusion of a synthetic fermentation medium into a mass spectrometer via ESI. The spectrum was acquired on a high-resolution TOF instrument and from the accurate mass data it was possible to confirm the identity of numerous metabolites from the medium. Table 5 lists the metabolites with their respective masses. Although several ions are identified in the mass spectrum, there are still a considerable number of ions that remain unknown. These might arise from solvent clusters, unpredicted ion clusters, ion fragmentation, redox reactions during ESI etc. The calculated errors are all within positive 10 mDa, which demonstrates the power of accurate mass spectrometry and reduces the molecular search space remarkably. Another observation is that the error is positive for all identified ions, which might indicate that there is a small off-set in the calibration since the mean error of 6.8 ($\pm$ 1.2) mDa is different from zero.

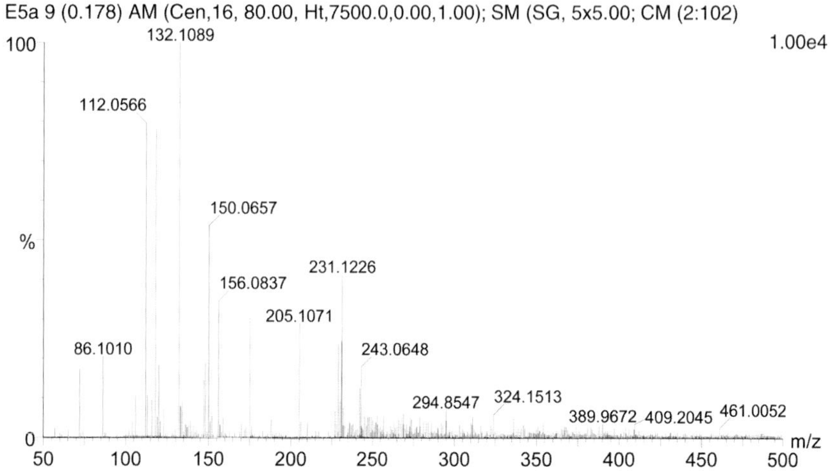

Figure 1.
Direct infusion MS of a synthetic fermentation medium. The spectrum is acquired on a high-resolution TOF instrument.

Table 5.
Identified ions from direct infusion MS of a fermentation medium

Metabolite	**Ion**	**Observed Mass**	**Calculated Mass**	**Error**
Serine	$[M + H]^+$	106.0550 Da	106.0504 Da	5.5 mDa
Cytosine	$[M + H]^+$	112.0567 Da	112.0511 Da	5.6 mDa
Valine	$[M + H]^+$	118.0927 Da	118.0868 Da	5.9 mDa
Threonine	$[M + H]^+$	120.0726 Da	120.0660 Da	6.6 mDa
Leucine	$[M + H]^+$	132.1089 Da	132.1024 Da	6.5 mDa
Aspartic acid	$[M + H]^+$	134.0511 Da	134.0453 Da	5.8 mDa
Lysine	$[M + H]^+$	147.1203 Da	147.1133 Da	7.0 mDa
Glutamic acid	$[M + H]^+$	148.0679 Da	148.0610 Da	6.9 mDa
Methionine	$[M + H]^+$	150.0658 Da	150.0588 Da	7.0 mDa
Histidine	$[M + H]^+$	156.0838 Da	156.0773 Da	6.5 mDa
Arginine	$[M + H]^+$	175.1269 Da	175.1195 Da	7.4 mDa
Tryptophane	$[M + H]^+$	205.1071 Da	205.0977 Da	9.4 mDa
	$[M + Na]^+$	227.0884 Da	227.0797 Da	8.7 mDa

In a functional genomic context Allen et al. [12] analyzed the extracellular metabolite profiles of single knockout strains of the yeast *Saccharomyces cerevisiae* by direct infusion MS. The results proved that mutants with related genotypes express similar extracellular metabolite profiles and that this method was thus applicable for assignment of gene functions through guilt-by-association. Expanding this strategy, it was demonstrated that metabolic footprinting also can be used to determine mode-of-action of antifungal compounds [13]. Quantitative analysis by direct infusion MS is rare, but Nagy et al. [33] analyzed amino acids in blood spots by direct infusion tandem MS, where addition of isotope-labeled internal standards allowed quantification of 19 native amino acids.

Conformational isomers cannot be resolved by MS alone simply because they will have the same mass, but tandem MS or coupling of separation techniques prior to MS analysis can help to identify conformational isomers. Combination of separation techniques with MS tremendously improves the resolution of complex samples.

2.1.2 Gas chromatography coupled to MS

Any chromatographic technique is based on equilibrium between a stationary phase and a mobile phase. In gas chromatography (GC), the mobile phase is a gas and therefore the molecules that are to be analyzed must be volatile. Although this part of the metabolome has often been neglected, it does provide insight into metabolism and taxonomy [34]. On the other hand, many metabolites are small polar molecules that not are readily evaporated into the gas phase. This can be overcome by derivatization that converts the functional polar groups in such molecules into non-polar groups. A classical derivatization reaction is silylation, where active hydrogen atoms from hydroxyl, amine, thiol and carboxylic acid groups are typically substituted by silyl groups, e.g., trimethylsilyl [$-Si(CH_3)_3$] or tert-butyldimethylsilyl [$-Si(CH_3)_2C_4H_9$]. The reactions proceed under strictly anhydrous conditions at slightly elevated temperature and produces derivates that are generally less polar, more volatile, and thermally more stable than the parent compound. The derivatization reaction is very versatile and covers most primary metabolites although not all of them will end up being volatile. [19, 35, 36]. Alternatively, alkylation can be used for derivatization of functional groups with acidic or basic hydrogen atoms, e.g., carboxylic acids, and primary and secondary amines. Chloroformates have been suggested as a good alternative for silylation and have been successfully applied in analysis of amino and organic acids in blood [37, 38] and in metabolite extracts [39, 40]. One of the major advantages of the chloroformate reaction is that it can be performed under partly aqueous conditions and at room temperature, but it does not enable analysis of sugars and sugar derived compounds. One thing to keep in mind is that the derivatization reaction rarely results in a single product, and multiple byproducts can be formed. This complicates the chromatograms and makes the data analysis more cumbersome, since one peak does not necessarily correspond to one metabolite.

Coupling of capillary GC and MS combines two robust technologies. GC offers high resolution between similar compounds and MS produces compound-specific mass spectra that may further resolve co-eluting compounds. An electron impact (EI) ionization source is often used for interfacing the GC and the MS. EI is a classic technique within the field of MS and is frequently used in connection with GC. The EI process takes place *in vacuo* where the analyte molecule is ionized by passing through a beam of electrons. The electrons are accelerated through a potential of 70 eV and when an electron hits the molecule it results in ionization. The EI process is considered a hard ionization process since the ionization energy of 70 eV is high compared to the energy of a covalent bond (3–7 eV). This leaves excess energy in the ions and frequently results in fragmentation of the ionized molecule, yielding a specific fingerprint of the molecule. This fragmentation is compound specific and makes the EI spectra suited for identification based on reference spectra. The ionization is very robust and gives reproducible fragmentation patterns over time and with different instruments. This allows construction of libraries for searching and identification of metabolites [36, 41]. Metabolite profiling of plants has significantly contributed to the field of metabolite profiling by GC-MS [1, 2, 35] and the methodologies can readily be transferred to microbial metabolite profiling [42].

Recently, two-dimensional GC (GC×GC)-TOF-MS instruments have been applied for metabolite profiling and this is currently the most comprehensive GC-based technology available. Two-dimensional GC enables very high chromatographic resolution and this, coupled with high scan rates from the TOF mass spectrometer, makes it possible to resolve very complex samples with high sensitivity [16, 43].

2.1.3 Liquid chromatography coupled to MS

The introduction of API techniques opened up new possibilities for metabolite profiling by enabling the coupling of liquid chromatography (LC) to MS. LC-MS instrumentation is now standard equipment in many labs. To date, the major applications of LC-MS have been within the analysis of pharmaceuticals and profiling of biofluids. Although liquid chromatography (LC)-MS has not been as widely applied for primary metabolite profiling it has a major potential to complement GC-MS. Derivatization is not required and low separation temperatures compared to GC-MS reduces the degradation of heat labile compounds. Metabolites from the central carbon metabolism [44–46] as well as nucleotides [47] can be analyzed by LC-MS. Separation of highly polar and ionized metabolites can be achieved by ion-exchange chromatography that includes gradient elution at high salt concentrations. This is not readily compatible with ESI, but insertion of a desalting device in between the LC and the MS is a solution for improved sensitivity and robustness. Reversed phase ion-pair chromatography is another option for separation of ionic metabolites. The only requirement is that the counter-ion used for ion-pairing should be volatile, e.g., alkyl amines and perfluoro-carboxylic acids, such compounds minimize, but do not eliminate the problem of contamination of the ion-source.

The ESI process is known to be prone to matrix effects that change the ionization efficiency and lead to suppression or amplification of the ionization. One of the major reasons for this phenomena is that changes in the ion strength of the liquid will affect the charge distribution in the droplet and on its surface due to co-eluting substances [48, 49]. High concentrations of buffers and especially non-volatile buffers are incompatible with ESI and will result in low signals, if any at all. The buffer will simply snatch the charge from the molecules of interest. Application of volatile buffers consisting of, e.g., formic or acidic acid and ammonia are however a way to reduce the ion suppression caused by buffers [50].

Matrix effects are especially critical for quantitative studies. Although tandem MS allows highly specific and sensitive detection of metabolites, matrix effects during ionization are deleterious to quantification. Addition of isotopic-labeled internal standards can overcome the discrimination observed during ionization. The labeled standard is ionized together with the compound of interest and the ions will be separated by the mass spectrometer [51]. The only drawback is that only a limited number of labeled metabolites are commercially available and they tend to be expensive; however, *in vivo* synthesis by feeding labeled substrates is an option [52–54].

Derivatization is also an option for LC-MS in order to change the chromatographic selectivity or improve the sensitivity [36]. Furthermore, advances in LC column technologies pose new possibilities through novel stationary phases and improved resolution. One of the most recent technologies is ultrahigh pressure liquid chromatography. Here reduction of the particle size of the column material to sub-2 μm and high linear flow rates have significantly improved the chromatographic resolution to levels only seen for GC previously [55].

2.1.4 Capillary electrophoresis coupled to MS

Separation by capillary electrophoresis (CE) relies on differential migration of ions in an electrical field and is performed in a buffer-filled capillary of fused silica. The capillary is placed in two separate buffer reservoirs with a potential difference of up to 30 kV. The potential over the capillary mediates an electroosmotic flow that carries the analytes along while they are separated by differential migration. The electroosmotic flow can be varied by changing the applied potential and the ion strength in the buffer. The migration velocity is determined by the charge-to-volume ratio of the ion and the overall migration velocity will be a sum of the electroosmotic flow and the migration of the individual ions.

CE offers high separation efficiencies, which makes it powerful for analysis of complex samples although sensitivity might be limited by fairly small injection volumes of 1–30 nL. Coupling of CE to mass spectrometry is possible, but currently not that widespread. This might change in the future though. Due to the low flow rates the ionization is mostly performed by ESI, and the interface between the CE instrument and the ESI source often includes a coaxial sheath flow to maintain a stable spray. A thorough review of CE-MS has been written by Schmitt-Kopplin and Frommberger [56].

There is no requirement for derivatization and many different compound classes can be analyzed, e.g., organic acids, amino acids, nucleotides and carbohydrates with indirect UV detection [57]. Soga et al. [58] coupled CE to MS enabling analysis of 32 central anionic metabolites from glycolysis and TCA cycle, and in a study of the bacteria *Bacillus subtilis* more than 1,500 metabolites were detected [59]. This was done by combining three different CE methods that covered cationic metabolites, anionic metabolites, and nucleotides and coenzymes, respectively.

2.2 Spectroscopy

Spectroscopy is another option for analysis of metabolites. All spectroscopy technologies are non-destructive in contrast to MS and therefore any analyzed sample can be recovered and analyzed by another technique if desired.

2.2.1 Ultraviolet and visible spectroscopy

The ultraviolet (UV; 200–400 nm) and visible (VIS; 400–780 nm) light absorption of most primary metabolites is unspecific and absent above 210 nm, which hinders widespread use for the profiling of primary metabolites in complex mixtures. Of course derivatization reactions that add UV-VIS active groups to the metabolites are an option to overcome this limitation. However, when it comes to profiling of secondary metabolites, e.g., polyketides, alkaloids and isoprenoids, the UV absorption can be quite distinct and useful for compound identification. The UV absorption relates to changes in energy levels of the electrons in the π-bonds and is characteristic for conjugated double bounds (chromophores). Thus, UV absorption spectra contain structural information of the electronic arrangement in the molecule and similar molecules have similar spectra. We will return to this later when we discuss natural products and drug discovery. UV-VIS detectors or diode-array-detectors (DADs) are usually coupled to LC that can be further coupled to MS to obtain increased specificity [60].

2.2.2 Nuclear magnetic resonance spectroscopy

Nuclear magnetic resonance (NMR) spectroscopy is a versatile technology and probably *the* technique of choice when it comes to detailed structure elucidation of metabolites. NMR relies on the nuclear spin of atoms. The nuclear spin is determined by unpaired protons and neutrons and makes the nuclei act like small magnets. Thus ^{1}H, ^{13}C, ^{15}N and ^{31}P can all be analyzed by NMR. When an external magnetic field is applied to nuclei that have a non-zero spin they will align according to the field. The nuclei can be flipped to a high-energy level by a radiation with a given frequency. The electrons around the nuclei affect the local magnetic field for the nuclei and therefore change the energy needed to flip the nuclei. The normalized frequency for flipping the nuclei is known as the chemical shift, which is specific for the nucleus dependent on the local chemical environment.

NMR is widely applied for metabolic profiling. The sensitivity is not as high as for MS; however, NMR does not discriminate between metabolites in the samples and therefore represents an unbiased technique for metabolite profiling. Nicholson and co-workers have pioneered the application of NMR for metabolite profiling [61, 62]. In particular, they have analyzed urine and blood by NMR and successfully identified biomarkers for diagnostics. Fingerprinting by ^{1}H-NMR of metabolite extracts from yeast was proposed for assignment of unknown gene functions. The analysis of six yeast knockout strains using NMR-based metabolite identification was utilized to classify and relate the genotypes by multivariate statistics, which has potential implications for the application of NMR-based metabolomics in functional genomics [11]. Another example is the investigation of mode-of-action of bioactive compounds in plants using NMR followed by spectral analysis using neural networks [63]. Furthermore, NMR is non-destructive and therefore *in vivo* analysis is possible. Insertion of a special probe into the NMR instrument makes it possible to grow microbial cell in suspension and hereby perform non-invasive studies of the metabolite concentrations in a dynamic state [64–67].

3 Novel drug discovery

From an evolutionary point of view, many natural products are produced to attract or eliminate other organisms, which make them of particular interest and a good hunting ground for new drugs or other bioactive compounds. This is especially clear from the significant contribution of natural products to the discovery of new drugs [68]. There is a large chemical diversity among natural products that in many cases is superior to what can be obtained by pure combinatorial chemistry. However, applying combinatorial chemistry on natural products can efficiently lead to new drug analogous that can be even more potent [69].

To explore natural products, metabolite profiling has a key position in the search for new drug candidates. Whenever a new drug candidate shows up it is relevant to clarify whether this compound is already known. This is done by dereplication in order to rapidly determine already known and trivial compounds – and basically answers the simple question: Have we seen this compound before? – and, if yes, what is it? This ensures that isolation, structure elucidation, and pharmacological investigations can be focused on novel compounds and thereby improves the efficiency of discovery and making discovery more cost-efficient. MS and especially high-resolution MS is a core technology for dereplication, since this can be used for deduction of molecular compositions. Tentative molecule compositions from accurate MS data along with UV data, chromatographic retention index etc. can be used for database searches in, e.g., SciFinder, Antibase or MarinLit to possibly identify the unknown compound [70].

As already mentioned UV-spectroscopy can also be used for guided screening of structurally similar compounds. Recently, Hansen et al. [71] proposed an algorithm, called X-hitting, for automatic dereplication (cross-hitting) and automatic finding of potentially new and similar compounds (new-hitting). X-hitting extracts UV-VIS spectra from HPLC-DAD (high pressure liquid chromatography with diode array detector) data and compares shapes of these spectra across samples using a similarity measure. Cross-hitting reports compounds with similar spectra and retention times, whereas new-hitting finds compounds with similar spectra, but different retention times indicating a new but related compound. This way, two novel spiro-quinazoline metabolites where tracked, isolated and structure elucidated as a proof of concept [72].

In a microbial context, filamentous fungi have a high potential of providing lead compounds, since they are known to produce a vast number of bioactive molecules [70]. To explore the chemical capabilities of microbes through biodiversity they first of all have to be viable in the lab and secondly the secondary metabolism has to be stimulated. Induction of the secondary metabolism is not trivial and typically the optimum conditions are rather different from the conditions optimal for growth and furthermore, the optimum varies from microbe to microbe [73]. Thus, the nutrient sources have major impact on the fluxes through the pathways producing secondary metabolites, and often there is carbon catabolite repression on secondary metabolite production.

4 *In vivo* metabolic fluxes

Quantification of metabolic fluxes is an important technique in terms of basic understanding of metabolism and metabolic activity (see also the chapter of Hornberg et al. in this volume). The actual cellular phenotype is closely related to fluxes whether it is simple growth or formation of a certain product [74]. Unfortunately, it is rare that there is a simple correlation between intracellular metabolite concentrations and metabolic fluxes, since a high concentration is not necessarily the result of high flux. This is simply because the flux is seldom determined by simple kinetics with one or two variables, but multiple variables affect the actual reaction rate in terms of multiple substrates and products as well as regulatory mechanisms may superimpose the influence of the metabolites. Thus, metabolic profiling cannot alone reveal actual metabolic fluxes (except when the *in vivo* enzyme kinetics is fully known), but analysis of isotope isomers – also know as isotopomers – is powerful in relation to *in vivo* metabolic flux calculations [75–77]. Typically flux estimation experiments are conducted by introducing substrates with specific isotopic labeling e.g., glucose labeled with a ^{13}C-atom in the first position ([1-^{13}C]glucose). The labeling will then be distributed throughout the metabolic network dependent on the fluxes through the different branches of the metabolic network. Dif-

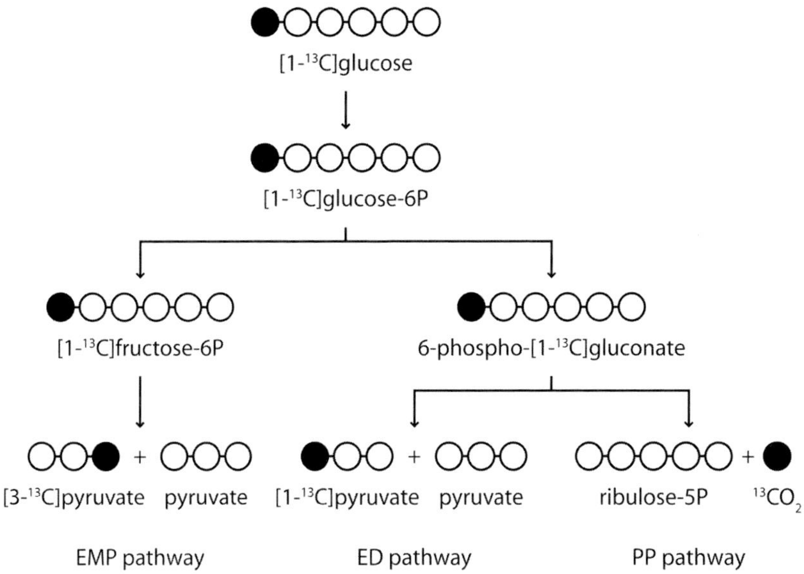

Figure 2.
Resulting labeling patterns when [1-^{13}C]glucose is metabolized through the Embden-Meyerhof-Parnas (EMP), Entner-Doudoroff (ED) or pentose phosphate (PP) pathway. ● indicates the ^{13}C-labeling position; ○ is the unlabeled C-atoms).

ferent metabolic routes result in different isotopomer distributions arising from different carbon atom transitions. To illustrate the concept, Figure 2 summarizes the labeling resulting from conversion of [1-^{13}C]glucose through the three glycolytic pathways: Embden-Meyerhof-Parnas (EMP), Entner-Doudoroff (ED) or pentose phosphate (PP) pathway. Pyruvate is the end-product of the EMP- and ED-pathway and the pyruvate ends up being 50% labeled in the 3rd and 1st position, respectively. When glucose is converted through the PP-pathway, the labeling is lost by decarboxylation of 6-phospho-gluconate to ribulose 5-phosphate. Thus, any pyruvate produced from the PP-pathway is unlabeled. The actual labeling patterns (isotopomers) are mostly determined by GC-MS [78–80] or NMR [81, 82], but there are a few examples using LC-MS [83, 84].

The mathematical formalism of flux analysis relies on simple mass balances of the metabolic reactions together with carbon atom balances that map the transitions of the individual carbon atoms throughout the metabolic reactions. This results in a set of bilinear equations that can be solved by an iterative algorithm, where the objective is to minimize the deviation between measured and calculated isotopomers [75].

5 Metabolites in systems biology

Moving into systems biology and integrating data from different cellular levels will surely improve the understanding of microorganisms, and this may be used to both guide the identification of new targets for antimicrobials as well as guiding the development of improved cell factories for production of bioactive compounds. Especially the unraveling of regulatory mechanisms will allow discovery of novel specific drug targets. In systems biology, dynamic experiments might even play a key role in elucidating specific functions in this context [15, 85]. Here dynamic experiments will be more likely to capture the cascade of changes arising from a system perturbation compared to a classical steady-state experiment of two conditions representing before and after perturbation.

Construction of genome-scale metabolic models has generated insight into the structure of metabolic networks [86, 87]. It turns out that metabolic reaction networks are highly connected and for *S. cerevisiae* [88] <30 % of the metabolites participate in two or fewer reactions, whereas 12 % of the metabolites are involved in >10 reactions and 4 % of the metabolites are involved in >20 reactions. Additionally, the majority of reactions includes more than one substrate and one product [89]. This shows the integrative information available in the metabolome, which makes the metabolome data valuable, but also highly convoluted, making the data interpretation challenging. Given the highly connected metabolic networks it is most likely that the metabolite concentrations will change rather than the fluxes and therefore to make metabolite data useful in relation to systems biology, emphasis should be placed on (semi-)quantitative data.

Mathematical models will be pivotal for deconvolution of metabolite data in order to infer biological functions [90]. The application of already known structural relationships can be represented as a graph which may serve as a scaffold for analysis of the data. Recently the use of metabolic graphs as a scaffold for analysis of microarray data was identified, and it was shown possible to identify parts of the metabolic network that are transcriptionally co-regulated and hence may be under some kind of global control [91]. The approach is extendable and can potentially be designed to cover protein and metabolite data, and even integration of these data.

Systems biology formulates a quantitative science and in order to apply metabolite data in a systems biology context, (semi)quantitative data is required [89]. This differentiates metabolite profiling in relation to systems biology from many of the previous applications, where metabolite data has mainly been used for classification (see examples above). The desire for quantitative data poses a schism in systems biology especially for metabolite data, because the accurate quantity of a certain metabolite is typically obtained at the cost of the number of metabolites detected. On the other hand, systems biology aims at understanding the whole, which implies a requirement for analysis of many metabolites. The schism arises from a trade-off between detected and quantified metabolites, which we illustrate in Figure 3. The more metabolites that are detected the fewer are quantified (or known). However, continuous advancement for analytical technologies will move the curve in Figure 3 to the right and thereby increase the impact of metabolite profiling in systems biology.

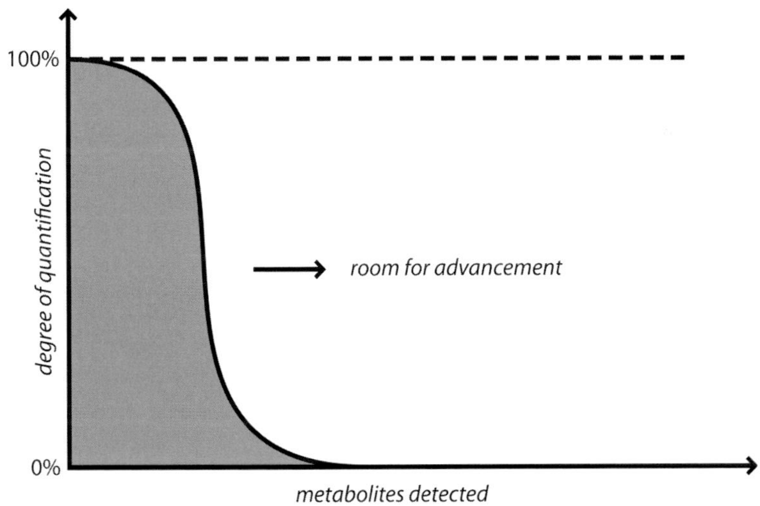

Figure 3.
The trade-off between (qualitative) detection and quantitative measurement of metabolites. The degree of quantification expresses the percentage of quantified metabolites relative to the detected metabolite.

Acknowledgements

We recognize the Danish Technical Research Council for support through the Center for Advanced Engineering: Center for Microbial Biotechnology.

References

1 Fiehn O, Kopka J, Dormann P, Altmann T, Trethewey RN, Willmitzer L (2000) Metabolite profiling for plant functional genomics. *Nat Biotechnol* 18: 1157–1161

2 Roessner U, Luedemann A, Brust D, Fiehn O, Linke T, Willmitzer L, Fernie A (2001) Metabolic profiling allows comprehensive phenotyping of genetically or environmentally modified plant systems. *Plant Cell* 13: 11–29

3 Trethewey RN (2001) Gene discovery via metabolic profiling. *Curr Opin Biotechnol* 12: 135–138

4 Trethewey RN, Krotzky AJ, Willmitzer L (1999) Metabolic profiling: a rosetta stone for genomics? *Curr Opin Plant Biol* 2: 83–85

5 Weckwerth W, Fiehn O (2002) Can we discover novel pathways using metabolomic analysis? *Curr Opin Biotechnol* 13: 156–160

6 Weckwerth W (2003) Metabolomics in systems biology. *Annu Rev Plant Biol* 54: 669–689

7 Oliver SG, Winson MK, Kell DB, Baganz F (1998) Systematic functional analysis of the yeast genome. *Trends Biotechnol* 16: 373–378

8 Tweeddale H, Notley-McRobb L, Ferenci T (1998) Effect of slow growth on metabolism of Escherichia coli, as revealed by global metabolite pool ("Metabolome") analysis. *J Bacteriol* 180: 5109–5116

9 Fiehn O (2002) Metabolomics – the link between genotypes and phenotypes. *Plant Mol Biol* 48: 155–171

10 Schmidt CW (2004) Metabolomics: what's happening downstream of DNA. *Environ Health Perspect* 112: A410–A415

11 Raamsdonk LM, Teusink B, Broadhurst D, Zhang N, Hayes A, Walsh MC, Berden JA, Brindle KM, Kell DB, Rowland JJ et al (2001) A functional genomics strategy that uses metabolome data to reveal the phenotype of silent mutations. *Nat Biotechnol* 19: 45–50

12 Allen J, Davey HM, Broadhurst D, Heald JK, Rowland JJ, Oliver SG, Kell DB (2003) High-throughput classification of yeast mutants for functional genomics using metabolic footprinting. *Nat Biotechnol* 21: 692–696

13 Allen J, Davey HM, Broadhurst D, Rowland JJ, Oliver SG, Kell DB (2004) Discrimination of modes of action of antifungal substances by use of metabolic footprinting. *Appl Environ Microbiol* 70: 6157–6165

14 Aranibar N, Singh BK, Stockton GW, Ott KH (2001) Automated mode-of-action detection by metabolic profiling. *Biochem Biophys Res Commun* 286: 150–155

15 Nicholson JK, Holmes E, Lindon JC, Wilson ID (2004) The challenges of modeling mammalian biocomplexity. *Nat Biotechnol* 22: 1268–1274

16 Kell DB, Brown M, Davey HM, Dunn WB, Spasic I, Oliver SG (2005) Metabolic footprinting and systems biology: The medium is the message. *Nat Rev Microbiol* 3: 557–565

17 Dunn WB, Bailey NJ, Johnson HE (2005) Measuring the metabolome: current analytical technologies. *Analyst* 130: 606–625

18 Fiehn O (2001) Combining genomics, metabolome analysis, and biochemical modelling to understand metabolic networks. *Comp Funct Genom* 2: 155–168

19 Villas-Boas SG, Mas S, Akesson M, Smedsgaard J, Nielsen J (2005) Mass spectrometry in metabolome analysis. *Mass Spectrom Rev* 24: 613–646

20 Villas-Boas SG, Rasmussen S, Lane GA (2005) Metabolomics or metabolite profiles? *Trends Biotechnol* 23: 385–386

21 Hajjaj H, Blanc PJ, Goma G, Francois J (1998) Sampling techniques and comparative extraction procedures for quantitative determination of intra- and extracellular metabolites in filamentous fungi. *FEMS Microbiol Lett* 164: 195–200

22 Maharjan RP, Ferenci T (2003) Global metabolite analysis: the influence of extraction methodology on metabolome profiles of *Escherichia coli*. *Anal Biochem* 313: 145–154

23 Villas-Boas SG, Hojer-Pedersen J, Akesson M, Smedsgaard J, Nielsen J (2005) Global metabolite analysis of yeast: evaluation of sample preparation methods. *Yeast* 22: 1155–1169

24 Smedsgaard J (1997) Micro-scale extraction procedure for standardized screening of fungal metabolite production in cultures. *J Chromatogr A* 760: 264–270

25 van der Greef J, van der Heijden R, Verheij ER (2004) The role of mass spectrometry in systems biology: data processing and identification strategies in metabolomics. *Adv Mass Spectrom* 16: 145–165

26 Smedsgaard J, Frisvad JC (1996) Using direct electrospray mass spectrometry in taxonomy and secondary metabolite profiling of crude fungal extracts. *J Microbiol Meth* 25: 5–17

27 Smedsgaard J, Frisvad JC (1997) Terverticillate penicillia studied by direct electrospray mass spectrometric profiling of crude extracts .1. Chemosystematics. *Biochem Syst Ecol* 25: 51–64

28 Smedsgaard J, Hansen ME, Frisvad JC (2004) Classification of terverticillate Penicillia by electrospray mass spectrometric profiling. *Stud Mycol* 243–251

29 Smedsgaard J, Nielsen J (2005) Metabolite profiling of fungi and yeast: from phenotype to metabolome by MS and informatics. *J Exp Bot* 56: 273–286

30 Vaidyanathan S, Kell DB, Goodacre R (2002) Flow-injection electrospray ionization mass spectrometry of crude cell extracts for high-throughput bacterial identification. *J Am Soc Mass Spectrom* 13: 118–128

31 Aharoni A, de Vos CHR, Verhoeven HA, Maliepaard CA, Kruppa G, Bino R, Goodenowe DB (2002) Nontargeted metabolome analysis by use of Fourier Transform Ion Cyclotron Mass Spectrometry. *OMICS* 6: 217–234

32 Sleno L, Volmer DA, Marshall AG (2005) Assigning product ions from complex MS/MS spectra: The importance of mass uncertainty and resolving power. *J Am Soc Mass Spectrom* 16: 183–198
33 Nagy K, Takats Z, Pollreisz F, Szabo T, Vekey K (2003) Direct tandem mass spectrometric analysis of amino acids in dried blood spots without chemical derivatization for neonatal screening. *Rapid Commun Mass Spectrom* 17: 983–990
34 Karlshoj K, Larsen TO (2005) Differentiation of species from the *Penicillium roqueforti* group by volatile metabolite profiling. *J Agri Food Chem* 53: 708–715
35 Roessner U, Wagner C, Kopka J, Trethewey RN, Willmitzer L (2000) Simultaneous analysis of metabolites in potato tuber by gas chromatography-mass spectrometry. *Plant J* 23: 131–142
36 Halket JM, Waterman D, Przyborowska AM, Patel RK, Fraser PD, Bramley PM (2005) Chemical derivatization and mass spectral libraries in metabolic profiling by GC/MS and LC/MS/MS. *J Exp Bot* 56: 219–243
37 Husek P (1998) Chloroformates in gas chromatography as general purpose derivatizing agents. *J Chromatogr B* 717: 57–91
38 Husek P (1995) Simultaneous profile analysis of plasma amino and organic acids by capillary gas chromatography. *J Chromatogr B* 669: 352–357
39 Villas-Boas SG, Delicado DG, Akesson M, Nielsen J (2003) Simultaneous analysis of amino and nonamino organic acids as methyl chloroformate derivatives using gas chromatography-mass spectrometry. *Anal Biochem* 322: 134–138
40 Villas-Boas SG, Moxley JF, Akesson M, Stephanopoulos G, Nielsen J (2005) High-throughput metabolic state analysis: the missing link in integrated functional genomics of yeasts. *Biochem J* 388: 669–677
41 Schauer N, Steinhauser D, Strelkov S, Schomburg D, Allison G, Moritz T, Lundgren K, Roessner-Tunali U, Forbes MG, Willmitzer L et al (2005) GC-MS libraries for the rapid identification of metabolites in complex biological samples. *FEBS Lett* 579: 1332–1337
42 Strelkov S, von Elstermann M, Schomburg D (2004) Comprehensive analysis of metabolites in *Corynebacterium glutamicum* by gas chromatography/mass spectrometry. *Biol Chem* 385: 853–861
43 Jover E, Adahchour M, Bayona JM, Vreuls RJJ, Brinkman UAT (2005) Characterization of lipids in complex samples using comprehensive two-dimensional gas chromatography with time-of-flight mass spectrometry. *J Chromatogr A* 1086: 2–11
44 Buchholz A, Takors R, Wandrey C (2001) Quantification of intracellular metabolites in *Escherichia coli* K12 using liquid chromatographic-electrospray ionization tandem mass spectrometric techniques. *Anal Biochem* 295: 129–137
45 van Dam JC, Eman MR, Frank J, Lange HC, van Dedem GW, Heijnen SJ (2002) Analysis of glycolytic intermediates in *Saccharomyces cerevisiae* using anion exchange chromatography and electrospray ionization with tandem mass spectrometric detection. *Anal Chim Acta* 460: 209–218
46 Huck JH, Struys EA, Verhoeven NM, Jakobs C, van der Knaap MS (2003) Profiling of pentose phosphate pathway intermediates in blood spots by tandem mass spectrometry: application to transaldolase deficiency. *Clin Chem* 49: 1375–1380

47 Xing J, Apedo A, Tymiak A, Zhao N (2004) Liquid chromatographic analysis of nucleosides and their mono-, di- and triphosphates using porous graphitic carbon stationary phase coupled with electrospray mass spectrometry. *Rapid Commun Mass Spectrom* 18: 1599–1606

48 Taylor PJ (2005) Matrix effects: The Achilles heel of quantitative high-performance liquid chromatography-electrospray-tandem mass spectrometry. *Clin Biochem* 38: 328–334

49 Matuszewski BK, Constanzer ML, Chavez-Eng CM (2003) Strategies for the assessment of matrix effect in quantitative bioanalytical methods based on HPLC-MS/MS. *Anal Chem* 75: 3019–3030

50 McCalley DV (2003) Comparison of peak shapes obtained with volatile (mass spectrometry-compatible) buffers and conventional buffers in reversed-phase high-performance liquid chromatography of bases on particulate and monolithic columns. *J Chromatogr A* 987: 17–28

51 Stokvis E, Rosing H, Beijnen JH (2005) Stable isotopically labeled internal standards in quantitative bioanalysis using liquid chromatography/mass spectrometry: necessity or not? *Rapid Commun Mass Spectrom* 19: 401–407

52 Birkemeyer C, Luedemann A, Wagner C, Erban A, Kopka J (2005) Metabolome analysis: the potential of *in vivo* labeling with stable isotopes for metabolite profiling. *Trends Biotechnol* 23: 28–33

53 Mashego MR, Wu L, van Dam JC, Ras C, Vinke JL, van Winden WA, van Gulik WM, Heijnen JJ (2004) MIRACLE: mass isotopomer ratio analysis of U-^{13}C-labeled extracts. A new method for accurate quantification of changes in concentrations of intracellular metabolites. *Biotechnol Bioeng* 85: 620–628

54 Wu L, Mashego MR, van Dam JC, Proell AM, Vinke JL, Ras C, van Winden WA, van Gulik WM, Heijnen JJ (2005) Quantitative analysis of the microbial metabolome by isotope dilution mass spectrometry using uniformly C-13-labeled cell extracts as internal standards. *Anal Biochem* 336: 164–171

55 Plumb R, Castro-Perez J, Granger J, Beattie I, Joncour K, Wright A (2004) Ultra-performance liquid chromatography coupled to quadrupole-orthogonal time-of-flight mass spectrometry. *Rapid Commun Mass Spectrom* 18: 2331–2337

56 Schmitt-Kopplin P, Frommberger M (2003) Capillary electrophoresis – mass spectrometry: 15 years of developments and applications. *Electrophoresis* 24: 3837–3867

57 Soga T, Imaizumi M (2001) Capillary electrophoresis method for the analysis of inorganic anions, organic acids, amino acids, nucleotides, carbohydrates and other anionic compounds. *Electrophoresis* 22: 3418–3425

58 Soga T, Ueno Y, Naraoka H, Ohashi Y, Tomita M, Nishiokat T (2002) Simultaneous determination of anionic intermediates for *Bacillus subtilis* metabolic pathways by capillary electrophoresis electrospray ionization mass spectrometry. *Anal Chem* 74: 2233–2239

59 Soga T, Ohashi Y, Ueno Y, Naraoka H, Tomita M, Nishioka T (2003) Quantitative metabolome analysis using capillary electrophoresis mass spectrometry. *J Proteome Res* 2: 488–494

60 Nielsen KF, Smedsgaard J (2003) Fungal metabolite screening: database of 474 mycotoxins and fungal metabolites for dereplication by standardised liquid chromatography-UV-mass spectrometry methodology. *J Chromatogr A* 1002: 111–136
61 Bollard ME, Stanley EG, Lindon JC, Nicholson JK, Holmes E (2005) NMR-based metabonomic approaches for evaluating physiological influences on biofluid composition. *Nmr in Biomedicine* 18: 143–162
62 Lindon JC, Holmes E, Nicholson JK (2003) So whats the deal with metabonomics? Metabonomics measures the fingerprint of biochemical perturbations caused by disease, drugs, and toxins. *Anal Chem* 75: 384A–391A
63 Ott KH, Aranibar N, Singh BJ, Stockton GW (2003) Metabonomics classifies pathways affected by bioactive compounds. Artificial neural network classification of NMR spectra of plant extracts. *Phytochemistry* 62: 971–985
64 Weuster-Botz D, de Graaf AA (1996) Reaction engineering methods to study intracellular metabolite concentrations. *Adv Biochem Eng Biotechnol* 54: 75–108
65 Neves AR, Pool WA, Kok J, Kuipers OP, Santos H (2005) Overview on sugar metabolism and its control in *Lactococcus lactis* – The input from *in vivo* NMR. *FEMS Microbiol Rev* 29: 531–554
66 Gmati D, Chen JK, Jolicoeur M (2005) Development of a small-scale bioreactor: Application to *in vivo* NMR measurement. *Biotechnol Bioeng* 89: 138–147
67 Gonzalez B, de Graaf A, Renaud M, Sahm H (2000) Dynamic *in vivo* P-31 nuclear magnetic resonance study of *Saccharomyces cerevisiae* in glucose-limited chemostat culture during the aerobic-anaerobic shift. *Yeast* 16: 483–497
68 Butler MS (2004) The role of natural product chemistry in drug discovery. *J Nat Prod* 67: 2141–2153
69 Ganesan A (2004) Natural products as a hunting ground for combinatorial chemistry. *Curr Opin Biotechnol* 15: 584–590
70 Larsen TO, Smedsgaard J, Nielsen KF, Hansen ME, Frisvad JC (2005) Phenotypic taxonomy and metabolite profiling in microbial drug discovery. *Nat Prod Rep* 22: 672–695
71 Hansen ME, Smedsgaard J, Larsen TO (2005) X-hitting: A new algorithm for novelty detection and de-replication by UV spectra of complex mixtures of natural products. *Anal Chem* 77: 6805–6817
72 Larsen TO, Petersen BO, Duus JO, Sorensen D, Frisvad JC, Hansen ME (2005) Discovery of new natural products by application of X-hitting, a novel algorithm for automated comparison of full UV spectra, combined with structural determination by NMR spectroscopy. *J Nat Prod* 68: 871–874
73 Knight V, Sanglier JJ, DiTullio D, Braccili S, Bonner P, Waters J, Hughes D, Zhang L (2003) Diversifying microbial natural products for drug discovery. *Appl Microbiol Biotechnol* 62: 446–458
74 Nielsen J (2003) It is all about metabolic fluxes. *J Bacteriol* 185: 7031–7035
75 Christensen B, Nielsen J (2000) Metabolic network analysis. A powerful tool in metabolic engineering. *Adv Biochem Eng Biotechnol* 66: 209–231
76 Stephanopoulos GN, Aristidou AA, Nielsen J (1998) *Metabolic engineering. Principles and methodologies*. Academic Press, San Diego

77 Wiechert W (2001) ^{13}C metabolic flux analysis. *Metab Eng* 3: 195–206
78 Christensen B, Nielsen J (1999) Isotopomer analysis using GC-MS. *Metab Eng* 1: 282–290
79 Wittmann C, Heinzle E (1999) Mass spectrometry for metabolic flux analysis. *Biotechnol Bioeng* 62: 739–750
80 Dauner M, Sauer U (2000) GC-MS analysis of amino acids rapidly provides rich information for isotopomer balancing. *Biotechnol Prog* 16: 642–649
81 de Graaf AA, Mahle M, Mollney M, Wiechert W, Stahmann P, Sahm H (2000) Determination of full C-13 isotopomer distributions for metabolic flux analysis using heteronuclear spin echo difference NMR spectroscopy. *J Biotechnol* 77: 25–35
82 Schmidt K, Nielsen J, Villadsen J (1999) Quantitative analysis of metabolic fluxes in *Escherichia coli*, using two-dimensional NMR spectroscopy and complete isotopomer models. *J Biotechnol* 71: 175–189
83 Rantanen A, Rousu J, Kokkonen JT, Tarkiainen V, Ketola RA (2002) Computing positional isotopomer distributions from tandem mass spectrometric data. *Metab Eng* 4: 285–294
84 van Winden WA, van Dam JC, Ras C, Kleijn RJ, Vinke JL, van Gulik WM, Heijnen JJ (2005) Metabolic-flux analysis of *Saccharomyces cerevisiae* CEN.PK113-7D based on mass isotopomer measurements of C-13-labeled primary metabolites. *FEMS Yeast Res* 5: 559–568
85 Kell DB (2004) Metabolomics and systems biology: making sense of the soup. *Curr Opin Microbiol* 7: 296–307
86 Covert MW, Schilling CH, Famili I, Edwards JS, Goryanin II, Selkov E, Palsson BO (2001) Metabolic modeling of microbial strains *in silico*. *Trends Biochem Sci* 26: 179–186
87 Borodina I, Nielsen J (2005) From genomes to *in silico* cells via metabolic networks. *Curr Opin Biotechnol* 16: 350–355
88 Forster J, Famili I, Fu P, Palsson BO, Nielsen J (2003) Genome-scale reconstruction of the *Saccharomyces cerevisiae* metabolic network. *Genome Res* 13: 244–253
89 Nielsen J, Oliver SG (2005) The next wave in metabolome analysis. *Trends Biotechnol* 23: 544–546
90 Stelling J (2004) Mathematical models in microbial systems biology. *Curr Opin Microbiol* 7: 513–518
91 Patil KR, Nielsen J (2005) Uncovering transcriptional regulation of metabolism by using metabolic network topology. *Proc Natl Acad Sci USA* 102: 2685–2689
92 Castrillo JI, Hayes A, Mohammed S, Gaskell SJ, Oliver SG (2003) An optimized protocol for metabolome analysis in yeast using direct infusion electrospray mass spectrometry. *Phytochemistry* 62: 929–937

Progress in Drug Research, Vol. 64
(Helena I. Boshoff and Clifton E. Barry III, Eds)

A subsystems-based approach to the identification of drug targets in bacterial pathogens

By Andrei L. Osterman[1,2]
and Tadhg P. Begley[3]

[1]Burnham Institute for Medical Research,
Infectious and Inflammatory
Disease Center,
La Jolla, California, USA
<osterman@burnham.org>

[2]Fellowship for Interpretation
of Genomes (FIG),
Burr Ridge, Illinois, USA

[3]Cornell University,
Ithaca, New York, USA

Abstract

This chapter describes a three-stage approach to target identification based upon subsystem analysis. Subsystems analysis focuses on related metabolic pathways as a unit and is a biochemically-informed approach to target selection. The process involves three stages of analysis; the first stage, selection of the target subsystem, is guided by information about its essentiality and on the predicted vulnerability of the targeted pathway or enzyme to inhibition. The second stage involves analysis of the target subsystem by means of comparative genomics, including genome context analysis and metabolic reconstruction. The third stage evaluates the selection of the specific target genes within the subsystem by target prioritization and validation. The whole process allows for a careful consideration of spectrum, drugability, biological rationale and the metabolic role of the specific target within the context of an integrated circuit within a specific metabolic pathway.

1 Introduction

In this chapter we will outline the principles and the applications of comparative genomics for the identification of anti-infective drug targets. The approach described will use a collection of annotated *subsystems* projected across a variety of sequenced bacterial genomes. We use the term *subsystem* to refer to a compilation of functional roles (e.g., enzymes, transporters, etc.) that captures the existing knowledge of a biological process [1]. One may think of a subsystem as a generalization of the concept of a biochemical pathway, extended to include ancillary components and alternative reactions reflecting all *functional variants* [2] found in various species. The inclusive nature of subsystems allows us to capture a broader biological context and, most importantly, to cope with an emerging diversity of biological networks revealed by the growing body of sequenced genomes. Tools supporting subsystem annotation and a large collection of draft subsystems, reflecting upon many aspects of the central machinery of life, are provided within The SEED genomic platform (http://theseed.uchicago.edu/FIG/subsys.cgi and [1]).

A subsystems-based approach to the identification and prioritization of drug targets consists of three major stages (see Fig. 1):

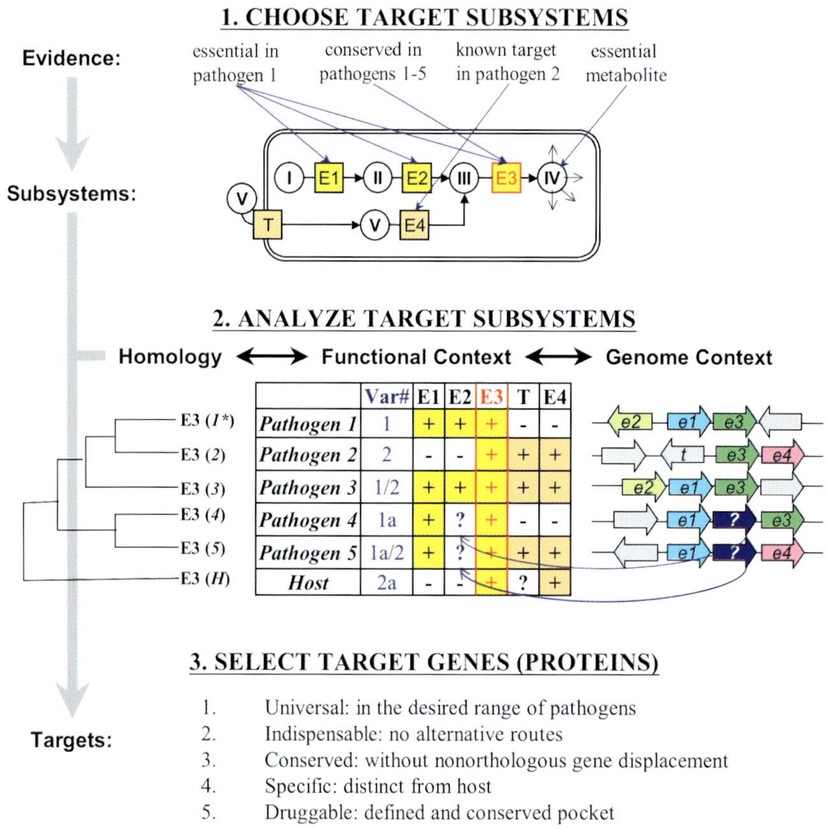

Figure 1.
Three stages of the subsystems-based approach to drug target identification and prioritization

1. Choosing target subsystems. The choice of target subsystem is dictated by the desired drug features (e.g., spectrum of target pathogens), and by various types of available implicating evidence (e.g., biochemical and functional genomics data).

2. Analyzing target subsystems. Subsystem annotation and cross-genome comparative analysis provides a detailed picture of species-to-species variations in the underlying biological process. This analysis usually reveals gaps in knowledge (e.g., *missing genes*), which may be addressed by genome context analysis followed by experimental validation of functional predictions.

3. Selecting target genes. Classification and analysis of subsystem functional variants leads to the identification of critical modules (enzymes, pathways, interactions), which may comprise actual drug targets. Prioritization of candidate target genes includes a combination of established criteria, such as expected essentiality and conservation in a set of target pathogens, distinction from the human host, etc.

The defining feature of this approach is that it begins with the selection and analysis of *target subsystems* instead of the direct selection of *target genes* (as in many described genomics-based strategies [3–9]). Therefore, the experimentally observed and computed characteristics of individual genes are used to implicate possible target subsystems. The dissection of the entire cellular network into quasi-independent sub-networks provides a viable strategy for the identification of novel targets and for the critical reevaluation of existing targets. Among the specific advantages of the subsystems-based approach are:

- The generalization of experimentally or computationally derived features of individual genes in the form of target subsystems makes the identification of target genes more robust and better protected against the inevitable false positives and false negatives. *Every target gene gets a 'second chance'.*
- Annotated subsystems provide a natural framework for the projection and comparative analysis of various types of data. *Subsystems provide a functional context for Functional Genomics.*
- While less rigorous than whole-cell modeling, the subsystems-based approach is more applicable to a large number of relatively poorly studied species. At the same time, it constitutes a significant step forward compared to the single-gene model for target identification. *Subsystems pave the way towards systems biology.*
- The detailed analysis of variations in a subsystem facilitates the identification of alternative pathways, genes and resistance mechanisms. *Subsystems contribute to the understanding of microbial physiology.*

In the following sections, we will describe in more detail the three-stage approach to target identification and analysis using selected examples. We will focus mostly on the second stage, which involves encoding and cross-genome comparative analysis of target subsystems. This analysis often reveals problems with gene assignment and with the reconstruction of pathways, especially for divergent and poorly characterized species. Application of genome context analysis, most notably chromosomal clustering of functionally coupled genes, predicts gene candidates for missing functional roles identified by subsystem analysis [10]. Such *missing genes* often emerge due to nonorthologous gene displacements [11, 12], which precludes the possibility of finding them by straightforward homology-based searches. Gene candidates predicted by a combination of bioinformatics techniques then become the subject of direct experimental validation.

Although this approach is, in principle, applicable to various types of biological processes, including those directly associated with virulence, here we will focus on universal metabolic subsystems, such as the biosynthesis of the essential cofactors. This focus will enable us to clearly describe target selection and unexplored opportunities for the development of new anti-infective therapies. The examples discussed will include several cases where 'missing genes' were predicted using genome context analysis and validated by biochemical and genetic experiments.

2 Stage I: Choosing target subsystems. Genome-scale essentiality and conservation analysis

Although the target-driven drug discovery paradigm is built around molecular targets (individual genes or proteins), the actual target of anti-infective therapy is, obviously, the whole organism. A subsystems-based approach is a first step towards target identification at the whole-organism scale. It is based on a hierarchical decomposition of the cellular machinery, which allows us to: (i) rationalize the possible impact of disrupting a subsystem at the whole-cell level, and (ii) evaluate the subsystem-level consequences of targeting its individual components. This approach efficiently supports application of comparative and functional genomics techniques. It provides a natural framework to analyze various types of implicating evidence generated by different techniques and in different species, and it allows us to project the accumulated knowledge across the whole spectrum of target pathogens.

The choice of possible target subsystems strongly depends on the specific goals, priorities and constraints of a particular drug development project. For example, different types of implicating evidence would be used, and different subsystems would be considered for niche-specific *versus* broad-spectrum targets. Likewise, prodrug-activating targets and virulence targets are unlikely to come from the same set of subsystems. Nevertheless, certain types of evidence and considerations are equally useful for implicating target subsystems of different kinds.

In general, we would expect a target subsystem to minimally meet the following criteria: (i) *essentiality* – it should play an essential role in pathogen survival and/or propagation in its natural niche; (ii) *vulnerability* – it should contain critical (non-redundant) components, whose inactivation would largely block this essential role, and (iii) *conservation* – at least some of these components should be present in the whole spectrum of target pathogens.

2.1 Collecting the evidence

The large body of biochemical, physiological, genetic, and functional genomics data on model bacteria is a rich source of information for the identification of candidate target subsystems. For example, in most bacteria, NAD(P) cannot be imported. This observation suggests that the NAD(P) biosynthetic subsystem is a potential source of anti-infective targets, without explicitly referring to any gene. Convincing evidence implicating a subsystem may also be deduced from the mechanism of action of an antibacterial agent (irrespective of its therapeutic value). For example, pyrazinamide and isoniazid manifest their anti-tuberculosis activity via interference with fatty acid biosynthesis [13]. This knowledge points to the possible target subsystem even if the exact protein target is unknown.

2.1.1 Metabolic modeling

The rapidly progressing techniques of metabolic modeling [14, 15] allow us to predict critical fluxes within the whole-cell network. This approach can be used for the tentative identification of essential genes, as was recently demonstrated in a number of model systems, including *Escherichia coli* [16], *Helicobacter pylori* [17], *Staphylococcus aureus* [18] and *Saccharomyces cerevisiae* [19]. It is important to emphasize the complementarity of the semi-quantitative whole-cell modeling and the qualitative subsystems analysis. An insufficient knowledge of metabolism, beyond a handful of model organisms, currently limits our ability to accurately model multiple diverse species. However, individual predictions generated by the analysis of model species may be efficiently projected over a wide spectrum of pathogens via implicated subsystems. At the same time, the annotation of multiple metabolic subsystems (as recently launched by the SEED project [1]), along with other community efforts [20–23] contributes to improving the accuracy of genome-scale modeling technology.

2.1.2 Comparative genomics: The minimal gene set

The most abundant data that can be used to identify candidate target subsystems derive from comparative genome analysis and from genome-scale gene inactivation studies. These data provide the initial evidence for conservation and essentiality, the key criteria for subsystem selection mentioned above. Each of these criteria has been broadly exploited by academic and industrial research groups for the direct identification and prioritization of drug targets (e.g., see [9, 24–28]).

Attempts to use genome comparison to define the *minimal gene set* that is required to support a prokaryotic life style began immediately after the appearance of the first pair of complete genomes [29], both of bacterial pathogens, *H. influenzae* [30] and *M. genitalium* [31]. Although the fundamental scope of this effort is distinct from drug target identification, its methodology has obvious implications for the subject of this chapter. In line with early expectations, a subset of protein families, broadly conserved in diverse microbial genomes, are substantially enriched with indispensable components of the Central Machinery, most notably of DNA replication, transcription and translation, which may constitute potential drug targets. Various criteria were applied for further prioritization of universally conserved genes, the absence of eukaryotic (human) homologs being the most common. This criterion, however, is not undisputable. For example, successful antibiotics such as trimetoprim and quinolones display selectivity towards bacterial targets despite the existence of their human homologs (as discussed in [4]).

2.1.3 Functional genomics: Essential genes

The importance of gene essentiality data was recognized long before genome-scale studies became feasible. Various gene inactivation techniques (such as chemical and transposon mutagenesis) have been used in numerous single-gene studies, and, hundreds of gene essentiality assignments have been accumulated for model microorganisms. The genomic revolution has triggered the development of genome-scale essentiality technology. After the first groundbreaking efforts in *Mycoplasma* species [32] and in *S. cerevisiae* [33, 34], several genome-scale essentiality studies were accomplished. Comprehensive data sets were published for: *H. influenzae* [35], *B. subtilis* [36], *E. coli* [37], *M. tuberculosis* [28], and *P. aeruginosa* [38]. For some of these and related species, the analysis of gene essentiality was also performed in the model of infection [39–41]. Although genome-scale essentiality studies of major clinical pathogens have been performed in many pharmaceutical and biotech companies, only partial data sets have been published for *S. aureus* [25, 27] and *S. pneumoniae* [26].

The various techniques used in these studies may be divided into two groups: 1) targeted disruption or deletion, and 2) random transposon mutagenesis followed by the analysis of individual viable clones or of the whole population after competitive outgrowth. Among other methods are: complementation of temperature-sensitive mutant collections [42], and gene 'knock-downs' by antisense RNA (reviewed in [43]). Due to the substantial differences in gene inactivation techniques and growth conditions, the exact meaning of *gene essentiality* inferred by different studies varies from 'strictly indispensable' to 'contributes to fitness'. Moreover, various pitfalls, as well as significant variations in sensitivity and accuracy of detection protocols, lead to technical failures, false positive and false negative essentiality assignments for a significant number of genes. Therefore, choosing drug targets directly from single-genome essentiality data, even if generated in one of the relevant pathogens, is a risky approach. In addition to technical limitations, lists of essential genes do not provide any indication of whether these genes should be essential or even present in other pathogens of the desired spectrum. The integration of essentiality data, acquired in different species, in a single database (such as [44]) provides us with a very useful resource for their comparative analysis.

2.2 Integrating the evidence

Combining essentiality data with gene conservation analysis is a powerful approach that helps to overcome some of the problems mentioned above. A strong correlation between essentiality and conservation, observed for a subset of core bacterial genes [36, 37, 45], leads to significant refinement of a list of potential targets. An early implementation of this approach was described for a small subset of essential and universally conserved genes with unknown functions [24]. Among more recent examples of large-scale integration of gene conservation and essentiality data are the *minimal gene set* surveys [46, 47]. A set of ~60 genes, derived by combining cross-taxon gene conservation with essentiality data in bacteria, yeast and worm, represents mostly genes involved in translation, transcription and replication [46]. Such a small set is a likely result of a high frequency of nonorthologous gene displacements, and is insufficient to support life in any conceivable form. Another derived set of ~206 conserved and essential bacterial genes was substantially refined via the reconstruction of minimal bacterial metabolism [47]. Although the latter analysis was geared more towards metabolic engineering, its methodology and some of the specific findings have implications for subsystems-based drug target analysis.

2.2.1 Case study: Broad spectrum target subsystems

A similar approach was applied to the analysis of ~620 *E. coli* genes shown to be required for the robust competitive growth in rich medium by applying transposon mutagenesis combined with genetic footprinting [37]. Here we use these data to illustrate the approach to selection of candidate subsystems expected to contain broad-spectrum antibacterial drug targets. This was accomplished by: (i) selection of a subset of essential *E. coli* genes conserved in a broad range of diverse bacterial genomes, and (ii) projection of this subset to a collection of annotated subsystems present in the first release of The SEED database [1]. Some of the results are illustrated in Table 1.

Table 1.
Target metabolic subsystems implicated by essentiality and conservation analysis

E.coli[1]	Annotation in SEED	ERI[2]	Essentiality[3]	Subsystem in SEED
Cofactors, Prosthetic Groups:				
ppnK	NAD kinase (EC 2.7.1.23)	**0.9**	MG, SP	**NAD and NADP cofactor biosynthesis**
nadE	NAD synthetase (EC 6.3.1.5)	**0.9**	BS, MG, SA	
nadD	Nicotinate-nucleotide adenylyltransferase (EC 2.7.7.18)	**0.8**	BS, SA, SP	
coaE	Dephospho-CoA kinase (EC 2.7.1.24)	**0.9**	BS, PA, SP	**Coenzyme A Biosynthesis**
coaD	Phosphopantetheine adenylyltransferase (EC 2.7.7.3)	**0.9**	HI, PA, SA, SP	
coaBC	Phosphopantothenoylcysteine decarboxylase (EC 4.1.1.36)-/-Phosphopantothenoylcysteine synthetase (EC 6.3.2.5)	**0.8**	SA	
ribF	Riboflavin kinase (EC 2.7.1.26)-/-FMN adenylyltransferase (EC 2.7.7.2)	**0.9**	MG, SA, SP	**FMN and FAD biosynthesis**
ribH	6,7-dimethyl-8-ribityllumazine synthase (EC 2.5.1.9)	**0.8**	HI	
ribA	GTP cyclohydrolase II (EC 3.5.4.25)	**0.8**	HI, PA	
ribE	Riboflavin synthase alpha chain (EC 2.5.1.9)	**0.8**	HI, PA	
ribD	Diaminohydroxyphosphoribosylaminopyrimidine deaminase (EC 3.5.4.26)-/-5-amino-6-(5-phosphoribosylamino)uracil reductase (EC 1.1.1.193)	**0.8**	PA	
folC	Dihydrofolate synthase (EC 6.3.2.12)-/-Folylpolyglutamate synthase (EC 6.3.2.17)	**0.9**	PA	**Folate Biosynthesis**
folK	2-amino-4-hydroxy-6-hydroxymethyldihydropteridine pyrophosphokinase (EC 2.7.6.3)	**0.8**	PA	
thyA	Thymidylate synthase (EC 2.1.1.45)	**0.8**	PA, SA	
ubiE	Ubiquinone/menaquinone biosynthesis methyltransferase UbiE/COQ5	**0.8**	BS	**Ubiquinone Biosynthesis**
metK	S-adenosylmethionine synthetase (EC 2.5.1.6)	**1.0**	BS, MG, SA	**SAM metabolism**
hemC	Porphobilinogen deaminase (EC 2.5.1.61)	**0.8**	SA	**Porphyrin, Heme, and Siroheme Biosynthesis**
hemH	Ferrochelatase, protoheme ferro-lyase (EC 4.99.1.1)	**0.8**	HI, PA	
Amino Acids and Derivatives:				
asd	Aspartate-semialdehyde dehydrogenase (EC 1.2.1.11)	**0.9**	BS, HI, PA	**Lysine Biosynthesis DAP Pathway**
dapA	Dihydrodipicolinate synthase (EC 4.2.1.52)	**0.8**	BS, HI, PA	
dapB	Dihydrodipicolinate reductase (EC 1.3.1.26)	**0.8**	BS, HI, SP	
dapF	Diaminopimelate epimerase (EC 5.1.1.7)	**0.8**	BS, HI	
dapE	N-succinyl-L,L-diaminopimelate desuccinylase (EC 3.5.1.18)	**0.8**	HI	
glyA	Serine hydroxymethyltransferase (EC 2.1.2.1)	**1.0**	BS, PA	**Glycine synthesis**
aroK	Shikimate kinase I (EC 2.7.1.71)	**0.8**	HI	**Chorismate Synthesis**

Table 1 (continued)

Nucleotides and Derivatives:				
adk	Adenylate kinase (EC 2.7.4.3)	**1.0**	BS, MG, SA	**Purine conversions**
gmk	Guanylate kinase (EC 2.7.4.8)	**0.9**	BS, HI, MG	
apt	Adenine phosphoribosyltransferase (EC 2.4.2.7)	**0.8**	HI, MG, SA	
pyrG	CTP synthase (EC 6.3.4.2)	**0.9**	BS, HI, PA	**Pyrimidine conversions**
pyrH	Uridylate kinase (EC 2.7.4.-)	**0.9**	HI, MG, PA	
cmk	Cytidylate kinase (EC 2.7.4.14)	**0.9**	BS, HI, MG, PA	
tmk	Thymidylate kinase (EC 2.7.4.9)	**0.9**	BS, HI, MG, PA	
ndk	Nucleoside diphosphate kinase (EC 2.7.4.6)	**0.8**	PA	
nrdA	Ribonucleotide reductase of class Ia, alpha subunit (EC 1.17.4.1)	**0.9**	BS, HI, PA	**Ribonucleotide reduction**
nrdB	Ribonucleotide reductase of class Ia), beta subunit (EC 1.17.4.1)	**0.8**	HI, PA	
spoT	GTP pyrophosphokinase (EC 2.7.6.5)/-Guanosine-3',5'-bis(diphosphate) 3'-pyrophosphohydrolase (EC 3.1.7.2)	**0.9**	HI, SP	**ppGpp biosynthesis**
Central carbohydrate metabolism:				
pgk	Phosphoglycerate kinase (EC 2.7.2.3)	**1.0**	BS, HI, MG, SP	**Embden-Meyerhof and Gluconeogenesis**
eno	Enolase (EC 4.2.1.11)	**1.0**	BS, MG, SA	
gapA	NAD-dependent glyceraldehyde-3-phosphate dehydrogenase (EC 1.2.1.12)	**1.0**	MG, SA	
tktA	Transketolase (EC 2.2.1.1)	**0.9**	BS, HI, MG, SA	**Pentose phosphate pathway**
rpe	Ribulose-phosphate 3-epimerase (EC 5.1.3.1)	**0.9**	HI, MG, PA, SP	
prsA	Ribose-phosphate pyrophosphokinase (EC 2.7.6.1)	**0.9**	BS, HI, MG	
zwf	Glucose-6-phosphate 1-dehydrogenase (EC 1.1.1.49)	**0.8**	SA	
lpdA	Dihydrolipoamide dehydrogenase (EC 1.8.1.4)	**0.8**	HI, SA	**TCA cycle**
Fatty Acids and Lipids:				
fabG	3-oxoacyl-[acyl-carrier protein] reductase (EC 1.1.1.100)	**0.9**	BS, HI, PA, SP	**Fatty Acid Biosynthesis FASII**
birA	Biotin-protein ligase (EC 6.3.4.15)/-Biotin operon repressor	**0.9**	BS, HI	
acpP	Acyl carrier protein	**0.9**	BS, MG, PA	
accD	Acetyl-coenzyme A carboxyl transferase beta chain (EC 6.4.1.2)	**0.8**	BS, HI, PA, SA, SP	
fabD	Malonyl CoA-acyl carrier protein transacylase (EC 2.3.1.39)	**0.8**	BS, HI, SP	
fabH	3-oxoacyl-[acyl-carrier-protein] synthase, KASIII (EC 2.3.1.41)	**0.8**	HI	
accC	Biotin carboxylase of acetyl-CoA carboxylase (EC 6.3.4.14)	**0.8**	BS, HI, SP	
fabZ	(3R)-hydroxymyristoyl-[acyl carrier protein] dehydratase (EC 4.2.1.-)	**0.8**	HI, PA, SP	
acpS	Holo-[acyl-carrier protein] synthase (EC 2.7.8.7)	**0.8**	BS	
accA	Acetyl-coenzyme A carboxyl transferase alpha chain (EC 6.4.1.2)	**0.8**	BS, HI, PA, SP	
accB	Biotin carboxyl carrier protein of acetyl-CoA carboxylase	**0.8**	BS, SP	

Table 1 (continued)

pgsA	CDP-diacylglycerol--glycerol-3-phosphate 3-phosphatidyltransferase (EC 2.7.8.5)	**0.9**	BS, HI, MG, PA	**Glycerolipid and glycerphospholipid metabolism**
cdsA	Phosphatidate cytidylyltransferase (EC 2.7.7.41)	**0.9**	BS, PA, SA	
plsC	1-acyl-sn-glycerol-3-phosphate acyltransferase (EC 2.3.1.51)	**0.9**	BS, HI, SA, SP	
Cell Wall and Capsule:				
uppS	Undecaprenyl pyrophosphate synthetase (EC 2.5.1.31)	**1.0**	PA	**Isoprenoid and Polyisoprenoid Biosynthesis**
dxs	1-deoxy-D-xylulose 5-phosphate synthase (EC 2.2.1.7)	**0.9**	BS, HI, PA	
ispA	Geranyltranstransferase (EC 2.5.1.10)	**0.8**	BS, HI, PA	
ispB	Octaprenyl-diphosphate synthase (EC 2.5.1.-)	**0.8**	BS, HI, PA	
ispG	1-hydroxy-2-methyl-2-(E)-butenyl 4-diphosphate synthase (EC 1.17.4.3)	**0.8**	BS, PA	
ispE	4-diphosphocytidyl-2-C-methyl-D-erythritol kinase (EC 2.7.1.148)	**0.8**	BS, HI, PA	
dxr	1-deoxy-D-xylulose 5-phosphate reductoisomerase (EC 1.1.1.267)	**0.8**	BS, HI, PA	
ispH	4-hydroxy-3-methylbut-2-enyl diphosphate reductase (EC 1.17.1.2)	**0.8**	BS, HI, PA	
murB	UDP-N-acetylenolpyruvoylglucosamine reductase (EC 1.1.1.158)	**1.0**	BS, PA, SA	**UDP-N-acetylmuramate from Fructose-6-phosphate Biosynthesis**
murA	UDP-N-acetylglucosamine 1-carboxyvinyltransferase (EC 2.5.1.7)	**1.0**	BS, SA, SP	
glmS	Glucosamine--fructose-6-phosphate aminotransferase [isomerizing] (EC 2.6.1.16)	**0.9**	BS, SA, SP	
glmU	N-acetylglucosamine-1-phosphate uridyltransferase (EC 2.7.7.23) / Glucosamine-1-phosphate N-acetyltransferase (EC 2.3.1.157)	**0.9**	BS, SP	
mrsA	Phosphoglucosamine mutase (EC 5.4.2.10)	**0.8**	BS, HI, SP	
murD	UDP-N-acetylmuramoylalanine--D-glutamate ligase (EC 6.3.2.9)	**1.0**	BS, HI	**Peptidoglycan Biosynthesis**
murC	UDP-N-acetylmuramate--alanine ligase (EC 6.3.2.8)	**1.0**	BS, HI, PA, SA	
murG	UDP-N-acetylglucosamine--N-acetylmuramyl-(pentapeptide) pyrophosphoryl-undecaprenol N-acetylglucosamine transferase (EC 2.4.1.227)	**1.0**	BS, HI, PA, SA	
murE	UDP-N-acetylmuramoylalanyl-D-glutamate--2,6-diaminopimelate ligase (EC 6.3.2.13)	**1.0**	BS, HI, PA, SP	
mraY	Phospho-N-acetylmuramoyl-pentapeptide-transferase (EC 2.7.8.13)	**1.0**	BS, PA, SP	
ftsI	Cell division protein ftsI [Peptidoglycan synthetase] (EC 2.4.1.129)	**0.9**	BS, HI	
murF	UDP-N-acetylmuramoylalanyl-D-glutamyl-2,6-diaminopimelate--D-alanyl-D- alanyl ligase (EC 6.3.2.15)	**0.9**	BS, HI, PA	
ddlB	D-alanine--D-alanine ligase B (EC 6.3.2.4)	**0.9**	BS, HI, SA	
murI	Glutamate racemase (EC 5.1.1.3)	**0.8**	BS, PA	

1. E. coli genes implicated by genome-scale essentiality analysis [37]. To compensate for technically failed or ambiguous assignments, several essential genes were added from the compilation of historic single-gene studies (http://www.shigen.nig.ac.jp/ecoli/pec/index.jsp).
2. ERI = Evolutionary Retention Index, a parameter introduced in [37], reflects a tendency of genes to be broadly conserved in diverse bacterial genomes on the scale from 0 to 1. Genes in this tables are selected at ERI >0.75, i.e. conserved in >75% or at least in 24 out of 32 representative bacterial genomes selected for this analysis.
1. Organisms where orthologous genes were deemed essential by the published genome-scale studies are shown by two-letter abbreviations: MG – Mycoplasma species [32]; HI – H. influenzae [35]; BS – B. subtilis [36], PA – P. aeruginosa [38], SA – S. aureus [25] and S. pneumoniae [26]).

The original set of essential genes was supplemented by essentiality assignments from previous studies (http://www.shigen.nig.ac.jp/ecoli/pec/index.jsp) to minimize the effect of false negatives and to compensate for the ~10% technical failure in the genetic footprinting experiment [37]. Gene conservation was approximated using the evolutionary retention index (ERI) as in [37]. A total of 250 genes with ERI >0.75 (e.g., having putative orthologs in >75% of 32 bacterial genomes selected to represent maximum phylogenetic diversity) were further analyzed. Remarkably, orthologs of all but 15 genes in this set (94%) were found to be essential by at least one of the genome-scale studies in other bacteria as indicated in Table 1. Of no less importance, ~95% of these genes have well-defined functional roles (annotations), most of which (>85%) map to our collection of subsystems. Not surprisingly, a significant fraction of the mapped genes (total of 115, not shown) belong to non-metabolic subsystems related to replication, transcription, translation, protein folding, secretion and cell division. At the same time, a comparable fraction of ~90 genes can be mapped to core metabolic subsystems, and 80 of them (implicated by an additional essentiality screen in at least one more organism) are listed in Table 1.

2.2.2 Essential and conserved metabolic subsystems: An unexplored target landscape

Altogether, these genes implicate a very limited number of metabolic subsystems (total of 22) with some remarkable features. From this list, 16 subsystems are implicated by more than one gene and about half of those by three genes or more, providing additional prioritization criteria. The derived list of broad-spectrum target subsystems covers <10% of the bacterial Central Machinery. Even before considering *what is* in this list, it is worth noting *what is not*. For example, it does not contain *de novo* biosynthesis of amino acids (except lysine, see below), purines or pyrimidines, as these can be replaced by salvage. The absence of catabolic pathways such as utilization of exogenous carbon sources, is due to their redundancy and variability between species. On the other hand, this list contains subsystems involved with biogenesis of indispensable cofactors (NAD, Coenzyme A, FAD) and nucleotides (of note, all of them being phosphorylated compounds, which, in general, cannot be imported from the medium). Not surprisingly, the largest component of the list is a set of subsystems related to cell wall biogenesis, including the biosynthesis of fatty acids, lipids, isoprenoids and peptidoglycan. The importance of the latter process provides the rationale for the apparent essentiality of the lysine biosynthetic pathway. While lysine requirement *per se* may be satisfied by salvage from the host, diaminopimelate (DAP), a penultimate intermediate of the same biosynthetic pathway is a common essential component of peptidoglycan. Not surprisingly, only the last step of this pathway, conversion of DAP to lysine, appears to be dispensable for the growth of *E. coli* in a regular rich medium (as discussed in [37]).

Overall, one may notice a surprising consistency in the results obtained by this unbiased and strictly formal analysis with the previously accumulated knowledge of microbial physiology. Moreover, almost all of the known targets of antibiotics and other antibacterial compounds appear in the subsystems revealed by this approach. Although most of these targets occur in the information processing subsystems (not shown), including DNA replication and transcription (e.g., quinolones, ofloxacin, rifampin groups) and protein synthesis (indolmycin, kirromycin, mupirocin groups), others occur in implicated metabolic subsystems, e.g., fatty acid (isoniazid, cerulenin, triclosan) and folate (trimetoprim, sulfonamides) synthesis.

Although it is tempting to perceive the *list of genes* in Table 1 as a *list of targets*, in our approach we use it for the sole purpose of compiling the '*list of target subsystems*'. Therefore, even if some of the subsystem components were missed in the initial analysis, due to a technical failure or redundancy in the model organism, they would still be considered at the next stage. That is what we mean by saying that *every target gets a second chance*. For example, the *nadD* gene was deemed nonessential in our genetic footprinting studies in *E. coli* [48]. Nevertheless, a subsystem analysis strongly implicated it as a good target candidate. This was later confirmed by a single-gene knockout experiment and by essentiality studies in other species. Likewise, some of the implicated genes may be 'downgraded' by the subsequent subsystem analysis. For example, all of the genes of riboflavin *de novo* biosynthesis (*ribH, ribA, ribD* and *ribE* in Table 1), which are essential in *E. coli* and *H. infuenzae*, should be dispensable in many Gram-positive pathogens due to the existence of active transport of exogenous vitamin B_2. Therefore, only one of the five initially listed genes of the FMN and FAD biosynthesis subsystem (*ribF*) should be considered as a prospective broad-spectrum drug target.

A detailed subsystem analysis across the whole spectrum of target species (see next section) provides a solid foundation for prioritizing individual targets depending on many criteria, which will vary between drug development projects (as discussed in the last section of this chapter).

3 Stage II: Analyzing target subsystems. Metabolic reconstruction and functional predictions

A preliminary notion of the subsystems corresponding to experimentally identified essential genes or other types of evidence (discussed in the Section I) may be obtained from a variety of sources, including biochemical textbooks (such as [49]) and web-resources, such as KEGG pathways [21], GO terms [22], and functional categories of COGs [50]. An insightful integration of functional and genomic context, in the format of *genome properties,* was recently described [20]. The breadth and the depth of genomic annotations in a growing collection of subsystems within The SEED database is gradually improving due to a community effort and the contributions by experts [1]. While expecting that this and similar developments will soon provide us with substantial coverage of many target subsystems, we realize that for any new drug development project, an additional subsystem analysis may be in order. The scope of such analysis may range from the extension and refinement of existing subsystems in order to accommodate new genomes and experimental data, up to *de novo* encoding of subsystems implicated by new data and not present in the existing collection.

Therefore, in this section we will briefly outline the key principles and practical steps of subsystem development and analysis. We will illustrate this process, as implemented in the SEED environment, using NAD(P) biosynthesis as an example. An early analysis of this target subsystem identified by essentiality and conservation data (see Tab. 1), allowed us to select nicotinic acid mononucleotide adenylyltransferase (NAMNAT, encoded by *nadD* gene in *E. coli*) as the most attractive drug target for follow-up studies [48] (see Section III for more details). This subsystem, covering >270 diverse genomes, and a shorter version focusing on bacterial pathogens, is a part of The SEED subsystem collection available on-line (http://theseed.uchicago.edu/FIG/subsys.cgi).

Subsystem encoding uses the inference of pathways and individual reactions based on the presence of respective genes [51, 52]. A subsystem is initially defined by a set of functional roles (e.g., enzymes), based on available knowledge. Genes in the analyzed genomes are connected to these roles via tentative annotations. An initial set of annotations is generated by homology-based projections from a limited number of genes with experimentally confirmed function. These semi-automated annotations are further refined using additional evidence provided by *genome context* (e.g., clustering on the chromosome) and *functional context* (pathway reconstruction) analysis.

Homology and genome context analysis are established techniques, and they are supported by a number of advanced tools [53], including tools in the SEED. Functional context-based reasoning is less formalized and includes a significant element of subjective judgment. This amounts to reconciling an observed pattern of relevant genes with biochemical transformations within established or inferred pathways. Classification and consistency analysis of subsystem variants [2], over a wide range of diverse genomes, has at least three important implications: (i) it significantly improves the quality and the reliability of genomic annotations; (ii) it allows us to infer novel pathway variants, and (iii) it efficiently reveals *missing genes* [10, 54]. In some cases, the apparent absence of a gene ortholog for a functional role inferred by metabolic reconstruction is due to 'technical' reasons, such as Open Reading Frame (ORF) identification problems or gaps in genome sequence/assembly. Individual occurrences of such technical problems are randomly spread in genomes, and they are usually easy to diagnose and reconcile. However, the appearance of a missing gene in the middle of an 'almost complete' pathway (functional variant) in a number of related species often points to a nonorthologous gene displacement.

3.1 The NAD(P) biosynthesis subsystem

A *table of functional roles*, which are known to be involved in the biogenesis of NAD and NADP in various species is shown in Table 2. A general *subsystem diagram,* illustrating respective biochemical transformations, is shown in Figure 2. Once the initial set of functional roles is defined and matched with annotations from model organisms, the system automatically fills in gene identifiers (IDs) in the respective cells of a *subsystem spreadsheet.* This spreadsheet is a key representation of a subsystem, showing functional roles as columns and organisms as rows. Populating a subsystem amounts to the gradual expansion of the initial spreadsheet by adding genomes and by carefully projecting annotations. Table 3 provides a condensed form of the original NAD(P) subsystem spreadsheet. It reflects the gene occurrence patterns of all functional variants identified in the ~100 genomes of pathogens, commensals and related bacteria in The SEED database. In this condensed presentation, gene IDs are replaced by symbols, and each *functional variant* is illustrated by a single representative species.

The NAD(P) subsystem can be divided into six modules: two distinct *de novo* pathways – one from aspartate as in many bacterial pathogens and the other from tryptophan as in humans; three alternative salvage pathways – two involving either the deamidating or the non-deamidating salvage of niacin (vitamin B_3) and the third involving the utilization of nicotinamide ribose. The final module is the 'universal' pathway for the conversion of nicotinic acid mononucleotide (NaMN) to NAD and NADP (see Fig. 2 and Tab. 3). Different combinations of these modules, along with some nonorthologous gene displacements, results in the substantial diversity reflected here involving >20 distinct functional variants clustered in five major groups (see Tab. 3). None of the organisms contain all six modules. *E. coli* and *H. sapiens* are among the richest functional variants, while some obligate intracellular pathogens such as *Chlamydia* and *Rickettsia* spp., manifest extreme pathway truncation. These organisms may have developed a unique transport machinery to scavenge the NAD cofactor from the host [48], and the recent identification of a possible NAD transporter in one of the plant-borne *Chlamydia* provides the first experimental evidence supporting this prediction [55].

The most common type of *incomplete functional variants* involves a missing gene for the Gln-amidotransferase component (GAT) of NAD synthetase (NADS), as indicated by '?' in the respective cells of the spreadsheet. This component was experimentally identified as an N-terminal nitrilase-like domain of a two-domain ('long') form of NADS in eukaryotes [56] and some bacteria [57]. At the same time, many other bacterial NADS homologs lack the corresponding amidotransferase domain, and they are unable to utilize glutamine as an amide donor *in vitro* [58–61]. Among other missing gene problems in this subsystem are possible nonorthologous gene displacements of aspartate oxidase (AOX) and NAD kinase (NADK) in a limited number of species (marked by '?' in Tab. 3).

Table 2.
Functional roles and subsets (pathways) in NAD (P) biosynthesis subsystem

Abbrev	Functional role	Subset (pathway)
TDO	Tryptophan 2,3-dioxygenase (EC 1.13.11.11)	*De novo* biosynthesis I, from tryptophane (includes QAPRT)
IDO	Indoleamine 2,3-dioxygenase (EC 1.13.11.42)	
KFA_e	Kynurenine formamidase (EC 3.5.1.9)	
KFA_b	Kynurenine formamidase, bacterial (EC 3.5.1.9)	
KMO	Kynurenine 3-monooxygenase (EC 1.14.13.9)	
KYN	Kynureninase (EC 3.7.1.3)	
HAD	3-hydroxyanthranilate 3,4-dioxygenase (EC 1.13.11.6)	
ASPOX	L-aspartate oxidase (EC 1.4.3.16)	*De novo* biosynthesis II, from aspartate
QSYN	Quinolinate synthetase (EC 4.1.99.-)	
QAPRT	Quinolinate phosphoribosyltransferase (EC 2.4.2.19)	
NAMNAT	**Nicotinate-nucleotide adenylyltransferase (EC 2.7.7.18)**	Universal pathway
NADS	**NAD synthetase (EC 6.3.1.5)**	
GAT	Glutamine amidotransferase chain of NAD synthetase	
NADK	**NAD kinase (EC 2.7.1.23)**	
NAM	Nicotinamidase (EC 3.5.1.19)	Nicotinamide salvage I, deamidating pathway
NAPRT	Nicotinate phosphoribosyltransferase (EC 2.4.2.11)	
NMPRT	Nicotinamide phosphoribosyltransferase (EC 2.4.2.12)	Nicotinamide salvage II, nondeamidating pathway
NMNAT	Nicotinamide-nucleotide adenylyltransferase (EC 2.7.7.1)	
PNUC	Ribosyl nicotinamide transporter, pnuC-like	Salvage/recycling of nicotinamide ribose (includes NMNAT)
RNK_b	Ribosylnicotinamide kinase (EC 2.7.1.22)	
RNK_e	Ribosylnicotinamide kinase, ekaryotic (EC 2.7.1.22)	

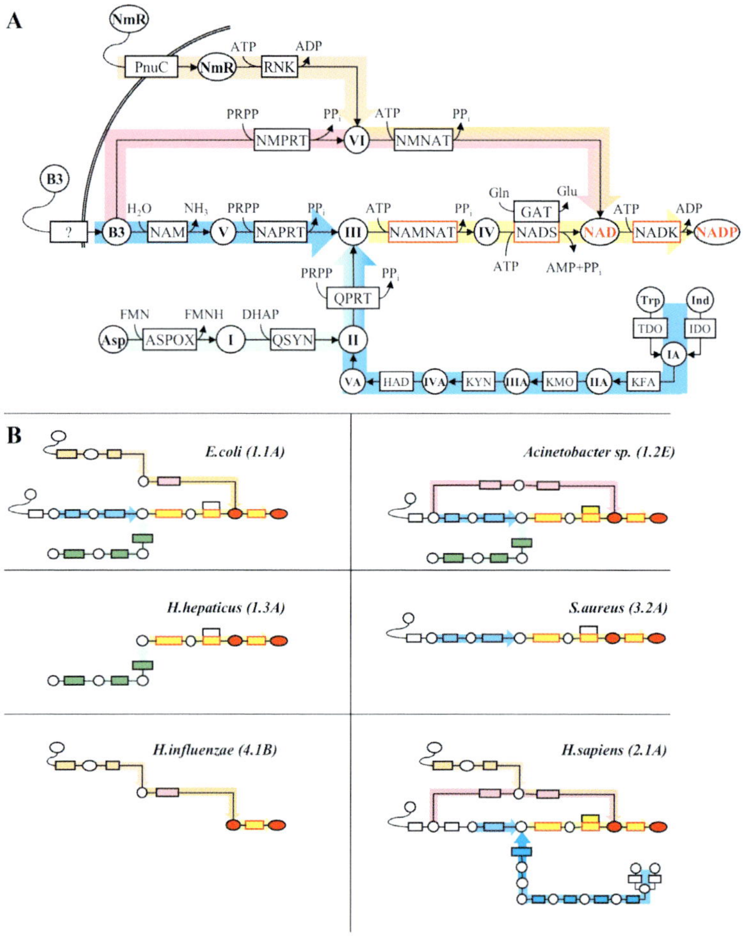

Figure 2.
NAD(P) biosynthesis subsystem diagram. A) A general map of possible biochemical transformations. Functional roles (mostly enzymes) are shown by boxed abbreviations (as defined in Tab. 2). Boxes with red borders correspond to possible broad-spectrum, drug targets (as in Tab. 1). The reactions are shown by thin lines and arrows. Main intermediates are shown in circles: Asp – L-Aspartate; I – Iminoaspartate; II – Quinolinic acid; III – Nicotinate mononucleotide; IV – Deamido-NAD; B3 – Nicotinamide; V – Nicotinic acid; NmR – N-Ribosylnicotinamide; VI – Nicotinamide mononucleotide; Trp – L-tryptophan, Ind – Indoleamine; IA – N-formylkynurenine ; IIA – Kynurenine; IIIA – 3-hydroxykynurenine ; IVA – 3-hydroxyanthranilate; VA – alpha-amino-beta-carboxymuconic semialdehyde. Other intermediates are shown using standard abbreviations including: PRPP – 5-Phosphoribosyl 1-pyrophosphate; DAHP – Dihydroxyacetone-P. Subsets of roles (pathways) are outlined by thick arrows using the same color-coding as in Tables 2 and 3. B) Examples of six functional variants, which are schematically shown by the presence of functional roles highlighted by a respective color.

Table 3.
Distribution of functional variants of NAD biosynthesis subsystem in bacterial pathogens and related species

EXAMPLES	Variant codes	TDO	KFA	KMO	KYN	HAD	ASPOX	QSYN	QAPRT	NAMNAT	NADS	GAT	NADK	NAM	NAPRT	NMPRT	NMNAT	PNUC	RNK	Total genomes
		De novo pathways								Universal				Salvage/recycling						
Group 1. *De novo* pathway from Asp and the universal pathway:																				
Escherichia coli	1.1A	*B3 and V-factor salvage*					*nadB*	*nadA*	*nadC*	*nadD*	*nadE*	?	*nadK*	*pncA*	*pncB*		*nadR*	*pnuC*	*nadR*	15
Yersinia pestis	1.1B						+	+	+	+	+	+	+	+	+		+	+	+	9
Pseudomonas aeruginosa	1.1C	±	±		±		+	+	+	+	+	?	+	+	+			+	+	2
Bacillus anthracis	1.2A	±	±		±		+	+	+	+	+	?	+	+	+					23
Burkholderia pseudomallei	1.2B	*B3 salvage*					+	+	+	+	+	+	+	+	+					8
Fusobacterium nucleatum	1.2C						+	+	+	+	+	?	+		+					2
Coxiella burnetii	1.2D						+	+	+	+	+	+	+		+					4
Acinetobacter sp.	1.2E						+	+	+	+	+	+	+	+	+	+	+			9
Francisella tularensis	1.2F						+	+	+	?	+	?	+			+	+			1
Helicobacter hepaticus	1.3A	*No B3 salvage*					+	+	+	+	+	?	+							1
Mycobacterium leprae	1.3B						+	+	+	+	+	+	+							1
Leptospira interrogans	1.3C						+	+	+	+	+	+	?							2
Shigella flexneri	1.4A	*Missing ASPOX*					?	+	+	+	+	?	+	+	+		+	+	+	2
Corynebacterium efficiens	1.4B						?	+	+	+	+	?	+	+	+		+			2
Helicobacter pylori	1.4C						?	+	+	+	+	?	+				+			2
Ehrlichia canis	1.4D						?	+	+	+	+	+	+				+			1
Group 2. *De novo* biosynthesis from tryptophan (mostly in eukaryotes):																				
Homo sapiens	2.1A	+	+	+	+	+			+	+	+	+	+	+	+	+	+		+	
Group 3. Universal pathway without *de novo* biosynthesis:																				
Proteus mirabilis	3.1A									+	+	+	+	+	+		+	+	+	1
Staphylococcus epidermidis	3.2A									+	+	?	+	+	+					33
Brucella melitensis	3.2B									+	+	+	+	+	+					11
Mycoplasma penetrans	3.2C									+	+	?	+		+					3
Treponema denticola	3.2D									+	+	+	+		+					2
Streptococcus suis	3.2E									+	+	?	?		+					2
Mycoplasma genitalium	3.2F									+	+	?	+			+				2
Group 4. No universal pathway (NMN shunt, bypassing NADS):																				
Mannheimia haemolytica	4.1A												+			+	+	+	+	5
Haemophilus influenzae	4.1B												+				+	+	+	5
Group 5. Salvage of NAD and/or NADP:																				
Rickettsia prowazekii	5.1A												+							5
Chlamydia trachomatis	none																			9

A condensed subsystem spreadsheet (modified from "NAD and NADP biosynthesis in pathogens" subsystem at http://theseed.uchicago.edu/FIG/subsys.cgi) shows gene patterns characteristic of functional variants identified in ~160 complete bacterial genomes (and in the human genome). Presence of genes assigned with respective functional roles (abbreviation are as in Tab. 2) is indicated by: '+' – required to implement a functional variant; '±' – optional; '?' – inferred by pathway analysis but a gene is unknown (cannot be projected by homology). Representative genomes and a total number of genomes implementing each variant are shown in the last and in the first columns. Background colors correspond to subsystem modules (pathways).

Despite a few remaining problems, this example reveals a very clear picture, which allows us to reliably predict the phenotype and even the details of the NAD(P) biosynthetic sub-network in hundreds of species. For example, we can predict that ~50 diverse bacterial species, which implement functional variants clustered in Group 3 (Tab. 3), are strictly dependent on exogenous nicotinamide or nicotinic acid (vitamin B_3). Straightforward conjectures of this type may have immediate implications for the development of new therapies, and for the reevaluation of existing therapies.

The most substantial difference between the human and bacterial variants of the subsystem is related to the *de novo* biosynthesis of quinolinate (see Fig. 2). Although for many years the pathway from tryptophan to quinolinate was thought to be a eukaryotic pathway, it was recently identified in a small group of bacteria by a comparative genomics study followed by experimental verification [62, 63]. None of the analyzed human pathogens belong to this group, although some of them (e.g., *P. aeruginosa* and *B. anthracis,* see Tab. 3) contain a 'nonfunctional' variant of this pathway leading to anthranilate instead of quinolinate [64].

The observed picture of conservation and nonrandom variations in the NAD(P) biosynthesis subsystem is consistent with an emerging understanding of the intrinsic *modularity of cellular networks* and the *conservation of functional modules* in the Central Machinery of Life [65–68]. A crucial aspect of this cross-species subsystem analysis is the identification of the most conserved modules, which potentially contain possible drug targets. For the NAD(P) subsystem, such a module is the three-step 'universal' pathway (see Fig. 2 and Tab. 3), since: (i) it is conserved in most bacterial pathogens; (ii) its indispensable role is supported by the observed essentiality of all three enzymes involved (see Tab. 1); and (iii) this essentiality is in agreement with the fact that all of the intermediates and products of this pathway are phosphorylated compounds (see Fig. 2), which cannot be directly imported from the medium.

Comparative genomics helped to fill in many gaps in our knowledge of NAD(P) biosynthesis. Several 'missing' genes were identified using a combination of bioinformatics techniques such as long-range homology and genome context analysis. These techniques and their applications in gene discovery have been discussed in a number of recent surveys [10, 20, 23, 67, 69]. Here, we will briefly illustrate the gene discovery aspect of subsystems analysis using selected examples immediately related to drug target development.

3.1.1 Example 1: Nicotinic acid mononucleotide adenylyltransferase

Although, this enzymatic activity was for a long time known to play a central role in NAD biosynthesis [70], a respective gene was only recently identified by bioinformatics techniques followed by experimental verification. This was accomplished using a combination of its approximate chromosomal location with long-range similarity searches [71], and, independently, based on the observation of chromosomal clustering of a putative nucleotidyl transferase gene with other NAD biosynthetic genes in a number of analyzed genomes (see Fig. 3). The latter approach, which allows us to infer functional coupling of genes based on their operon-like clustering on the prokaryotic chromosome, is one of the most powerful techniques of genome context analysis. It was pioneered by R. Overbeek and colleagues [72, 73], later implemented in a number of web-based tools, including The SEED, and successfully applied to the identification of several missing genes [10]. Although the *E. coli nadD* gene, as well as its orthologs in most bacterial pathogens, is not involved in any 'suggestive' chromosomal clustering, its assignment was a straightforward homology-based expansion of the implicated protein family. These assignments were directly verified by the cloning overexpression and characterization of several representatives of this family from divergent bacterial pathogens, including *S. aureus*, *H. pylori* and *F. nucleatum* [48]. In addition, a long-range similarity analysis allowed us to expand this new family to include previously missing enzymes playing the same role in human NAD biosynthesis. Three identified human isoforms were experimentally verified and characterized [74–78], revealing a number of fundamental differences between these enzymes and their bacterial counterparts (as reviewed by [79]). Some of these findings, relating to the development of NadD as a potential anti-infective drug target, are further discussed in the next Section.

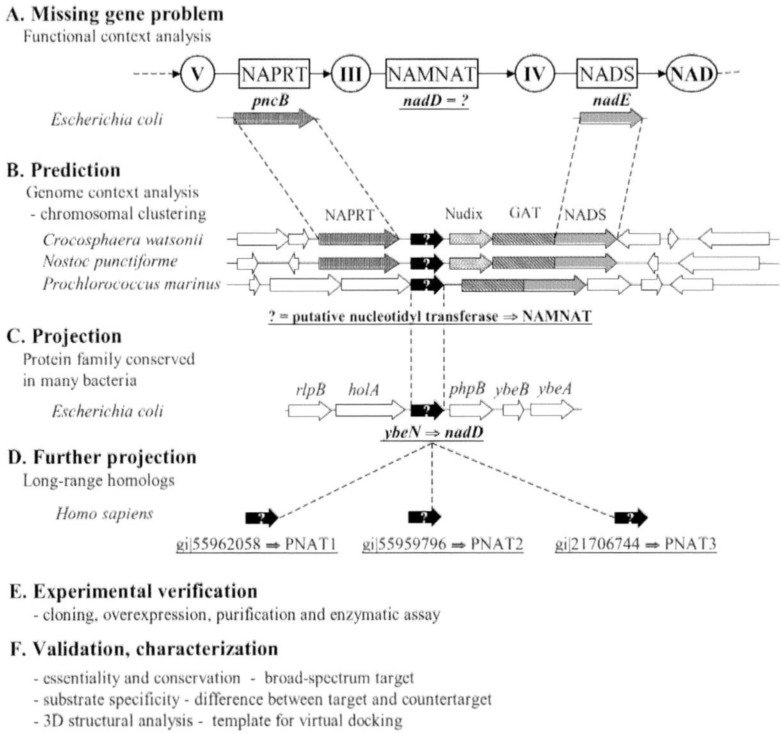

Figure 3.
Missing genes and genome context analysis. Example 1: Nicotinic acid mononucleotide adenylyltransferase (NAMNAT), a possible broad-spectrum drug target. A) Until recently, a gene encoding NAMNAT remained unknown. In addition to biochemical and genetic data in some model species, the presence of this enzyme could be inferred by metabolic reconstruction of NAD biosynthesis in most bacterial genomes (see Tab. 3). A shown segment of NAD subsystem (as in Fig. 2) includes the two known genes (*pncB* and *nadE* in *E. coli*), which constitute a functional context of the missing gene (designated *nadD*). B) A chromosomal cluster conserved in many cyanobacterial genomes, contained a previously uncharacterized putative nucleotidyl transferase of HIGH-superfamily. A respective gene (black arrow marked by '?') was predicted to encode the missing NAMNAT. C) This tentative assignment was projected to putative orthologs in most other bacteria, including gene *ybeN* of *E. coli.* D) Three isoforms of putative human NAMNAT were identified by homology searches. E) The predicted activity was verified for several representatives of the family, including recombinant enzymes of *E. coli, H. pylori, S. aureus* and *H. sapiens.* F) Essentiality of NAMNAT was confirmed by directed gene knockout experiments in *E. coli* and *S. aureus.* Steady state kinetic analysis revealed a strong preference of bacterial NAMNAT for NaMN over NMN, in contrast with a dual specificity of human NAMNAT/NMNAT enzymes. Topological differences in the active sites of bacterial and human enzymes were employed to design a structural template for *in silico* screening of a small molecule compound library.

3.1.2 Example 2: The bi-functional nicotinamide mononucleotide adenylyltransferase/ribosylnicotinamide kinase (NMNAT/RNK, NadR family)

The inference of functional coupling, based on protein domain fusion events, is another important strategy of genome context analysis [80]. This approach played a critical role in the prediction and verification of the previously unknown gene encoding bacterial ribosylnicotinamide kinase (RNK) (see Fig. 4) [81]. This prediction was triggered by the analysis of one of the extremely truncated NAD biosynthesis subsystem variants (Group 4 in Tab. 3) – an NADS-independent salvage of nicotinamide ribose, which is essential for the survival of *H. influenzae* [82] and related Pasteurellaceae. Remarkably, both essential enzymatic activities, RNK and NMNAT, were found within a single fusion protein, a homolog of *E. coli* NadR, originally described as a transcriptional regulator of the *nadA-pnuC* operon [83], and later shown to possess NMNAT activity [84]. An additional RNK activity was predicted based on the presence of a domain with unknown function containing Walker A and B motifs characteristic of many kinases. Both activities were experimentally verified, and confirmed to be essential for the survival of *H. influenzae* in culture [81], and later, *in vivo* [85, 86]. However, only one of these activities, namely NMNAT, is expected to be essential in *H.ducreyi*, a related bacterial representative of the V-factor independent Pasteurellaceae, which contain an additional gene (nadV) encoding nicotinamide phosphoribosyl transferase (NMPRT) [87]. The addition of this enzyme enables the non-deamidating salvage of exogenous vitamin B_3, bypassing the requirement for V-factors and RNK activity. More representatives of this functional variant, which include *Manheimia haemolytica* (see Tab. 3) and *Actinobacillus actinomycetemcomitans*, are predicted by the subsystem analysis. This is another example illustrating the importance of subsystem analysis for drug target identification and evaluation. The 3D structure of the *H. influenzae* NadR protein was solved, providing more insights into the structure-function relations in the NaMNAT/NMNAT superfamily [88] and setting the stage for niche-specific drug development.

Two additional examples provide a brief illustration of using similar techniques for the analysis of Coenzyme A and Fatty acid biosynthesis (see Tab. 1).

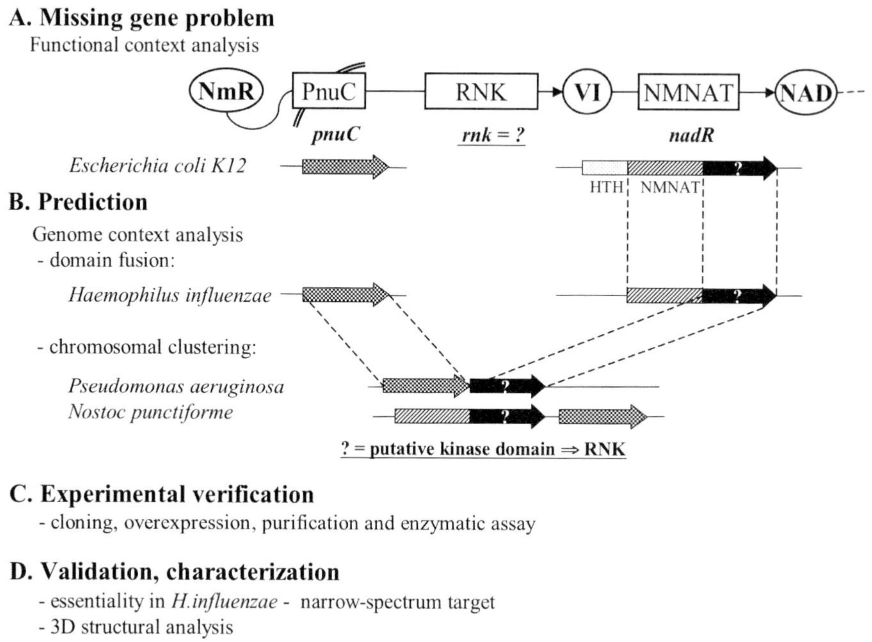

Figure 4.
Missing genes and genome context analysis. Example 2: Nicotinamide mononucleotide adenylyltransferase/ribosylnicotinamide kinase (NaMNAT/RNK) a possible drug target in *H. influenzae.* A) A gene encoding RNK activity, which is required for the Nicotinamide Ribose (NmR) salvage pathway was unknown. This pathway is the only route of NAD biogenesis in *H. influenzae* (see Fig. 2). B) A putative kinase domain fused with NMNAT-domain of NadR protein was predicted to constitute a missing RNK. This conjecture is additionally supported by chromosomal clustering of NadR and PnuC homologs in several bacterial genomes. C) Both enzymatic activities, RNK and NMNAT, were verified and characterized for recombinant NadR proteins of *H. influenzae* and *S. enterica.* Essentiality of *nadR* gene in *H. influenzae* was confirmed by transposon mutagenesis.

3.1.3 Example 3: The human bi-functional phosphopantetheine adenylyltransferase/dephospho-CoA kinase/(PPAT/DPCK)

The host/pathogen comparative analysis of the universal subsystems (such as many of those in Tab. 1) plays an important role in target prioritization. In addition to that, this analysis helps to significantly refine our knowledge of the human variants of subsystems, which is still incomplete. For example, until recently, four of the five genes in the human CoA biosynthetic pathways were unknown, and even the relative order of the biosynthetic steps in this pathway remained controversial. The identification of the complete set of genes implementing this pathway in *E. coli* [89–91] and its homology-based projection across the collection of genomes, allowed us to reliably predict three out of the four unidentified human genes. The last missing gene, encoding a nonorthologous human PPAT enzyme, was identified using the same domain fusion analysis technique as described in the previous example. An uncharacterized human protein containing a domain of unknown function with a nucleotidyl transferase signature fused with another domain homologous to bacterial DPCK, was predicted and experimentally verified to be a bi-functional PPAT/DPCK enzyme [92]. The four-step human CoA biosynthetic pathway from phosphopantothenate was verified by reconstitution *in vitro* using a mixture of purified recombinant enzymes. This analysis contributed to the selection of bacterial PPAT as a high-priority drug target [48]. Functional variants and remaining unsolved problems in the Coenzyme A biosynthesis subsystem were briefly discussed in [2].

3.1.4 Example 4: The nonorthologous displacement of enoyl-ACP reductase (FabI) in *Streptococcus pneumoniae*

Sequence analysis of the first *S. pneumoniae* genome provided an immediate rationale for its resistance to triclosan: an apparent loss of the target, enoyl-ACP reductase, which is encoded by an essential gene (*fabI)* in *E. coli* and many other bacteria. Considering the absolute requirement for this enzymatic step in the elongation cycle of fatty acid biosynthesis, nonorthologous gene displacement was the most likely explanation for the missing *fabI*. Indeed, a putative oxidoreductase gene embedded in a large chromosomal cluster of FAS genes, was predicted and experimentally confirmed as an alternative FMN-dependent and triclosan-insensitive enoyl-ACP reductase [93]. Although, initially, the replacement of *fabI* with a nonorthologous gene termed *fabK* appeared to be a characteristic feature of *Streptococci*, our recent analysis of the FAS subsystem in the SEED database revealed a substantial number of diverse bacteria carrying *fabK* instead of, or in addition, to *fabI*. Such an analysis of distribution of nonorthologous gene displacements allows us to rapidly assess which species may be sensitive or resistant to a particular antibacterial agent.

4 Stage III: Selecting target genes. Target prioritization and validation

The comparative analysis of functional variants helps to reveal critical components of subsystems that may constitute potential targets, as illustrated for the example of NAD(P) biosynthesis. The selection and prioritization of drug targets is dictated by a combination of criteria, most of which are widely used and have been extensively discussed in a number of surveys (see Section I). Here we will briefly illustrate their application using the NAD(P) subsystem as an example.

The *spectrum of target species* defined by the specific goals of a drug development project is one of the most important and straightforward prioritization criteria. The strategy described in this chapter for the identification of targets for broad-spectrum drug development can also be applied to a narrower spectrum (e.g., Gram-positive) or niche pathogens (e.g., *H. influenzae* or *H. pylori*). The growing availability of genomes, including avirulent and attenuated strains and isolates, improves the quality of subsystem analysis and facilitates the selection of optimal drug targets.

4.1 Biological rationale and subsystem topology

A detailed analysis of metabolic subsystems, including all biochemical transformations, transport as well as the availability of precursors and intermediates in the cell and at the site of infection, makes it possible to assess the relative importance of the subsystem components. The analysis of functional variants of a subsystem enables us to make reliable projections across species, even in the absence of physiological data. As mentioned above, we may expect the three-step universal pathway of the NAD(P) subsystem to be essential for most of the bacterial species due to: (i) the strict requirement of NAD(P) for a large number of redox reactions in all types of living cells; (ii) the anticipated inability of the cell to import NAD(P) or phosphorylated intermediates, (iii) the merging of the most common *de novo* and salvage pathways at the start of the universal pathway, (iv) the non-redundance of this pathway. The existence of the non-deamidating salvage pathways, which in some species may generate enough NAD for cell survival, implicates NAD kinase (NADK) as the most universal drug target candidate (see Fig. 2).

4.2 Projection of gene essentiality

Despite some similar aspects, the scope of gene essentiality analysis at this stage is quite different from the initial subsystem selection process (Stage I). As already mentioned, two sets of genes – one that provided evidence implicating a target subsystem, and another one, representing selected targets, may not fully overlap. Although in the specific example of NAD(P) biosynthesis, both sets happened to be identical, in general it may not be the case, depending on the quality of essentiality data, the choice of filtration strategy, etc. While a certain level of 'noise' in the data, has almost no effect on the selection of target subsystems, it may not be acceptable for the evaluation of individual targets. For the broad-spectrum targets, this problem can be addressed by the integration of several essentiality data sets in different species or by single-gene disruption experiments. Emerging efforts in systematic targeted gene knockouts, such as the *E. coli* projects in Japan (http://ecoli.aist-nara.ac.jp/) and the USA (http://www.genome.wisc.edu/functional/tnmutagenesis.htm), open excellent opportunities for acquiring reliable gene essentiality assignments at the whole-genome scale. The biggest challenge however is the projection of gene essentiality across the entire spectrum of target pathogens. Comparative analysis of subsystem functional variants, including alternative routes and nonorthologous displacements, provides a natural framework for the tentative projection and even prediction of essentiality of certain genes. For example, the essentiality of the *nadD* gene, projected from *E. coli* to *S. aureus*, was confirmed by a directed knockout experiment [48]. In another example discussed in Section II, orthologs of *nadR* and *pnuC* (nicotinamide transporter), which are dispensable in *E. coli,* were predicted and experimentally proven to be essential in *H. influenzae* [81]. Likewise, analysis of the subsystem leads to the prediction of essentiality for the *de novo* pathway genes in *H. pylori,* and for the niacin salvage genes in *S. aureus* (see Fig. 2B). Such predictions, if proven experimentally, would allow us to consider these genes as possible drug targets in a number of pathogens implementing the respective functional variants of the NAD(P) biosynthesis subsystem.

4.3 Target conservation

Two aspects of target conservation play a role in target prioritization. The first is the requirement for the presence of the corresponding orthologs across the entire spectrum of target pathogens. Instead of the global homology screening, which was used for the initial subsystem selection (Stage I), target prioritization requires more stringent orthology analysis supported by subsystem-based functional assignments. Likewise, the threshold used in the initial conservation analysis (ERI >0.75) is irrelevant when selecting a common target for a strictly defined set of pathogens. The absence of a target in a pathogen would automatically exclude this organism from the spectrum, which may or may not be acceptable, depending on the scope of a particular drug development project. For example, two of the three potential targets in the universal pathway of NAD(P) biosynthesis, NaMNAT and NADS, are not present in a relatively small but important group of pathogens, including *H. influenzae* (see Tab. 3). That alone may exclude both of these, otherwise attractive, targets from a high-priority list of anti-respiratory drug development programs.

The second and a more subtle aspect of conservation analysis is the level of sequence similarity within the target protein family. The structural compactness of a protein family may be roughly assessed by building an HMM consensus profile and by computing the relative distance of each representative from this profile, as described in [48]. This analysis, however, may be used only for preliminary target prioritization, for the detection of outliers and the evaluation of the range of susceptible pathogens. Since the scope of sequence conservation analysis is to assess the likelihood of developing a universal inhibitor, the actual comparison should focus on the topology of the active site (or, more generally, binding pocket), rather than on the overall sequence conservation. The availability of a 3D structure for at least one target in a complex with substrate(s), product(s) or their analogs substantially improves the quality of such analysis. For example, 3D structures are available for two, rather divergent bacterial NAMNAT of the NadD family, one from *E. coli* [94] and the other from *B. subilis* [95].The comparative analysis of their active sites (revealed by co-crystallization with substrates) supports the selection of this enzyme family as a potential drug target for a relatively broad spectrum of bacterial pathogens.

4.4 Target validation and drugability

The most important aspect of target validation is the experimental confirmation of essentiality in representative pathogens. Functional comparison of divergent representatives of a target family, e.g., substrate specificity profiling, provides an additional assessment of the conservation of their active sites. For example, both analyzed representatives of the NadD family from gram-negative (*E. coli*) and gram-positive (*S. aureus*) bacteria, displayed a strong preference for NaMN over NMN in the adenylyl transferase reaction [48]. A steady state kinetic analysis indicated that this preference was manifested mostly at the level of substrate binding, contributing to the likelihood of finding a common inhibitor. The importance of structural data for conservation analysis was already emphasized. In addition to that, the availability of 3D structure opens up the possibility of assessing the 'drugability' of a target. This is another validation criterion, which requires a well-defined binding site on the protein suitable for the development of bioavailable, synthetically accessible small molecule inhibitors. While some non-metabolic targets do not meet this requirement, it is a characteristic feature of most metabolic enzymes with active sites that have evolved to interact with small molecule substrates and cofactors. The results of the 3D structural analysis of the *E. coli* NaMNAT were in line with such expectations and enabled us to define a structural template for the virtual screening of a small molecule library.

4.5 Comparison with human countertargets

While the absence of human homologs has been perceived as a very important target prioritization criterion, the existence of successful counterexamples suggests that this point of view needs to be refined. These counterexamples, [4] include trimetoprim, which specifically inhibits bacterial dihydrofolate reductase despite 28% sequence identity with its human ortholog, and quinolones, which specifically inhibit bacterial gyrase A despite 20% sequence similarity with human topoisomerase II. However, ideally, a target that has a minimal sequence similarity with its human counterpart is preferable. Mostly based on this consideration, of the three possible targets in NAD(P) biosynthesis, NaMNAT of the NadD family was preferred over NADS and NADK [48]. In our example, both, the functional and structural comparison of the bacterial and human enzymes provided support for this choice of target. In agreement with previous data, and in contrast to the bacterial NAMNAT, all three isoforms of the human enzyme displayed an almost equal preference for NMN and NaMN. This dual specificity of the human bifunctional NAMNAT/NMNAT is consistent with its biological role in the deamidating and non-deamidating pathways inferred by metabolic reconstruction (see Fig. 2). Although sequence comparison alone reveals almost no appreciable similarity between the *E. coli* NAMNAT and the human NAMNAT/NMNAT, their overall 3D structures are quite similar [75]. At the same time, substantial differences in the regions of the active site, presumably responsible for the difference in substrate specificity, provided an opportunity for selective targeting.

5 Concluding remarks: From targets to drugs

The central paradigm of target-based drug discovery is the development of small molecules that disrupt the functional activity of a target protein via specific binding with its active (or allosteric) site. To that end, various high-throughput screening strategies are usually applied, including *in silico* screening of virtual compound libraries. The latter approach is dependent on the availability of a high-quality 3D structure of at least one representative target. The rapidly improving efficiency of virtual docking algorithms, including freely available or affordable software packages (such as AutoDock, http://www.scripps.edu/mb/olson/doc/autodock/), access to growing electronic libraries of compounds (such as ZINC, http://blaster.docking.org/zinc/) and to new chemical web-resources (such as PubChem, http://pubchem.ncbi.nlm.nih.gov/), are factors that strongly affect the routines and perceptions in the field. For example, in contrast to a traditional high-throughput screening, a virtual screening of millions of compounds, followed by experimental testing of ~100 of the best-scoring compounds (available from several providers) is perfectly feasible for academic research groups. Moreover, this rapid and rather inexpensive procedure may become a routine aspect of target validation. The goal of such a prescreening effort would be to evaluate the drugability of a selected target, not to find actual lead compounds. Structural analysis of the target, complexed with some of the identified compounds, may provide very useful information for adjusting a screening template, various docking parameters and constraints.

Finally, it is worth noting that the small molecule library screening (virtual or experimental) is not the only strategy of target-driven drug development. Alternative approaches include rational inhibitor design based on the substrate or product structure or on the reaction mechanism. Covalent, enzyme-activated (or suicide) inhibitors represent a particularly sophisticated version of this approach. For example, difluoromethyl ornithine efficiently kills *Trypanosoma brucei* by covalently binding at the active site of ornithine decarboxylase. A similar but distinct strategy involves pathway-activated prodrugs. Previously we described pyrazinamide, an antituberculosis prodrug that is converted to pyrazinoic acid by NAM, the first enzyme of the niacin salvage pathway. Another interesting example related to NAD biosynthesis beyond anti-infective disease research, is the anticancer prodrug tiazofurin. This nicotinamide ribose analog is known to hijack the RNK/NMNAT-dependent salvage pathway in human cells, which leads to formation of tiazofurin adenine dinucleotide (TAD), a toxic analog of NAD. The latter is known to inhibit IMP dehydrogenase, a key enzyme in purine biosynthesis, ultimately suppressing the growth of certain cancer cells [96]. Although the notion of target for these pathway-activated antimetabolites is quite different from the main drug development paradigm, even in this case, certain techniques of target selection discussed in this chapter may be applicable. For example, both activities (subsystems), responsible for prodrug activation and the actual target of the ultimate antimetabolite, should be conserved and essential in the desired spectrum of pathogens.

The impact of subsystem analysis on the development of pathway-activated antibacterial agents, may also be illustrated by the mechanism of action of pantothenate analogs, such as N-pentylpantothenamide. The antibacterial activity of this compound was initially thought to be a result of inhibition of some of the CoA biosynthetic enzymes [97]. However, in a series of recent studies, it was shown that this compound is a prodrug activated by the CoA biosynthetic pathway, leading to formation of the toxic ethyldethia-CoA [90]. The latter ultimately inhibits fatty acid biosynthesis through the formation of the nonfunctional holo-acyl carrier protein [94]. While N-pentylpantothenamide does not appear to be a likely drug candidate due to its rather modest antibacterial activity, its mechanism of action provides an illustration of an alternative drug development strategy.

Acknowledgements

The authors are grateful to Ross Overbeek and other members of the SEED development team for their help in bioinformatics analysis. Gene essentiality analysis would not be possible without enthusiastic and highly professional guidance by Svetlana Gerdes. We are indebted to Oleg Kurnasov, Hong Zhang, Leonardo Sorci and Alex McKerrel for their critical role in the ongoing NAMNAT target development project. This project is supported by the NIAID grant to AO aimed at targeting cofactor biosynthesis in bacterial pathogens.

References

1 Overbeek R, Begley T, Butler RM, Choudhuri JV, Chuang HY, Cohoon M, de Crecy-Lagard V, Diaz N, Disz T, Edwards R et al (2005) The subsystems approach to genome annotation and its use in the project to annotate 1000 genomes. *Nucleic Acids Res* 33: 5691–5702

2 Ye Y, Osterman A, Overbeek R, Godzik A (2005) Automatic detection of subsystem/pathway variants in genome analysis. *Bioinformatics* 21: i1–i9

3 Schmid MB, Kapur N, Isaacson DR, Lindroos P, Sharpe C (1989) Genetic analysis of temperature-sensitive lethal mutants of *Salmonella typhimurium*. *Genetics* 123: 625–633

4 Moir DT, Shaw KJ, Hare RS, Vovis GF (1999) Genomics and antimicrobial drug discovery. *Antimicrob Agents Chemother* 43: 439–446

5 Galperin MY, Koonin EV (1999) Searching for drug targets in microbial genomes. *Curr Opin Biotechnol* 10: 571–578

6 Read TD, Gill SR, Tettelin H, Dougherty BA (2001) Finding drug targets in microbial genomes. *Drug Discovery Today* 6: 887–892

7 Ji Y (2002) The role of genomics in the discovery of novel targets for antibiotic therapy. *Pharmacogenomics* 3: 315–323

8 Lehoux DE, Sanschagrin F, Levesque RC (2001) Discovering essential and infection-related genes. *Curr Opin Microbiol* 4: 515–519

9 Yin D, Fox B, Lonetto ML, Etherton MR, Payne DJ, Holmes DJ, Rosenberg M, Ji Y (2004) Identification of antimicrobial targets using a comprehensive genomic approach. *Pharmacogenomics* 5: 101–113

10 Osterman A, Overbeek R (2003) Missing genes in metabolic pathways: a comparative genomics approach. *Curr Opin Chem Biol* 7: 238–251

11 Koonin EV, Mushegian AR, Bork P (1996) Non-orthologous gene displacement. *Trends Genet* 12: 334–336

12 Galperin MY, Koonin EV (2001) Chapter 15: Comparative Genome Analysis. In: A Baxevanis, F Ouellette (eds): *Bioinformatics: A Practical Guide to the Analysis of Genes and Proteins*. Second Edition. Wiley-Liss Inc. pp 359–392

13 Kremer LS, Besra GS (2002) Current status and future development of antitubercular chemotherapy. *Expert Opin Investig Drugs* 11: 1033–1049

14 Palsson BO, Price ND, Papin JA (2003) Development of network-based pathway definitions: the need to analyze real metabolic networks. *Trends Biotechnol* 21: 195–198

15 Burgard AP, Nikolaev EV, Schilling CH, Maranas CD (2004) Flux coupling analysis of genome-scale metabolic network reconstructions. *Genome Res* 14(2): 301–312

16 Edwards JS, Palsson BO (2000) Metabolic flux balance analysis and the in silico analysis of *Escherichia coli* K-12 gene deletions. *BMC Bioinformatics* 1: 1

17 Thiele I, Vo TD, Price ND, Palsson BO (2005) Expanded metabolic reconstruction of *Helicobacter pylori* (iIT341 GSM/GPR): an in silico genome-scale characterization of single- and double-deletion mutants. *J Bacteriol* 187: 5818–5830

18 Becker SA, Palsson BO (2005) Genome-scale reconstruction of the metabolic network in *Staphylococcus aureus* N315: an initial draft to the two-dimensional annotation. *BMC Microbiol* 5: 8

19 Forster J, Famili I, Palsson BO, Nielsen J (2003) Large-scale evaluation of in silico gene deletions in *Saccharomyces cerevisiae*. *Omics* 7: 193–202

20 Haft DH, Selengut JD, Brinkac LM, Zafar N, White O (2005) Genome Properties: a system for the investigation of prokaryotic genetic content for microbiology, genome annotation and comparative genomics. *Bioinformatics* 21: 293–306

21 Kanehisa M, Goto S, Kawashima S, Okuno Y, Hattori M (2004) The KEGG resource for deciphering the genome. *Nucleic Acids Res* 32 Database issue: D277–280

22 (2005) Get ready to GO! A biologist's guide to the Gene Ontology. *Brief Bioinform* 6: 298–304

23 Krieger CJ, Zhang P, Mueller LA, Wang A, Paley S, Arnaud M, Pick J, Rhee SY, Karp PD (2004) MetaCyc: a multiorganism database of metabolic pathways and enzymes. *Nucleic Acids Res* 32: D438–442

24 Arigoni F, Talabot F, Peitsch M, Edgerton MD, Meldrum E, Allet E, Fish R, Jamotte T, Curchod ML, Loferer H (1998) A genome-based approach for the identification of essential bacterial genes. *Nat Biotechnol* 16: 851–856

25 Ji Y, Zhang B, Van SF, Horn, Warren P, Woodnutt G, Burnham MK, Rosenberg M (2001) Identification of critical staphylococcal genes using conditional phenotypes generated by antisense RNA. *Science* 293: 2266–2269

26 Thanassi JA, Hartman-Neumann SL, Dougherty TJ, Dougherty BA, Pucci MJ (2002) Identification of 113 conserved essential genes using a high-throughput gene disruption system in *Streptococcus pneumoniae*. *Nucleic Acids Res* 30: 3152–3162

27 Forsyth RA, Haselbeck RJ, Ohlsen KL, Yamamoto RT, Xu H, Trawick JD, Wall D, Wang L, Brown-Driver V, Froelich JM et al (2002) A genome-wide strategy for the identification of essential genes in *Staphylococcus aureus*. *Mol Microbiol* 43: 1387–1400

28 Sassetti CM, Boyd DH, Rubin EJ (2003) Genes required for mycobacterial growth defined by high density mutagenesis. *Mol Microbiol* 48: 77–84

29 Mushegian AR, Koonin EV (1996) A minimal gene set for cellular life derived by comparison of complete bacterial genomes. *Proc Natl Acad Sci USA* 93: 10268–10273

30 Fleischmann RD, Adams MD, White O, Clayton RA, Kirkness EF, Kerlavage AR, Bult CJ, Tomb JF, Dougherty BA, Merrick JM et al (1995) Whole-genome random sequencing and assembly of *Haemophilus influenzae* Rd. *Science* 269: 496–512

31 Fraser CM, Gocayne JD, White O, Adams MD, Clayton RA, Fleischmann RD, Bult CJ, Kerlavage AR, Sutton G, Kelley GM et al (1995) The minimal gene complement of *Mycoplasma genitalium*. *Science* 270: 397–403

32 Hutchison CA, Peterson SN, Gill SR, Cline RT, White O, Fraser CM, Smith HO, Venter JC (1999) Global transposon mutagenesis and a minimal *Mycoplasma* genome. *Science* 286: 2165–2169

33 Ross-Macdonald P, Coelho PS, Roemer T, Agarwal S, Kumar A, Jansen R, Cheung KH, Sheehan A, Symoniatis D, Umansky L et al (1999) Large-scale analysis of the yeast genome by transposon tagging and gene disruption. *Nature* 402: 413–418

34 Winzeler EA, Shoemaker DD, Astromoff A, Liang H, Anderson K, Andre B, Bangham R, Benito R, Boeke JD, Bussey H et al (1999) Functional characterization of the *S. cerevisiae* genome by gene deletion and parallel analysis. *Science* 285: 901–906

35 Akerley BJ, Rubin EJ, Novick VL, Amaya K, Judson N, Mekalanos JJ (2002) A genome-scale analysis for identification of genes required for growth or survival of *Haemophilus influenzae*. *Proc Nat Acad Sci USA* 99: 966–971

36 Kobayashi K, Ehrlich SD, Albertini A, Amati G, Andersen KK, Arnaud M, Asai K, Ashikaga S, Aymerich S, Bessieres P et al (2003) Essential *Bacillus subtilis* genes. *Proc Natl Acad Sci USA* 100: 4678–4683

37 Gerdes SY, Scholle MD, Campbell JW, Balazsi G, Ravasz E, Daugherty MD, Somera AL, Kyrpides NC, Anderson I, Gelfand MS et al (2003) Experimental determination and system level analysis of essential genes in *Escherichia coli* MG1655. *J Bacteriol* 185: 5673–5684

38 Jacobs MA, Alwood A, Thaipisuttikul I, Spencer D, Haugen E, Ernst S, Will O, Kaul R, Raymond C, Levy R et al (2003) Comprehensive transposon mutant library of *Pseudomonas aeruginosa*. *Proc Nat Acad Sci USA* 100: 14339–14344

39 Sassetti CM, Rubin EJ (2003) Genetic requirements for mycobacterial survival during infection. *Proc Nat Acad Sci USA* 100: 12989–12994

40 Potvin E, Lehoux DE, Kukavica-Ibrulj I, Richard KL, Sanschagrin F, Lau GW, Levesque RW (2003) *In vivo* functional genomics of *Pseudomonas aeruginosa* for high-throughput screening of new virulence factors and antibacterial targets. *Environ Microbiol* 5: 1294–1308

41 Herbert MA, Hayes S, Deadman ME, Tang CM, Hood DW, Moxon ER (2002) Signature tagged mutagenesis of *Haemophilus influenzae* identifies genes required for *in vivo* survival. *Microb Pathog* 33: 211–223

42 Schmid MB (1998) Novel approaches to the discovery of antimicrobial agents. *Curr Opin Chem Biol* 2: 529–534

43 Yin D, Ji Y (2002) Genomic analysis using conditional phenotypes generated by antisense RNA. *Curr Opin Microbiol* 5: 330–333

44 Zhang R, Ou HY, Zhang CT (2004) DEG: a database of essential genes. *Nucleic Acids Res* 32 Database issue: D271–272

45 Jordan IK, Rogozin IB, Wolf YI, Koonin EV (2002) Essential genes are more evolutionarily conserved than are nonessential genes in bacteria. *Genome Res* 12: 962–968

46 Koonin EV (2003) Comparative genomics, minimal gene-sets and the last universal common ancestor. *Nature Rev Microbiol* 1: 127–136

47 Gil R, Silva FJ, Pereto J, Moya A (2004) Determination of the core of a minimal bacterial gene set. *Microbiol Mol Biol Rev* 68: 518–537, table of contents

48 Gerdes SY, Scholle MD, D'Souza M, Bernal A, Baev MV, Farrell M, Kurnasov OV, Daugherty MD, Mseeh F, Polanuyer BM et al (2002) From genetic footprinting to antimicrobial drug targets: examples in cofactor biosynthetic pathways. *J Bacteriol* 184: 4555–4572

49 Michal G (1999) *Biochemical pathways: An atlas of biochemistry and molecular biology*. John Wiley & Sons, Inc. New York, USA

50 Tatusov RL, Natale DA, Garkavtsev IV, Tatusova TA, Shankavaram UT, Rao BS, Kiryutin B, Galperin MY, Fedorova ND, Koonin EV (2001) The COG database: new developments in phylogenetic classification of proteins from complete genomes. *Nucleic Acids Res* 29: 22–28

51 Selkov E, Maltsev N, Olsen GJ, Overbeek R, Whitman WB (1997) A reconstruction of the metabolism of *Methanococcus jannaschii* from sequence data. *Gene* 197: GC11–26

52 Bono H, Ogata H, Goto S, Kanehisa M (1998) Reconstruction of amino acid biosynthesis pathways from the complete genome sequence. *Genome Res* 8: 203–210

53 Galperin MY (2004) The Molecular Biology Database Collection: 2004 update. *Nucleic Acids Res* 32 Database issue: D3–22

54 Green ML, Karp PD (2004) A Bayesian method for identifying missing enzymes in predicted metabolic pathway databases. *BMC Bioinformatics* 5: 76

55 Haferkamp I, Schmitz-Esser S, Linka N, Urbany C, Collingro A, Wagner M, Horn M, Neuhaus HE (2004) A candidate NAD+ transporter in an intracellular bacterial symbiont related to Chlamydiae. *Nature* 432: 622–625

56 Bieganowski P, Pace HC, Brenner C (2003) Eukaryotic NAD+ synthetase Qns1 contains an essential, obligate intramolecular thiol glutamine amidotransferase domain related to nitrilase. *J Biol Chem* 278: 33049–33055

57 Bellinzoni M, Buroni S, Pasca MR, Guglierame P, Arcesi F, De Rossi E, Riccardi G (2005) Glutamine amidotransferase activity of NAD+ synthetase from *Mycobacterium tuberculosis* depends on an amino-terminal nitrilase domain. *Res Microbiol* 156: 173–177

58 Willison JC, Tissot G (1994) The *Escherichia coli* efg gene and the *Rhodobacter capsulatus* adgA gene code for NH3-dependent NAD synthetase. *J Bacteriol* 176: 3400–3402

59 Bieganowski P, Brenner C (2003) The reported human NADsyn2 is ammonia-dependent NAD synthetase from a pseudomonad. *J Biol Chem* 278: 33056–33059

60 Rizzi M, Nessi C, Mattevi A, Coda A, Bolognesi M, Galizzi A (1996) Crystal structure of NH3-dependent NAD+ synthetase from *Bacillus subtilis*. *Embo J* 15: 5125–5134

61 Kang GB, Kim YS, Im YJ, Rho SH, Lee JH, Eom SH (2005) Crystal structure of NH3-dependent NAD+ synthetase from *Helicobacter pylori*. *Proteins* 58: 985–988

62 Kurnasov O, Goral V, Colabroy K, Gerdes S, Anantha S, Osterman A, Begley TP (2003) NAD biosynthesis: identification of the tryptophan to quinolinate pathway in bacteria. *Chem Biol* 10: 1195–1204

63 Colabroy KL, Zhai H, Li T, Ge Y, Zhang Y, Liu A, Ealick SE, McLafferty FW, Begley TP (2005) The mechanism of inactivation of 3-Hydroxyanthranilate-3,4-dioxygenase by 4-Chloro-3-hydroxyanthranilate. *Biochemistry* 44: 7623–7631

64 Kurnasov O, Jablonski L, Polanuyer B, Dorrestein P, Begley T, Osterman A (2003) Aerobic tryptophan degradation pathway in bacteria: novel kynurenine formamidase. *FEMS Microbiol Lett* 227: 219–227

65 Ravasz E, Somera AL, Mongru DA, Oltvai ZN, Barabasi AL (2002) Hierarchical organization of modularity in metabolic networks. *Science* 297: 1551–1555

66 von Mering C, Zdobnov EM, Tsoka S, Ciccarelli FD, Pereira-Leal JB, Ouzounis CA, Bork P (2003) Genome evolution reveals biochemical networks and functional modules. *Proc Natl Acad Sci USA* 100: 15428–15433

67 Huynen MA, Snel B, von Mering C, Bork P (2003) Function prediction and protein networks. *Curr Opin Cell Biol* 15: 191–198

68 Dandekar T, Sauerborn R (2002) Comparative genome analysis and pathway reconstruction. *Pharmacogenomics* 3: 245–256

69 Koonin EV, Galperin MY (2002) SEQUENCE – EVOLUTION – FUNCTION. Computational approaches in comparative genomics. Kluwer Academic Publishers, Boston, USA

70 Penfound T, Foster JW (1996) Biosynthesis and Recycling of NAD. In: Neihardt (ed.): *Escherichia Coli and Salmonella*. ASM pp 721–730

71 Mehl RA, Kinsland C, Begley TP (2000) Identification of the *Escherichia coli* nicotinic acid mononucleotide adenylyltransferase gene. *J Bacteriol* 182: 4372–4374

72 Overbeek R, Fonstein M, D'Souza M, Pusch GD, Maltsev N (1999) The use of gene clusters to infer functional coupling. *Proc Natl Acad Sci USA* 96: 2896–2901

73 Overbeek R, Fonstein M, D'Souza M, Pusch GD, Maltsev N (1999) Use of contiguity on the chromosome to predict functional coupling. *In Silico Biol* 1: 93–108
74 Zhang X, Kurnasov OV, Karthikeyan S, Grishin NV, Osterman AL, Zhang H (2003) Structural characterization of a human cytosolic NMN/NaMN adenylyltransferase and implication in human NAD biosynthesis. *J Biol Chem* 278: 13503–13511
75 Zhou T, Kurnasov O, Tomchick DR, Binns DD, Grishin NV, Marquez VE, Osterman AL, Zhang H (2002) Structure of human nicotinamide/nicotinic acid mononucleotide adenylyltransferase. Basis for the dual substrate specificity and activation of the oncolytic agent tiazofurin. *J Biol Chem* 277: 13148–13154
76 Berger F, Lau C, Dahlmann M, Ziegler M (2005) Subcellular compartmentation and differential catalytic properties of the three human nicotinamide mononucleotide adenylyltransferase isoforms. *J Biol Chem* 280(43): 36334–36341
77 Garavaglia S, D'Angelo I, Emanuelli M, Carnevali F, Pierella F, Magni G, Rizzi M (2002) Structure of human NMN adenylyltransferase. A key nuclear enzyme for NAD homeostasis. *J Biol Chem* 277: 8524–8530
78 Raffaelli N, Sorci L, Amici A, Emanuelli M, Mazzola F, Magni G (2002) Identification of a novel human nicotinamide mononucleotide adenylyltransferase. *Biochem Biophys Res Commun* 297: 835–840
79 Magni G, Amici A, Emanuelli M, Orsomando G, Raffaelli N, Ruggieri S (2004) Structure and function of nicotinamide mononucleotide adenylyltransferase. *Curr Med Chem* 11: 873–885
80 Marcotte EM, Pellegrini M, Ng HL, Rice DW, Yeates TO, Eisenberg D (1999) Detecting protein function and protein–protein interactions from genome sequences. *Science* 285: 751–753
81 Kurnasov OV, Polanuyer BM, Ananta S, Sloutsky R, Tam A, Gerdes SY, Osterman AL (2002) Ribosylnicotinamide kinase domain of NadR protein: Identification and implications in NAD biosynthesis. *J Bacteriol* 184: 6906–6917
82 Kemmer G, Reilly TJ, Schmidt-Brauns J, Zlotnik GW, Green BA, Fiske MJ, Herbert M, Kraiss A, Schlor S, Smith A et al (2001) NadN and e (P4) are essential for utilization of NAD and nicotinamide mononucleotide but not nicotinamide riboside in *Haemophilus influenzae*. *J Bacteriol* 183: 3974–3981
83 Zhu N, Roth JR (1991) The nadI region of *Salmonella typhimurium* encodes a bifunctional regulatory protein. *J Bacteriol* 173: 1302–1310
84 Raffaelli N, Lorenzi T, Mariani PL, Emanuelli M, Amici A, Ruggieri S, Magni G (1999) The *Escherichia coli* NadR regulator is endowed with nicotinamide mononucleotide adenylyltransferase activity. *J Bacteriol* 181: 5509–5511
85 Merdanovic M, Sauer E, Reidl J (2005) Coupling of NAD + biosynthesis and nicotinamide ribosyl transport: Characterization of NadR ribonucleotide kinase mutants of *Haemophilus influenzae*. *J Bacteriol* 187: 4410–4420
86 Sauer E, Merdanovic M, Mortimer AP, Bringmann G, Reidl J (2004) PnuC and the utilization of the nicotinamide riboside analog 3-aminopyridine in *Haemophilus influenzae*. *Antimicrob Agents Chemother* 48: 4532–4541

87 Martin PR, Shea RJ, Mulks MH (2001) Identification of a plasmid-encoded gene from *Haemophilus ducreyi* which confers NAD independence. *J Bacteriol* 183: 1168–1174

88 Singh SK, Kurnasov OV, Chen B, Robinson H, Grishin NV, Osterman AL, Zhang H (2002) Crystal structure of *Haemophilus influenzae* NadR protein. A bifunctional enzyme endowed with NMN adenyltransferase and ribosylnicotinimide kinase activities. *J Biol Chem* 277: 33291–33299

89 Geerlof A, Lewendon A, Shaw WV (1999) Purification and characterization of phosphopantetheine adenylyltransferase from *Escherichia coli*. *J Biol Chem* 274: 27105–27111

90 Strauss E, Kinsland C, Ge Y, McLafferty FW, Begley TP (2001) Phosphopantothenoylcysteine synthetase from *Escherichia coli*. Identification and characterization of the last unidentified coenzyme A biosynthetic enzyme in bacteria. *J Biol Chem* 276: 13513–13516

91 Mishra P, Park PK, Drueckhammer DG (2001) Identification of yacE (coaE) as the structural gene for dephosphocoenzyme A kinase in *Escherichia coli* K-12. *J Bacteriol* 183: 2774–2778

92 Daugherty M, Polanuyer B, Farrell M, Scholle M, Lykidis A, de Crecy-Lagard V, Osterman A (2002) Complete reconstitution of the human coenzyme A biosynthetic pathway via comparative genomics. *J Biol Chem* 277: 21431–21439

93 Heath RJ, Rock CO (2000) A triclosan-resistant bacterial enzyme. *Nature* 406: 145–146

94 Zhang YM, Frank MW, Virga KG, Lee RE, Rock CO, Jackowski S (2004) Acyl carrier protein is a cellular target for the antibacterial action of the pantothenamide class of pantothenate antimetabolites. *J Biol Chem* 279: 50969–50975

95 Olland AM, Underwood KW, Czerwinski RM, Lo MC, Aulabaugh A, Bard J, Stahl ML, Somers WS, Sullivan FX, Chopra R (2002) Identification, characterization, and crystal structure of *Bacillus subtilis* nicotinic acid mononucleotide adenylyltransferase. *J Biol Chem* 277: 3698–3707

96 Jayaram HN, Cooney DA, Grusch M, Krupitza G (1999) Consequences of IMP dehydrogenase inhibition, and its relationship to cancer and apoptosis. *Curr Med Chem* 6: 561–574

97 Clifton G, Bryant SR, Skinner CG (1970) N′-(substituted) pantothenamides, antimetabolites of pantothenic acid. *Arch Biochem Biophys* 137: 523–528

Progress in Drug Research, Vol. 64
(Helena I. Boshoff and Clifton E. Barry III, Eds)

Metabolic control analysis to identify optimal drug targets

By Jorrit J. Hornberg[1,4],
Frank J. Bruggeman[1,2],
Barbara M. Bakker[1]
and Hans V. Westerhoff[1,2,3]

[1]Department of Molecular Cell Physiology,
Institute for Molecular Cell Biology,
Faculty of Earth and Life Sciences,
Vrije Universiteit,
Amsterdam, The Netherlands

[2]Manchester Centre for Integrative
Systems Biology,
Manchester Interdisciplinary BioCentre,
Faculty of Engineering and Physical
Sciences,
University of Manchester,
Manchester, UK

[3]Department of Mathematical
Biochemistry,
University of Amsterdam,
Amsterdam, The Netherlands

[4](presently at)
NV Organon,
Molecular Parmacology Unit,
Oss, The Netherlands
<jorrit.hornberg@organon.com>

Abstract

This chapter describes the basic principles of Metabolic Control Analysis (MCA) which is a quantitative methodology to evaluate the importance and relative contribution of individual metabolic steps in the overall functioning of a particular system. The control on the flux through a metabolic pathway or subsystem can be quantified by the control coefficients of the individual enzymes or components which reflects the extent to which the component is rate-limiting. The perturbation of an individual step is measured by its elasticity coefficient. The effect of perturbation of a single step on the entire pathway or subsystem is, in turn, measured by the response coefficient. Differential control analysis can be used to compare flux through a single metabolic pathway in a pathogen with the same pathway in its host to identify uniquely vulnerable steps with the greatest potential for specifically inhibiting flux through the pathogen metabolic pathway. The utility of this methodology is illustrated with the glycolysis in Trypanosomes and with oncogenic signaling.

1 Introduction

With the development and application of high-throughput techniques in the molecular biosciences, the amount of information on the components of living organisms is growing rapidly. The sequences of entire genomes have become available in recent years and measurements of gene-expression profiles as mRNA abundances, protein concentrations, fluxes and metabolite concentrations are now possible. More and more they are or will be carried out on a genome-, transcriptome-, proteome- or metabolome-wide scale. As a result, biological science is currently moving from a molecular biology era into a systems biology era [1]. One of the major tasks ahead is fulfillment of the high expectations that this next era will lead to a quantitative understanding of biological systems 'in disease as well as in health'.

Apart from being accessible to the administered drug, a successful drug target must be important for the functioning of the causative agent, both in an absolute (the drug must be *effective* against the disease) and in a relative sense (the drug must be *selective*, i.e., effective against the culprit of the disease but not against healthy processes in the patient) [2]. When searching for a good drug target, potential targets have to be screened for their absolute and relative importance. By applying Metabolic Control Analysis (MCA), one can quantify this importance. In this chapter, we introduce the basic principles of MCA and explain how MCA can be used to identify promising drug targets. Furthermore we discuss how this strategy can be used for the discovery of targets for drugs against parasitic diseases (in particular trypanosomiasis) and cancer.

2 Mathematical models: Assistants for the human brain

Biological systems often contain many components (e.g., enzymes) that jointly determine the behavior of the entire system. The concentrations and activities of those components are regulated at many hierarchical levels (transcription, translation, post-translational modification). The biochemical reactions they catalyze usually obey non-linear reaction kinetics, such as given by Michaelis-Menten type and Hill equations. Together, this complexity hampers our ability to understand large biological systems and to predict their behavior in response to perturbations. Such perturbations can include changes in the environment (e.g., extracellular glucose concentration), mutations (e.g., oncogenic K-Ras), epi-genetic alterations (e.g., loss of imprinting) or addition of an enzyme inhibitor (e.g., a drug). In order to understand complex biological systems, the human brain needs assistance. Systems biologists do therefore not only focus on collecting experimental data on a system or a part thereof, they additionally strive to integrate the knowledge obtained into mathematical models [3]. Many of those models can be used to run computer simulations of the behavior of a biological system. Models of some biological systems are available on the internet (www.siliconcell.net) such that they can be interrogated interactively [4], with the ultimate aim of merging them to construct a so-called Silicon Cell [5, 6].

Computer simulations can be helpful in several ways. First, by comparing the experimentally observed behavior of a system with the behavior of it's *in silico* counterpart, one can examine whether the available knowledge about the parts of a system (which are integrated in the model) is sufficient to explain the behavior of the system. In this way, the biochemical knowledge of the glycolytic enzymes in yeast has been integrated and compared with the empirical behavior of the pathway [7]. Other examples of such modeling exercises exist, dealing with systems ranging from metabolic pathways to signal transduction networks [6, 8]. The number is still limited however, mostly because it is rare that all kinetic properties required for the modeling have been determined experimentally. More often therefore models are hybrid, parts being known experimentally and parts being fitted to actual or suspected system behavior. Where model prediction and experimental results do not match, one may discover not yet observed regulatory [9] or catalytic processes, or of course fallacies in the experimental methodology. With present day complexities, the computational aspects of most biological modeling are not problematic.

Second, one can carry out *in silico* experiments, for instance to test the effects of perturbations made to the system (such as the administration of drugs or changes in nutrient levels). The advantages of such 'dry experiments' are that they have less experimental constraints. Some experiments are indeed only practicable in the computer [10]. In addition, they are generally less laborious and they require fewer resources than wet lab experiments. Clearly, if one requires an accurate description of the *in vivo* system, then results generated by computer simulations are only reliable when the model is accurate. As it is often difficult to know whether a model is 100% accurate, predictions that originate from the simulations should be tested in the lab as much as feasible. The simulations can guide the process of designing an experimental strategy, by providing indications as to which experiments (under which conditions) are most promising to lead to a satisfactory answer to the research question. In turn, the experimental results can be used to further optimize the model. Modern methods of analysis are now combined with the paradigms of MCA, which will be discussed below [11].

Third, by analyzing a model of a biological system, one can examine why a system behaves or responds as it does [10]. If for example, in the case of a network containing a negative feedback loop, removing that feedback loop from the model dramatically changes the adaptive behavior of the system, then this feedback loop explains the adaptation [12]. Such analyses enable the researcher to *understand* the behavior of the network in terms of its organization. Systems biologists thus combine wet lab experiments with mathematical modeling in cycles, resulting in a spiral towards better understanding of the system of interest.

A fourth point that argues for the use of mathematical models, is that it is impossible to know exactly how important a system component (gene, enzyme, pathway, etc.) is for the functioning of that system (pathway, cell, etc.), only by looking at the interaction map or reaction scheme of a biological network. Classical gene knockout studies cannot overcome this since they identify all essential components as important, without assigning a relative quantification to this importance. Likewise they classify all non-essential components as unimportant. If an essential function of an organism is carried out by two parallel processes, both processes will be classified as unimportant. MCA was developed for this purpose, in particular to quantify the extent to which individual enzymes control the flux through a metabolic pathway [13, 14]. This can be done by quantitative experimentation [16]. With a mathematical model of a system, one can calculate this control precisely.

3 Metabolic control analysis: Basic principles

In MCA the extent to which any system property (gene expression, metabolic flux, enzyme concentration, cell division rate, etc.) is controlled by a process of that system (catalytic conversion, transport, diffusion, etc.) is quantified in terms of a control coefficient. A control coefficient is defined as the relative change in a system property divided by the small relative change in the activity of the enzyme that catalyzes it [13–18]. The exact control of an enzyme over, for instance, the flux through an enzyme-catalyzed step in a network in steady state is quantified by a flux control coefficient. Hence C_i^J, i.e., the control of enzyme i over flux J, represents the fractional change in flux J that is caused by a fractional change in the rate v of the reaction catalyzed by enzyme i. Mathematically:

$$C_i^J = \frac{\dfrac{dJ}{dp_i}\Big/ J}{\dfrac{\partial v_i}{\partial p_i}\Big/ v_i} = \frac{\dfrac{d\ln J}{dp_i}}{\dfrac{\partial \ln v_i}{\partial p_i}} \qquad (1)$$

This is also often written in shorthand form as $\frac{d\ln J}{d\ln v_i}$, but this expression is equivocal: if the flux runs through the enzyme, then one might interpret this to be always equal to 1. The meaning of the definition is that one measures the extent to which the activation of an enzyme leads to a proportional increase in flux J. For enzymes that are not in physical association with others and catalyze only a single reaction, this extent is independent of the way in which the enzyme is activated [19]. A frequently used 'working definition' for a control coefficient is the percentage change in flux that is caused by a 1% change in the activity of the reaction. The change in reaction activity equals the change that would occur in the enzyme's reaction rate if all other factors around the enzyme were held constant. The latter condition is indicated by the symbols ∂ in equation 1.

Clearly, when an enzyme has a flux control coefficient of 0, it is not 'rate-limiting' for the flux. When the control coefficient is 1, then the change in flux is proportional to the change in the activity of the reaction. Then the reaction determines the flux completely. In principle, the values of flux control coefficients are not bounded. Depending on the structure of the network and on the kinetic properties of its enzymes, they can be negative and their absolute values larger than 1. For simple linear pathways however, flux control coefficients tend to range between 0 and 1. 'The' rate-limiting enzymes are the enzymes with the flux control coefficients equal to 1. Enzymes with higher control coefficients may be called super rate-limiting, if so desired. Interestingly, the sum of the flux control coefficients for all enzymes in the system with respect to any flux equals 1 [13, 14]:

$$\sum_{i=1}^{n} C_i^J = C_1^J + C_2^J \ldots + C_n^J = 1 \tag{2}$$

This summation theorem can be understood intuitively: if the activities of all enzymes involved in a metabolic pathway are increased by 1%, then the flux through that pathway will also increase by 1%. This has several interesting consequences. It shows for instance that there is always *at least* one enzyme that controls the flux. The flux through a metabolic pathway is thus always controlled, which is good news for those who wish to change a metabolic flux for biotechnological or medical applications. It is also possible, however, that all enzymes in the pathway control the flux to a certain extent, which implies that the flux is not necessarily dictated by one rate-limiting enzyme, but can be distributed over multiple enzymes. This is in fact what has been found for many systems, including mitochondrial respiration [20], trypanosome glycolysis [21] and mammalian signaling networks [22] such as Wnt/β-catenin [23], NF-κB [24] and MAPK [25]. Control coefficients have been defined in MCA for a wide variety of system properties and in many of those cases summation theorems have been derived [22, 26]. In some cases metabolic networks can be subdivided into mass flow connected modules, in an approach called modular control analysis [27]. In addition, MCA has been expanded to Hierarchical Control Analysis, which deals with networks involving gene expression, and signal transduction [27–30]. Here various levels are discerned which essentially do not share mass flux. This special aspect gives rise to a substantial number of additional principles and enables one to describe adaptation.

A control coefficient thus quantifies the change in flux (or another property) caused by a change in the activity of a process in the system. The activity of an enzyme can be regulated directly by a change in the concentration of the enzyme itself (e.g., as a result of gene induction or silencing), but also indirectly by a change in a variable or parameter addressing that enzyme. Such perturbations include changes in the concentration of a metabolite (e.g., the substrate or product of the reaction catalyzed by the enzyme) or modifier (e.g., an inhibitor or activator) or changes in the properties of the enzyme (e.g., a binding constant as a result of a mutation). In MCA, the relative extent to which the activity of an enzyme changes divided by the relative change in a parameter or variable metabolite concentration p that is the unique cause of that change, is termed an elasticity coefficient. Hence $\varepsilon_p^{v_i}$, i.e., the elasticity of the enzyme i towards parameter p (or equivalently, towards the concentration of a metabolite or modifier), represents the fractional change in the rate v of the reaction catalyzed by enzyme i that is caused by a fractional change in the parameter. In mathematical terms:

$$\varepsilon_p^{v_i} = \frac{\partial v_i / v_i}{\partial p / p} = \frac{\partial \ln v_i}{\partial \ln p} \tag{3}$$

Again the symbol ∂ refers to the condition that p is the only one of the factors that may affect the enzyme's rate, that is allowed to change here (in mathematics this is called a partial derivative).

In many cases, one is not ultimately interested in how the activity of an enzyme responds to a perturbation, but rather how such a perturbation percolates through the network eventually to bring about a change in a systemic property (e.g., flux). This can be quantified by a response coefficient, which is defined as the relative change in flux divided by the relative (small) change in the value of the perturbed parameter (or variable) that causes the change in flux. Hence R_p^J, i.e., the response of flux J to parameter p, represents the fractional change in flux J caused by the (small) fractional change in p. Mathematically,

$$R_p^J = \frac{dJ/_J}{dp/_p} = \frac{d\ln J}{d\ln p} \tag{4}$$

As an elasticity coefficient quantifies the effect of a change in a parameter on an enzyme activity (3) and a control coefficient quantifies how the flux is controlled by this enzyme activity (4), the response of the flux to a change in a parameter can be quantified by multiplying the elasticity coefficient by the control coefficient [31]:

$$R_p^J = C_i^J \cdot \varepsilon_p^{v_i} \tag{5}$$

Until now we have not described what is meant with flux J, as distinguished from rate v_i. A rate is a property of an individual enzyme; it exists independent of the existence of a steady state. A flux is a systems property; it typically runs through at least two consecutive enzymes in a metabolic pathway, and requires the rates of those two processes to be equal, i.e., to be at (quasi) steady state. Similarly all the 'straight' d's in the above definitions refer to differences between such steady states, where all metabolic variables are allowed to evolve from one steady state to another.

Taken together, MCA provides a theoretical framework for the (exact!) quantification of (i) the importance of a component for the functioning of the system (control coefficient) as well as of (ii) the effect of a perturbation (response coefficient) by taking into account the local effect of the perturbation on the affected component (elasticity coefficient) and the system effect of changes in activity of the latter. How such quantifications can be used for drug target discovery will be discussed in the next sections.

4 Effective drug target identification using MCA

As mentioned above, a good drug has to be effective against the cause of the disease. If a drug is administered that inhibits an enzyme to alter a particular metabolic flux, then the drug could be termed effective if it causes a relatively large change in this flux. In other words: for a drug to be effective it should have a high response coefficient. This response coefficient is the product of the elasticity coefficient of the enzyme towards the drug and the control coefficient of the enzyme on the flux. The effectiveness of the drug therefore depends not only on how efficient the drug inhibits the enzyme, but also on how important the enzyme is for the flux. Hence, a good drug target is a target that exerts much control on the system. One can thus determine the best drug target in a particular system by rank-ordering its components on the basis of the magnitude of their control coefficients on its function [32].

MCA has been applied to understand the onset and treatment of metabolic diseases. Impaired mitochondrial respiration during brain edema, for instance, can be treated by increasing succinate dehydrogenase activity with naftidrofuryl. This could be explained by the fact that succinate dehydrogenase was found to become a controlling step for mitochondrial oxidative phosphorylation during the onset of edema [33]. MCA also explains the so-called threshold effect often found in mitochondrial dysfunction, i.e., that deficiencies in enzyme complexes often need to be large to trigger metabolic disease. As flux control is distributed among multiple enzyme complexes, many complexes have low flux control coefficients [34].

5 Enhancing anti-parasite drug selectivity with differential control analysis

Apart from being effective, a drug must also be selective against the causative agent of the disease. This is particularly important when the drug is directed against a target that also functions in healthy cells of the host. An illustrative example is the case of the protozoan *Trypanosoma brucei*. This parasite resides in the bloodstream of a mammalian host and causes the fatal African sleeping sickness. As trypanosomes rely on glycolysis for their ATP production, a major strategy in drug design has been to decrease the glycolytic flux by enzyme inhibition [35]. The challenge of this effort is not reducing the glycolytic flux in the parasite such that it cannot survive: the bigger challenge is that glycolytic flux in the cells of the mammalian host must remain intact, such that the host is not affected (or at least not to a significant extent) by the drug [32]. This selectivity can be defined in terms of MCA as the ratio between the response coefficient of the glycolytic flux in the parasite towards the drug and the response coefficient of the glycolytic flux in the host towards the drug. If a drug inhibits enzyme i, this selectivity can be written mathematically as follows:

$$selectivity = \frac{R^{J(tryp)}_{drug}}{R^{J(host)}_{drug}} = \frac{C^{J(tryp)}_{i} \cdot \varepsilon^{v_i(tryp)}_{drug}}{C^{J(host)}_{i} \cdot \varepsilon^{v_i(host)}_{drug}} \qquad (6)$$

Part of this selectivity is determined by the ratio of the elasticity coefficients towards the drug of the respective equivalents of enzyme i in trypanosomes and in the host. Among other factors, this elasticity depends on the protein structure of enzyme i. The selectivity of anti-parasitic drugs can therefore be increased by designing drugs that specifically inhibit glycolytic enzymes of the parasite, based on structural differences with their mammalian equivalents [35]. Many enzyme inhibitors are, however, derivatives of a metabolic substrate of their target, and compete with this substrate both in the parasite and in the host. Applying the drug may increase the concentration of the competing substrate and thereby render the drug fairly ineffective [36]. Therefore, it is necessary to take the network differences between the parasite and the host into account, to increase drug selectivity beyond that based on the differences in protein structure of the drug target. This can be achieved by identifying a process that is relatively important for the glycolytic flux in the parasite but relatively unimportant for the glycolytic flux in the host. The approach in which the control distribution on the same biological system in two different organisms (or cell types) is compared is called *differential control analysis*.

In order to identify the most important steps in trypanosome glycolysis (Fig. 1), a detailed mathematical model was constructed containing measured kinetics for most enzymes in the pathway [37]. Predictions from model simulations regarding the metabolite concentrations and glycolytic flux accurately resembled experimental measurements. The model was used to calculate the flux control coefficients for all enzymes in the pathway. It turned out that the glucose transporter had the highest control, which is a prediction that this enzyme be a good target for a drug to influence the glycolytic flux [21]. Whereas the glucose transporter was fully rate-limiting at low (0.36 mM) extracellular glucose concentration, it lost some of its control to aldolase (ALD), glyceraldehydes-3-phosphate dehydrogenase (GAPDH), phosphoglycerate kinase (PGK) and glycerol-3-phosphate dehydrogenase (GDH) at a more physiological (5 mM) extracellular glucose concentration [38]. Interestingly, the model predicted hexokinase (HXK), phosphofructokinase (PFK) and pyruvate kinase (PYK) to have a very low control coefficients [21]. This was recently confirmed experimentally [39].

An interesting mammalian cell type to compare with the parasite, in terms of the distribution of the control on glycolytic flux, is the erythrocyte. Like the parasite, erythrocytes occur in the bloodstream and also depend on glycolysis for their ATP supply. Realistic computational models are available for glycolysis in the human erythrocyte [40–42]. Interestingly, the glycolytic flux in the erythrocyte appears to be mainly controlled by ATP utilization and not by the glucose transporter, ALD, GAPDH or PGK [42].

Taken together, the glucose transporter and to a lesser extent ALD, GAPDH and PGK, exert high control on glycolysis in the parasite but low control in the erythrocyte. This suggests that these enzymes should make effective and selective drug targets.

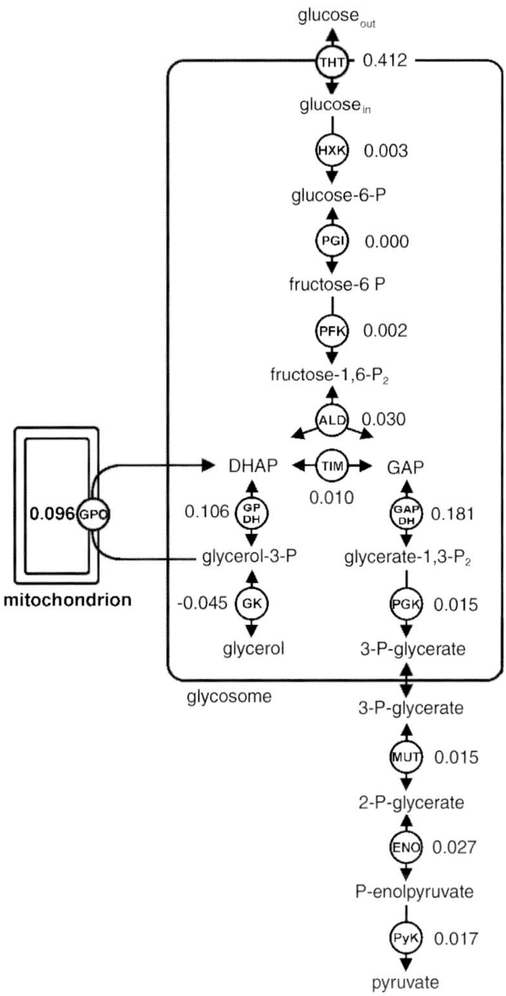

Figure 1.
Control of glycolysis in bloodstream form *Trypanosoma brucei*. The metabolites are converted by glycolytic enzymes, of which the abbreviated names are depicted in the circles. The control coefficients on the oxygen consumption flux, depicted for each enzyme by the number next to the respective enzymes, were calculated with a mathematical model of the system [21, 39]. Adenylate kinase was considered to be in equilibrium and is not indicated. ADP, ATP, Pi, NAD, NADH are also not indicated. THT, glucose transporter; HXK, hexokinase; PGI, phosphogluco-isomerase; PFK, phosphofructokinase; ALD, aldolase; TIM, triose phosphate isomerase; GAPDH, glyceraldehydes-3-phosphate dehydrogenase; PGK, phosphoglycerate kinase; GPDH, glycerol phosphate dehydrogenase; GK, glycerol kinase; GPO, glycerol-3-phosphate oxidase; MUT, phosphoglycerate mutase; ENO, enolase; PyK, pyruvate kinase.

6 Control of tumor cell growth

In addition to infectious diseases, MCA holds promise for identifying drug targets for treatment of multi-factorial diseases such as cancer, multiple sclerosis, diabetes type 2 and atherosclerosis. These diseases are complex by nature, hence difficult to understand. For cancer, for instance, many genes have been causally implicated in oncogenic transformation [43]. Most of these genes function in signal transduction pathways governing cell proliferation, apoptosis, angiogenesis, metastasis or invasion [44, 45]. Complicated network organization (regulatory circuitry, cross-talk between pathways, etc.) and non-linear kinetics of biochemical reactions and the multitude of factors involved, complicate understanding of signaling. Furthermore, interactions between tumor cells and other cell types generate a complex supra-cellular communication network. Therefore, even though many molecular differences have been identified between cancer cells and their healthy counterparts, the emerging picture is overwhelmingly complex. It has therefore been argued by us and others that cancer should be studied from a systems biology perspective, complementary to the current molecular and cellular biology research strategies [46–52]. Upon integration of the many pieces of knowledge on the biology of cancer, MCA can become a valuable tool to determine which components (genes, pathways, etc.) are important for the functioning of the system as a whole [51].

More than for infective diseases, drug target selectivity is an enormous problem for cancer treatment, because tumor cells are so very similar to their normal counterparts. Conventional cancer treatment relies on radiotherapy and chemotherapy, which is based on the generally higher susceptibility of cancer cells to damage induced by irradiation or chemical compounds than their normal non-transformed counterparts [53]. This therapeutic strategy, although successful to some extent, is rather nonspecific, leading to potentially severe side-effects and many cases where the disease becomes refractory to treatment. In addition, due to the increased mutation rates in many tumor cells, resistant cells often arise which, due to their selective advantage for growth during treatment, may out-compete their sensitive counterparts.

New therapies are currently emerging that aim to impair 'oncogenic' signal transduction by tyrosine kinase inhibitors or antibodies that block growth factor receptors [54–57]. The rationale behind this is that over-active signaling pathways, such as the mitogen-activated protein kinase (MAPK) pathway, are responsible for the transformed phenotype and that inhibition of those pathways should therefore reverse this. The question is however: which protein in a pathway would make the best drug target? Furthermore, the selectivity problem may remain, because some healthy cell types require the same enzymes and pathways for functional viability.

MCA may thus serve as a method to determine which reactions in a complex signaling network are actually controlling its behavior [51]. The control on the amplitude and duration of signaling (i.e., the extent to which a pathway is activated and the period of time this activation lasts, respectively) was found to be distributed over multiple enzymes, but not uniformly [22]. This means that inhibition of more than one enzyme might prove more effective than inhibition of a single enzyme. Recently, MCA was applied to the epidermal growth factor-induced MAPK pathway in order to calculate the extent to which the individual reactions and proteins control its output [25]. This was done on the basis of an updated version of a detailed kinetic model of this system [58]. An interesting observation was that most of the 148 studied reactions did not control the network at all (or to a very low extent). The activity of the Raf protein exerted the strongest control on the network, which may explain why mutated Raf confers a growth advantage to the affected cells and therefore why it is frequently reported to be mutated in cancer cells [25]. In line with what was discussed for trypanosomiasis, above, optimal drug targets could then be identified by differential control analysis, i.e., by comparing what controls the output of the network between normal cells and cancer cells.

Besides aberrant signal transduction, cancer cells also display alterations in metabolism. The enhanced proliferation rate, induced by oncogenic mutations, requires high glucose turnover for the synthesis of nucleotides. The resulting sensitivity of transformed cells to nutrient shortage could be exploited for therapeutic purposes [59]. As normal cells use glucose mainly for energy supply, it has been suggested to determine which enzymes in glucose metabolism strongly control nucleotide synthesis, hereby identifying these proteins as potential drug targets [60]. A good example would be transketolase, which was found to be enzyme exerting the most control in glucose metabolism over nucleotide synthesis [61].

Taken together, control analysis methods have a great potential in the discovery of targets for anti-cancer therapies, since controlling reactions in both signal transduction networks and metabolic pathways can be identified with MCA.

Acknowledgements

This work was supported in part by EU-FP6 (through BioSim, NucSys, EU-SYSBIO), NWO, and IBIVU, and by the Universitair Stimuleringsfonds Vrije Universiteit.

References

1 Westerhoff HV, Palsson BO (2004) The evolution of molecular biology into systems biology. *Nat Biotechnol* 22: 1249–1252
2 Bakker BM, Assmus HE, Bruggeman F, Haanstra JR, Klipp E, Westerhoff H (2002) Network-based selectivity of antiparasitic inhibitors. *Mol Biol Rep* 29: 1–5
3 Alberghina L, Westerhoff HV (2005) *Systems Biology. Definitions and Perspectives*, Springer, Berlin, Germany
4 Olivier BG, Snoep JL (2004) Web-based kinetic modelling using JWS Online. *Bioinformatics* 20: 2143–2144
5 Westerhoff HV (2001) The silicon cell, not dead but live! *Metab Eng* 3: 207–210
6 Snoep JL (2005) The Silicon Cell initiative: working towards a detailed kinetic description at the cellular level. *Curr Opin Biotechnol* 16: 336–343
7 Teusink B, Passarge J, Reijenga CA, Esgalhado E, van der Weijden CC, Schepper M, Walsh MC, Bakker BM, van Dam K, Westerhoff HV et al (2000) Can yeast glycolysis be understood in terms of in vitro kinetics of the constituent enzymes? Testing biochemistry. *Eur J Biochem* 267: 5313–5329
8 Tyson JJ, Chen K, Novak B (2001) Network dynamics and cell physiology. *Nat Rev Mol Cell Biol* 2: 908–916
9 Teusink B, Walsh MC, van Dam K, Westerhoff HV (1998) The danger of metabolic pathways with turbo design. *Trends Biochem Sci* 23: 162–169
10 Bakker BM, Mensonides FI, Teusink B, van Hoek P, Michels PA, Westerhoff HV (2000) Compartmentation protects trypanosomes from the dangerous design of glycolysis. *Proc Natl Acad Sci USA* 97: 2087–2092
11 Shulman RG, Rothman DL (2005) *Metabolomics by in vivo NMR*. John Wiley & Sons, Hoboken, NJ, USA

12 Bruggeman FJ, Boogerd FC, Westerhoff HV (2005) The multifarious short-term regulation of ammonium assimilation of *Escherichia coli*: dissection using an *in silico* replica. *Febs J* 272: 1965–1985
13 Kacser H, Burns JA (1973) The control of flux. *Symp Soc Exp Biol* 27: 65–104
14 Heinrich R, Rapoport TA (1974) A linear steady-state treatment of enzymatic chains. General properties, control and effector strength. *Eur J Biochem* 42: 89–95
15 Westerhoff HV, Van Dam K (1987) *Thermodynamics and Control of Biological Free-Energy Transduction*. Elsevier, Amsterdam, The Netherlands
16 Fell DA (1992) Metabolic control analysis: a survey of its theoretical and experimental development. *Biochem J* 286: 313–330
17 Fell DA (1997) *Understanding the control of metabolism*. Portland Press, London, UK
18 Heinrich R, Schuster S (1996) *The regulation of cellular systems*. Chapman & Hall, New York, USA
19 Kholodenko BN, Westerhoff HV (1993) Metabolic channelling and control of the flux. *FEBS Lett* 320: 71–74
20 Groen AK, Wanders RJ, Westerhoff HV, van der Meer R, Tager JM (1982) Quantification of the contribution of various steps to the control of mitochondrial respiration. *J Biol Chem* 257: 2754–2757
21 Bakker BM, Michels PA, Opperdoes FR, Westerhoff HV (1999) What controls glycolysis in bloodstream form *Trypanosoma brucei*? *J Biol Chem* 274: 14551–14559
22 Hornberg JJ, Bruggeman FJ, Binder B, Geest CR, Bij de Vaate AJM, Lankelma J, Heinrich R, Westerhoff HV (2005) Principles behind the multifarious control of signal transduction: ERK phosphorylation and kinase/phosphatase control. *FEBS J* 272: 244–258
23 Lee E, Salic A, Kruger R, Heinrich R, Kirschner MW (2003) The roles of APC and axin derived from experimental and theoretical analysis of the Wnt pathway. *PLoS Biology* 1: e10
24 Ihekwaba AE, Broomhead DS, Grimley RL, Benson N, Kell DB (2004) Sensitivity analysis of parameters controlling oscillatory signalling in the NF-kB pathway: the roles of IKK and IkBa. *Syst Biol* 1: 93–103
25 Hornberg JJ, Binder B, Bruggeman FJ, Schoeberl B, Heinrich R, Westerhoff HV (2005) Control of MAPK signalling: from complexity to what really matters. *Oncogene* 24: 5533–5542
26 Peletier MA, Westerhoff HV, Kholodenko BN (2003) Control of spatially heterogeneous and time-varying cellular reaction networks: a new summation law. *J Theor Biol* 225: 477–487
27 Schuster S, Kahn D, Westerhoff HV (1993) Modular analysis of the control of complex metabolic pathways. *Biophys Chem* 48: 1–17
28 Kahn D, Westerhoff HV (1991) Control theory of regulatory cascades. *J Theor Biol* 153: 255–285

29 Westerhoff HV, Koster JG, Van Workum M, Rudd KE (1989) On the control of gene expression. In: A Cornish-Bowden, ML Cardenas (eds): *Control of metabolic processes.* Plenum Press, New York, USA. pp. 399–413
30 Bruggeman F, Westerhoff H, Hoek J, Kholodenko B (2002) Modular response analysis of cellular regulatory networks. *J Theor Biol* 218: 507
31 Kholodenko BN (1988) How do external parameters control fluxes and concentrations of metabolites? An additional relationship in the theory of metabolic control. *FEBS Lett* 232: 383–386
32 Bakker BM, Westerhoff HV, Opperdoes FR, Michels PA (2000) Metabolic control analysis of glycolysis in trypanosomes as an approach to improve selectivity and effectiveness of drugs. *Mol Biochem Parasitol* 106: 1–10
33 Rigoulet M, Averet N, Mazat JP, Guerin B, Cohadon F (1988) Redistribution of the flux-control coefficients in mitochondrial oxidative phosphorylations in the course of brain edema. *Biochim Biophys Acta* 932: 116–123
34 Mazat JP, Rossignol R, Malgat M, Rocher C, Faustin B, Letellier T (2001) What do mitochondrial diseases teach us about normal mitochondrial functions that we already knew: threshold expression of mitochondrial defects. *Biochim Biophys Acta* 1504: 20–30
35 Verlinde CL, Hannaert V, Blonski C, Willson M, Perie JJ, Fothergill-Gilmore LA, Opperdoes FR, Gelb MH, Hol WG, Michels PA (2001) Glycolysis as a target for the design of new anti-trypanosome drugs. *Drug Resist Updat* 4: 50–65
36 Eisenthal R, Cornish-Bowden A (1998) Prospects for antiparasitic drugs. The case of *Trypanosoma brucei*, the causative agent of African sleeping sickness. *J Biol Chem* 273: 5500–5505
37 Bakker BM, Michels PA, Opperdoes FR, Westerhoff HV (1997) Glycolysis in bloodstream from *Trypanosoma brucei* can be understood in terms of the kinetics of the glycolytic enzymes. *J Biol Chem* 272: 3207–3215
38 Bakker BM, Walsh MC, ter Kuile BH, Mensonides FI, Michels PA, Opperdoes FR, Westerhoff HV (1999) Contribution of glucose transport to the control of the glycolytic flux in *Trypanosoma brucei. Proc Natl Acad Sci USA* 96: 10098–10103
39 Albert MA, Haanstra JR, Hannaert V, Van Roy J, Opperdoes FR, Bakker BM, Michels PA (2005) Experimental and *in silico* analyses of glycolytic flux control in bloodstream from *Trypanosoma brucei. J Biol Chem* 280: 28306–28315
40 Mulquiney PJ, Kuchel PW (1999) Model of 2,3-bisphosphoglycerate metabolism in the human erythrocyte based on detailed enzyme kinetic equations: equations and parameter refinement. *Biochem J* 342 Pt 3: 581–596
41 Joshi A, Palsson BO (1989) Metabolic dynamics in the human red cell. Part I–A comprehensive kinetic model. *J Theor Biol* 141: 515–528
42 Schuster R, Holzhutter HG (1995) Use of mathematical models for predicting the metabolic effect of large-scale enzyme activity alterations. Application to enzyme deficiencies of red blood cells. *Eur J Biochem* 229: 403–418
43 Futreal PA, Coin L, Marshall M, Down T, Hubbard T, Wooster R, Rahman N, Stratton MR (2004) A census of human cancer genes. *Nat Rev Cancer* 4: 177–183
44 Hanahan D, Weinberg RA (2000) The hallmarks of cancer. *Cell* 100: 57–70

45 Vogelstein B, Kinzler KW (2004) Cancer genes and the pathways they control. *Nat Med* 10: 789–799
46 Gatenby RA, Maini PK (2003) Mathematical oncology: cancer summed up. *Nature* 421: 321
47 Kitano H (2003) Cancer robustness: tumour tactics. *Nature* 426: 125
48 Butcher EC, Berg EL, Kunkel EJ (2004) Systems biology in drug discovery. *Nat Biotechnol* 22: 1253–1259
49 Christopher R, Dhiman A, Fox J, Gendelman R, Haberitcher T, Kagle D, Spizz G, Khalil IG, Hill C (2004) Data-driven computer simulation of human cancer cell. *Ann NY Acad Sci* 1020: 132–153
50 Khalil IG, Hill C (2005) Systems biology for cancer. *Curr Opin Oncol* 17: 44–48
51 Hornberg JJ, Bruggeman FJ, Westerhoff HV, Lankelma J (2006) Cancer: A Systems Biology Disease. *Biosystems* 83: 81–90
52 Alberghina L, Chiaradonna F, Vanoni M (2004) Systems biology and the molecular circuits of cancer. *Chembiochem* 5: 1322–1333
53 DeVita VT, Hellman S, Rosenberg SA (2001) *Cancer: Principles & Practice of Oncology*. 6th edition. Lippincott Williams & Wilkins, Philidelphia, PA, USA
54 Krause DS, Van Etten RA (2005) Tyrosine kinases as targets for cancer therapy. *N Engl J Med* 353: 172–187
55 Mendelsohn J, Baselga J (2000) The EGF receptor family as targets for cancer therapy. *Oncogene* 19: 6550–6565
56 Sebolt-Leopold JS, Herrera R (2004) Targeting the mitogen-activated protein kinase cascade to treat cancer. *Nat Rev Cancer* 4: 937–947
57 Shawver LK, Slamon D, Ullrich A (2002) Smart drugs: tyrosine kinase inhibitors in cancer therapy. *Cancer Cell* 1: 117–123
58 Schoeberl B, Eichler-Jonsson C, Gilles ED, Muller G (2002) Computational modeling of the dynamics of the MAP kinase cascade activated by surface and internalized EGF receptors. *Nat Biotechnol* 20: 370–375
59 Chiaradonna F, Magnani C, Sacco E, Manzoni R, Alberghina L, Vanoni M (2005) Acquired glucose sensitivity of k-ras transformed fibroblasts. *Biochem Soc Trans* 33: 297–299
60 Cascante M, Boros LG, Comin-Anduix B, de Atauri P, Centelles JJ, Lee PW (2002) Metabolic control analysis in drug discovery and disease. *Nat Biotechnol* 20: 243–249
61 Comin-Anduix B, Boren J, Martinez S, Moro C, Centelles JJ, Trebukhina R, Petushok N, Lee WN, Boros LG, Cascante M (2001) The effect of thiamine supplementation on tumour proliferation. A metabolic control analysis study. *Eur J Biochem* 268: 4177–4182

Progress in Drug Research, Vol. 64
(Helena I. Boshoff and Clifton E. Barry III, Eds)

The protein network as a tool for finding novel drug targets

By Michael Strong
and David Eisenberg

Howard Hughes Medical Institute,
UCLA-DOE Institute of Genomics and Proteomics,
University of California Los Angeles,
Los Angeles, California, USA
<strong@ucla.edu>

Abstract

Proteins are often referred to as the molecular workhorses of the cell since they are responsible for the majority of functions within a living cell. From the generation of energy, to the replication of DNA, proteins play a central role in most cellular functions. Because of their importance to cellular viability, proteins are commonly the target of therapeutic drugs, ranging from antimicrobial to anticancer drugs. With the rise of drug resistant and multi-drug resistant forms of many diseases, it has become increasingly important to develop new strategies to identify alternative drug targets. One such strategy arises from the analysis of protein networks. Protein networks help define individual proteins within the context of all other cellular proteins. In this chapter we discuss methods for the identification and analysis of genome-wide protein networks, and discuss how protein networks can be used to aid the identification of novel drug targets.

Keywords: protein network, protein interactions, protein linkages, drug targets

1 Protein linkages

Proteins can function together in many ways, ranging from direct physical associations among proteins in a complex, to transient interactions that occur among members of certain protein pathways. Proteins can also function as non-interacting members of the same pathway. As a result, it has been of great interest to develop methods to identify these protein associations, or protein linkages, on a genome-wide basis [1]. The detection of protein linkages has been aided by advances in both biochemical [2–6] and computational methods [7–15], which have yielded valuable insight into the underlying architecture of cellular networks [16–20].

2 Biochemical methods to identify protein-protein interactions

2.1 Yeast two-hybrid assay

One of the most widely used methods for identifying physically interacting proteins is the yeast two-hybrid assay (Y2H) [21]. The yeast two-hybrid assay enables the detection of physically interacting proteins, by exploiting the modular organization of transcriptional activators. Transcriptional activators contain two domains, a DNA binding domain and a transcriptional activator domain, which together can initiate transcription of a target gene. When separated, however, these domains cannot initiate transcription on their own, unless they are brought into close proximity by additional factors.

In the yeast two-hybrid assay, the DNA-binding domain (DBD) of a transcriptional activator is fused to one protein of interest. This fusion protein is known as the 'bait' protein. The transcriptional activating domain (AD) is fused to another protein, known as the 'prey' protein. If there is a physical interaction between the 'bait' protein and the 'prey' protein, then the DNA-binding domain and the transcriptional activating domain come into close proximity and activate a specific reporter gene [21]. If the bait protein and the prey protein do not interact, however, then the DNA-binding domain and the transcriptional activating domain do not come into close proximity, and thus do not activate the reporter gene. This method has been scaled up to enable the high-throughput detection of genome-wide protein–protein interactions [22], and has greatly aided the identification of protein interactions in organisms including yeast [2, 3], *C. elegans* [23], *Drosophila* [24], and humans [25].

2.2 Co-immunoprecipitation method

Another widely used method for detecting protein–protein interactions is the co-immunoprecipitation method (Co-IP) [26]. In the Co-IP method, an antibody is made to target a particular protein of interest. The antibody is then added to a mixture of proteins, often comprising the total cellular lysate of a particular cell type, and allowed to bind to the target protein. If the target protein interacts with additional proteins, then protein–protein interactions can be identified by capturing the antibody and all attached proteins on a solid support. After washing unbound proteins away, the antibody and attached proteins can be eluted and analyzed by a variety of methods ranging from gel electrophoresis to mass spectrometry. Proteins that interact with the target protein are identified in this manner [26].

2.3 Co-affinity purification coupled with mass spectrometry

Variations of the Co-IP method have also been employed to detect physically interacting proteins, including the co-affinity purification (Co-AP) method coupled with mass spectrometry (AP-MS) [4, 5]. In this strategy, a specific target protein is tagged with an affinity tag, expressed with other cellular proteins, and affinity purified. Protein–protein interactions are detected by the co-purification of additional proteins with the tagged protein. Mass spectrometry is then used to identify interacting proteins. This application has been applied to investigate the proteome of *Saccharomyces cerevisiae* [4, 5], where it has enabled the identification of hundreds of protein complexes [4, 5].

2.4 Protein–protein interaction databases

To date, over 50,000 protein–protein interactions have been reported in the literature and catalogued into various databases [27]. Among these databases are the Database of Interacting Proteins (DIP) [28], the Biomolecular Interaction Network Database (BIND) [29], and the Molecular Interactions Database (MINT) [30]. Additionally, a number of web servers have arisen to catalog both known and putative protein pathways. These servers include the Kyoto Encyclopedia of Genes and Genomes (KEGG) [31], the Encyclopedia of *E. coli* Genes and Metabolism (EcoCyc) [32], and the Munich Information Center for Protein Sequences (MIPS) [33]. Together these databases and web servers provide a useful source for investigating protein–protein interactions in organisms ranging from *E. coli* to human.

3 Computational methods to identify protein linkages

In addition to biochemical methods to identify linked proteins, a number of computational methods have been developed to identify functionally linked proteins, including the Rosetta Stone [8], Phylogenetic Profile [11], conserved Gene Neighbor [14, 15], and Operon/Gene Cluster [13, 34] methods. Each of these methods utilizes genomic sequence information garnered from genome sequencing efforts. Currently there are over 300 completed genomes available [35, 36], and over 1,000 ongoing genome sequencing efforts [35]. Together these efforts provide us with a tremendous amount of information regarding not only the genetic blueprint of hundreds of organisms, but also facilitate the computational inference of protein linkages and protein networks.

3.1 Rosetta Stone method

The Rosetta Stone method provides a means for inferring protein linkages based on genomic analyses [8]. The Rosetta Stone method identifies individual genes in one genome that occur as a single fusion gene in another genome. For example, the *leuC* and *leuD* genes of *Mycobacterium tuberculosis* (*Mtb*) occur as two separate genes [37], but in *Schizosaccharomyces pombe* these two genes occur as a single fused gene. Based on this observation, it can be inferred that the *M. tuberculosis leuC* and *leuD* genes are 'functionally linked'. Functionally linked genes may represent genes that encode members of a common protein complex, a common protein pathway, or proteins that serve related functions within the cell [1]. While the *leuC* and *leuD* example demonstrates a Rosetta Stone linkage between two genes of known function (both genes are involved in leucine biosynthesis), many Rosetta Stone linkages involve uncharacterized proteins [8].

3.2 Phylogenetic Profile method

A second method for inferring protein linkages is the Phylogenetic Profile method [11]. The Phylogenetic Profile method identifies genes that occur in a correlated manner across many genomes, specifically identifying genes that are present or absent in a correlated manner [11]. For example, the *fliC* and *fliG* genes of *E. coli* share similar Phylogenetic Profiles. Both *fliC* and *fliG* are present in genomes of flagellated motile bacteria, while both proteins are absent in genomes of non-motile bacteria. We might expect that genes that participate in a shared biochemical pathway or protein complex would share similar phylogenetic profiles.

3.3 Conserved Gene Neighbor method

A third method for inferring protein linkages is the conserved Gene Neighbor method [14, 15]. This method identifies genes that tend to be located in close chromosomal proximity in multiple genomes. For example, the *E. coli otsA* and *otsB* genes are both involved in trehalose biosynthesis, and are located in close chromosomal proximity in a number of genomes including *E. coli, S. typhi,* and *M. loti.* The close chromosomal positioning of genes across many genomes is a common feature of genes in bacterial operons, and suggests related functions. This is also observed in eukaryotic organisms, although to a lesser extent.

3.4 Operon/Gene Cluster method

The Operon method [13], also referred to as the Gene Cluster method [38], utilizes information from a single genome to identify putative operon members based on the distance between adjacent genes in the same orientation [13]. Genes that are separated by minimal intergenic distances are more likely to belong to common operons than genes separated by larger distances [10, 12, 39]. This method has been applied to identify linked genes in organisms ranging from *E. coli* [12] to *M. tuberculosis* [13], and this method is particularly useful in instances where no identifiable gene homologs are present. To date, most genome sequencing ventures have identified genes that are completely unique to a particular organism, and in these cases, the Operon/Gene Cluster method may be particularly useful for assigning putative function or linking uncharacterized genes to characterized genes.

3.5 Databases of inferred protein linkages

Collectively, the described computational methods provide a powerful tool to infer protein linkages, which can then be used to construct genome-wide protein networks. As the number of completed genomes continues to increase, these methods are likely to become more powerful. Currently the ProLinks Database [38] contains inferred protein linkages for over 160 sequenced genomes, and includes over 17 million high confidence linkages [38, 40] identified by the Rosetta Stone, Phylogenetic Profile, conserved Gene Neighbor, and Operon/Gene Cluster methods. Another useful database of inferred protein linkages is the EMBL STRING server [41].

4 Protein networks

Biochemical and computational methods have greatly facilitated the identification of protein linkages on a genome-wide scale. The next question we can ask is "How are these protein linkages organized on a genome-wide scale?" This question can be answered by the construction and analysis of protein networks. Protein networks provide a useful graphical method to investigate the connectivity of individual proteins, as well as sets of proteins [16–18]. Figure 1 depicts a protein network centered on the human cellular tumor antigen p53. p53 is an important tumor suppressor gene [42] that is frequently mutated or inactivated in human cancer cells [43]. As a result, this protein has been thoroughly studied at both the cellular and molecular level.

Figure 1a shows a list of proteins that p53 has been found to physically interact with, as retrieved from the Database of Interacting Proteins [28]. p53 interacts with a number of proteins, including other important cancer-related proteins such as the Breast cancer type 1 (BRCA1) and type 2 (BRCA2) susceptibility proteins, as shown in Figure 1a. Figure 1b depicts the same interactions listed in Figure 1a, but in this case the data are represented as a protein network. In the network, each protein is represented as a circular 'node', and each interaction is indicated as a connecting line, better known as an 'edge'. The p53 protein serves as the central node in this network. The network depicts proteins that interact directly with p53, as well as proteins that are linked by two edges. Protein networks facilitate the analysis of protein linkages and provide a useful graphical interface for analyzing and interpreting large amounts of data.

While the p53 protein network of Figure 1b was constructed using experimentally identified protein–protein interactions, protein networks can also be constructed using computationally inferred protein linkages [38]. Such methods have the advantage of providing information regarding organisms in which extensive biochemical or genetic experiments have not

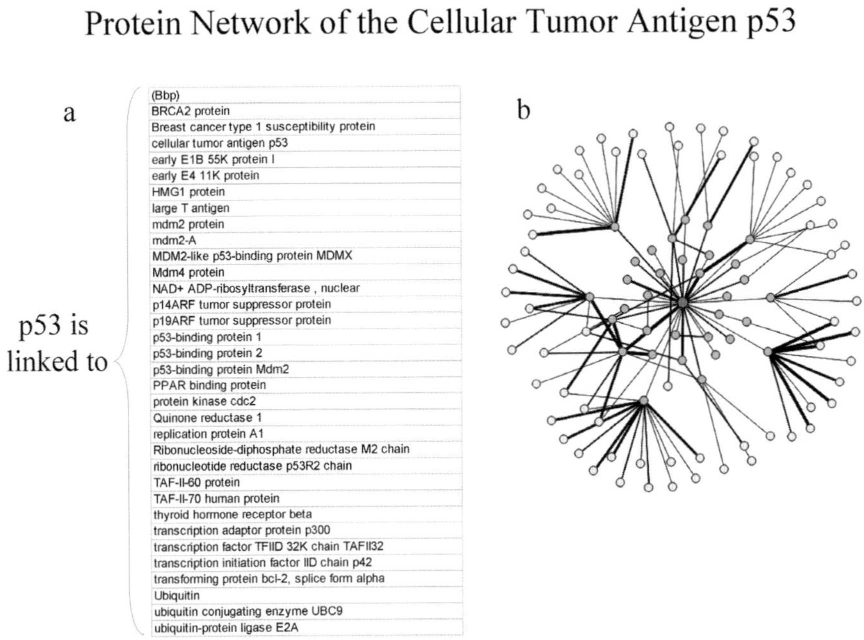

Figure 1.
Protein network of the cellular tumor antigen p53. a) List of proteins that p53 interacts with, as retrieved from the Database of Interacting Proteins [28]. b) p53 protein network. P53 serves as the central node in this network, with 1st and 2nd shell nodes depicted.

been done. Figure 2 depicts a computationally inferred protein network centered on the yeast prion protein Sup35. This network was constructed using a combination of the Phylogenetic Profile method (PP), the Rosetta Stone method (RS), the conserved Gene Neighbor (GN) method, and the Operon/Gene Cluster (GC) method [38].

The yeast prion protein, Sup35, has been shown to exhibit properties of prion-like infectivity [44, 45], resulting from the formation of amyloid-like fibrils [46–49]. The Sup35 network reveals a number of linkages to proteins involved in transcription and translation activities, which may be related to the natural cellular function of Sup35. The use of computationally inferred protein networks, such as the Sup35 network, as well as biochemical-based protein networks, such as the p53 network, may help us better understand the molecular framework in which normal and disease-

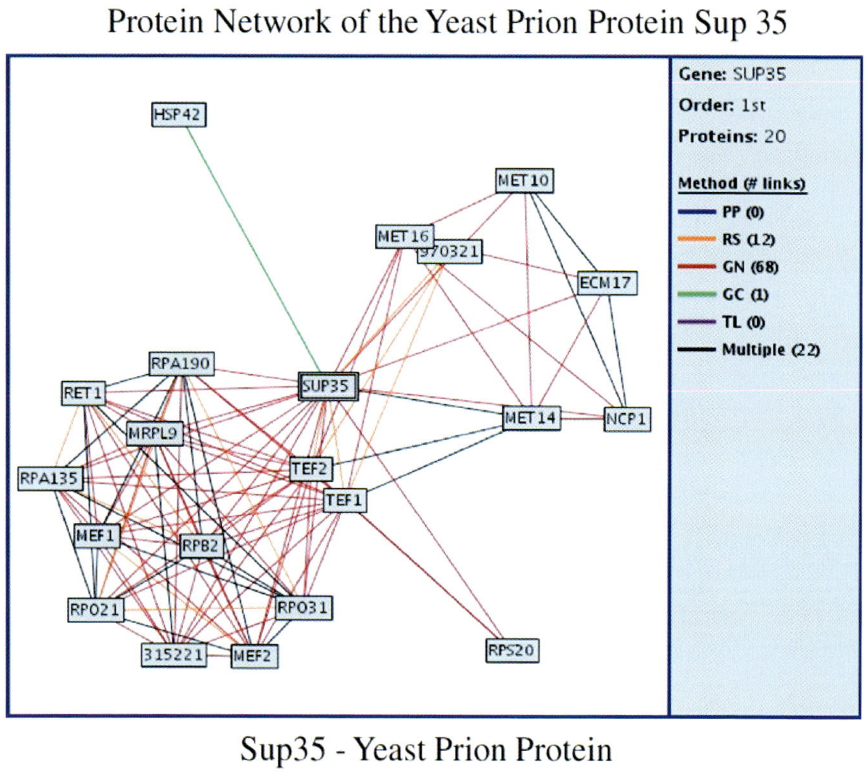

Figure 2.
Protein network of the yeast prion protein Sup35. Linkages indicated in this type of network are inferred by the Phylogenetic Profile (PP), Rosetta Stone (RS), conserved Gene Neighbor (GN), and Operon/Gene Cluster (GC) computational methods.

associated proteins function, and in turn may suggest new strategies to combat a variety of diseases.

Figures 1 and 2 represent somewhat simplified protein networks with only the 1st and 2nd shell nodes depicted. Many protein networks, however, exhibit higher complexity, as shown in Figure 3. In some cases, protein networks comprise hundreds or even thousands of linkages. While the classical method of protein network representation has relied on the node and edge type network (Fig. 3), recent work has demonstrated useful advantages of matrix-represented protein networks [19, 20, 50].

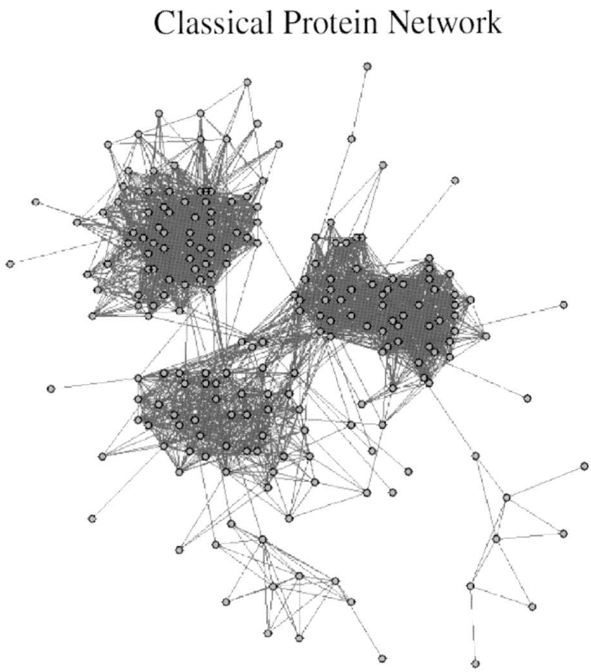

Figure 3.
Classical protein network depicting *M. tuberculosis* protein linkages. Figure adapted from Strong et al. [50].

4.1 Matrix-represented protein networks – genome maps

An alternative approach to represent genome-wide protein networks is shown in Figure 4. In this approach, each linked pair of proteins is indicated as a single point on a two dimensional matrix, corresponding to the position of the genes on the chromosome [50]. Each axis of the graph represents a monotonically ordered list of genes, starting at the origin of replication and proceeding along the chromosome. The *M. tuberculosis* genome has approximately 4,000 genes, as indicated on the x and y axis of the matrix in Figure 4c. Each point on this graph indicates a computationally inferred protein linkage between two proteins [50]. Figure 4a depicts a zoomed in region of the map, representing only the first 50 genes. The point at coordinate x=1, y=5 represents a linkage between the 1st gene on the *M. tuberculosis* chromosome (Rv0001, dnaA) and the 5th gene on

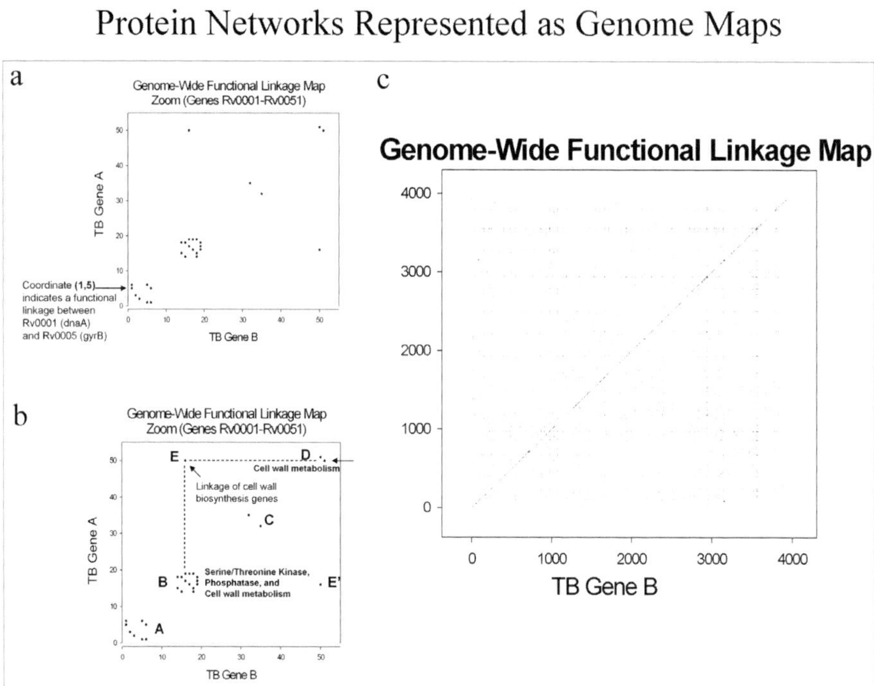

Figure 4.
Genome-wide functional linkage map. a) Zoomed in region of the genome-wide functional linkage map depicting the first 50 genes. Genes are organized according to the order on the chromosome. Each 'point' on the matrix represents a pair of functionally linked genes, for instance the point at coordinate x=1, y=5 indicates a linkage between the first gene, Rv0001 (dnaA) and the fifth gene, Rv0005 (gyrB). b) Functional categories of some of the proximal genes. c) Complete genome-wide functional linkage map depicting nearly 10,000 high confidence functional linkages in *M. tuberculosis*. Figure adapted from Strong et al. [50].

the chromosome (Rv0005, gyrB). Both these genes are involved in DNA replication or repair.

The representation of protein networks as two dimensional genome maps reveals certain characteristics that are not observable using traditional node and edge protein networks. Since information regarding chromosomal organization is maintained in the genome maps, we can analyze protein connectivity in relation to genome organization. One feature that is readily apparent in the genome map of Figure 4 is the local connectivity of genes that are located in close chromosomal proximity [50]. In many cases these clusters of highly connected genes correspond to known or putative operons. Often these clusters contain genes that perform related cellular functions. For instance in Figure 4b, cluster A, most of the genes are involved in DNA replication or repair. In cluster B, there are two genes encoding serine threonine kinases, one phosphatase, and two cell wall metabolism genes. Due to the functional connectivity among the genes of this region, it can be hypothesized that the genes of this cluster participate in a cell wall signaling cascade [50]. This hypothesis was further supported by the presence of a putative peptidoglycan-sensing domain on one of the serine-threonine kinase proteins [51].

The Genome-wide Functional Linkage Map represented in Figure 4c contains approximately 10,000 high confidence protein linkages, inferred by two or more computational methods. To further facilitate the analysis of these protein networks Strong et al. also developed a method to hierarchically cluster the genes of the matrix, based on the similarity of the functional linkage profiles [50]. A functional linkage profile indicates all genes a particular gene is linked to, represented as a bit vector. A '1' in the bit vector indicates a protein linkage and a '0' indicates the absence of a linkage. In the hypothetical example shown in Figure 5a, Gene A is linked to Gene B, Gene C, and Gene D, as indicated by the '1's in the profile. Profiles are then clustered using a hierarchical clustering algorithm, bringing together genes that share similar functional linkage profiles.

The resulting clustered map, shown in Figure 5b, reveals important characteristics of protein network connectivity and hierarchy. Many of the genes cluster into distinct modules, participating in related cellular functions [50]. Some of these modules correspond to protein pathways or complexes, while others contain genes that serve related cellular functions. Some of the functional modules are indicated in Figure 5b. Figure 5c depicts a zoomed-in region of the clustered map, indicated by the black square. Functional modules in this region correspond to genes involved in detoxification, polyketide synthesis, energy metabolism, and the degradation of fatty acids. This example illustrates how hierarchical clustering of genomic maps can enable the rapid identification of functional modules on a genome-wide basis [50].

Figure 6 shows ten representative clusters of the hierarchically clustered map. In some cases, the gene clusters can be used to infer protein

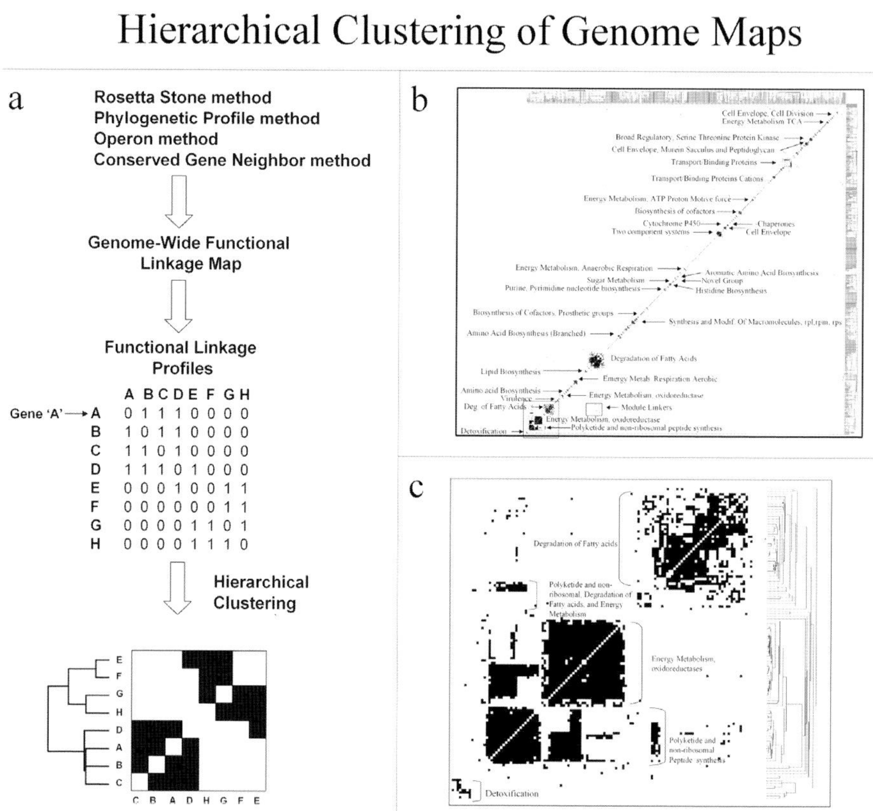

Figure 5.
Hierarchical clustering of the genome-wide functional linkage map. a) Outline of the method. b) Hierarchical clustering reveals the inherent modularity of the *M. tuberculosis* genome. c) Representative *M. tuberculosis* functional modules. Figure adapted from Strong et al. [50].

function for uncharacterized genes. In Figure 6a, a group of chaperone proteins cluster with a non-annotated gene, Rv2372c. Based on this observation, it can be inferred that Rv2372c has a function associated with that of the chaperones of this cluster. In Figure 6b, a number of genes involved in the synthesis and modification of polysaccharides cluster with the uncharacterized gene Rv0127. Based on this clustering, Rv0127 is hypothesized to be involved in polysaccharide synthesis or modification. In other cases, clusters contain a large percentage of non-annotated genes (Fig. 6d–j). These clusters may suggest previously uncharacterized mod-

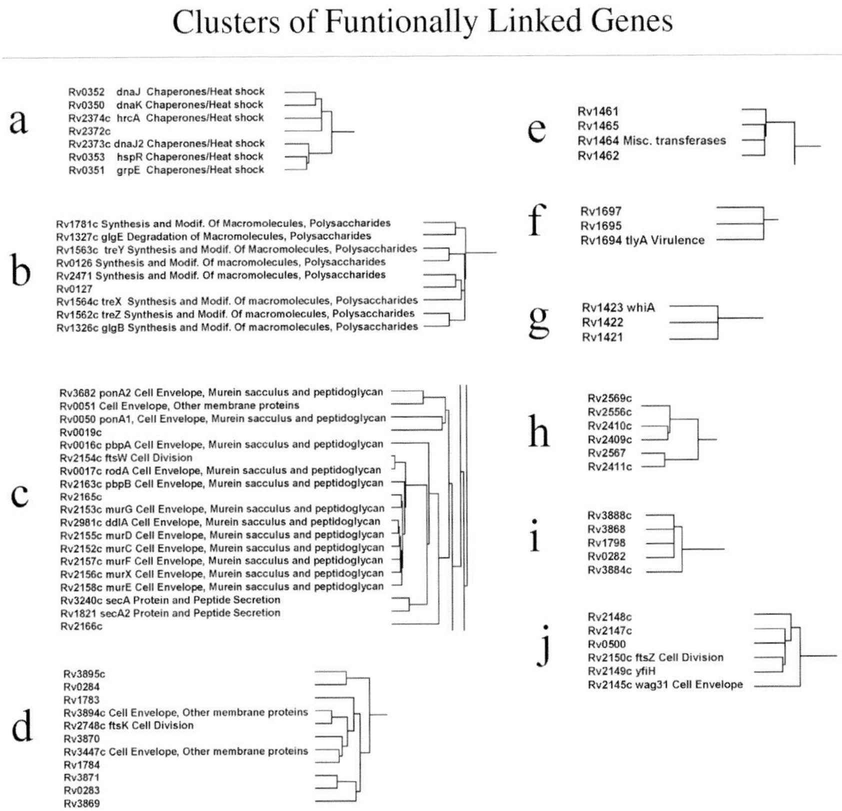

Figure 6.
Representative clusters of functionally linked genes. Gene clusters can aid the inference of gene function for uncharacterized genes as well as can identify novel groups of genes that may function together as a unit. Figure adapted from Strong et al. [50].

ules, possibly corresponding to members of common pathways or complexes, yet to be characterized. A more comprehensive understanding of the modularity of genome-wide protein networks in human pathogens may enable researchers to better devise strategies to combat the pathogenic effects that certain modules are responsible for.

Gene expression analyses have also become an essential tool to identify genes that play important roles during disease states or during infection. While gene expression analyses alone can be used to identify important genes, the examination of gene expression within the context of protein

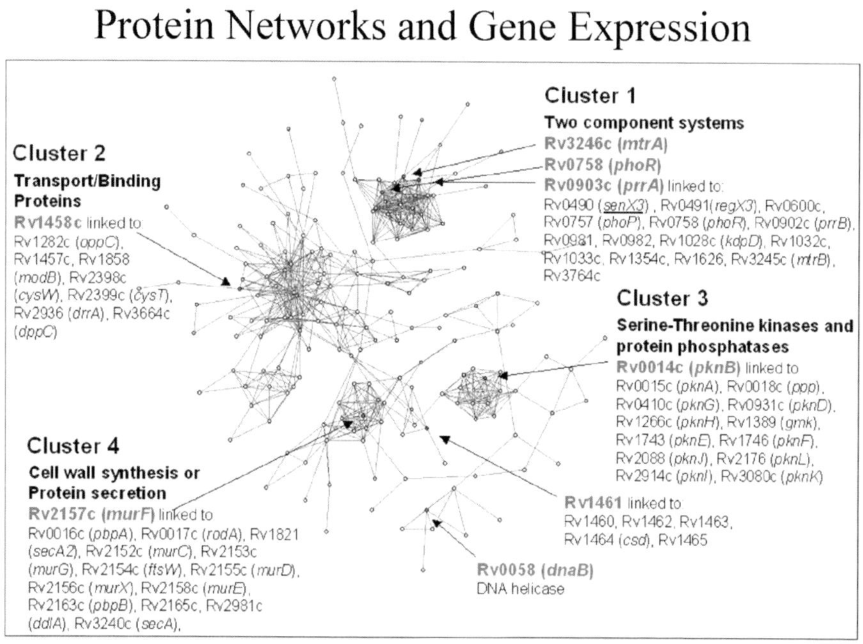

Figure 7.
Examination of gene expression patterns within the context of protein networks. Upregulated genes are indicated by the arrows. Figure adapted from Rachman et al. [52].

networks may further help us to understand the mechanisms by which certain systems are triggered during disease states or infection [52]. Figure 7 shows an example of *M. tuberculosis* gene expression profiling within the context of computationally inferred protein networks. In this case, *M. tuberculosis* genes that are upregulated during macrophage infection are indicated by arrows. Analyses such as these may aid the identification of modules that are important during infection, and may be useful in narrowing the field of potential drug targets.

5 Drug targets

One of the major challenges confronting many branches of infectious disease control is the emergence of drug resistant strains of many viral and bacterial pathogens [53]. Amplifying this concern is the emergence, in some cases, of multi-drug resistant strains [54]. As a result, there is a dire need for the identification of effective, alternative drug targets that may be used to combat these pathogens as they become resistant to current drugs. Often, drug resistance emerges as a result of specific amino acid alterations in targeted proteins [55]. In some cases, these mutations render drugs ineffective, while in other cases they decrease the efficiency of the drug. Resistance to penicillin, for example, is associated with specific amino acid mutations in the penicillin binding proteins [56].

While many drugs target a specific protein, the resulting activity of a drug is often the disruption of a particular cellular function, pathway, or complex. For example, fluoroquinolones inhibit the DNA unwinding activity of the gyraseAB complex, penicillin inhibits cell wall biosynthesis by targeting the penicillin binding proteins, rifampin inhibits the transcriptional activity of the RNA polymerase complex by targeting the RpoB protein, and streptomycin inhibits protein synthesis which can be alleviated by mutations in the *rpsL* gene [57]. In effect, each drug, by targeting a specific protein or small group of proteins, inhibits or disrupts an important cellular pathway, complex, or function. As protein targets become resistant, it may be useful to target other members of the same pathway or complex, as well as proteins that serve related cellular functions. In these cases, protein networks can be useful for the identification of new drug targets that are linked directly or indirectly to current drug targets.

Figure 8 shows computationally inferred protein networks involving four anti-tuberculosis drug targets, RpoB (the target of Rifampin), KasA (a target of Isoniazid), GyrA (the target of Fluoroquinolone drugs), and RpsL (the target of Streptomycin). Each of these networks was generated using the ProLinks server [38]. In each of these cases, we see that proteins of similar cellular function are linked. In the case of RpoB, the Rifampin drug target, there are linkages to other transcription related proteins such as RpoC (the RNA polymerase beta' subunit) and NusG (the transcription antitermination protein), as well as a number of ribosomal proteins.

In the GyrA protein network, GyrA is linked to GyrB (the other member of the DNA gyrase AB complex), the DNA replication initiator DnaA, the DNA replication and repair protein RecF, and the DNA polymerase III protein DnaN. GyrA is also linked to the uncharacterized gene Rv0007.

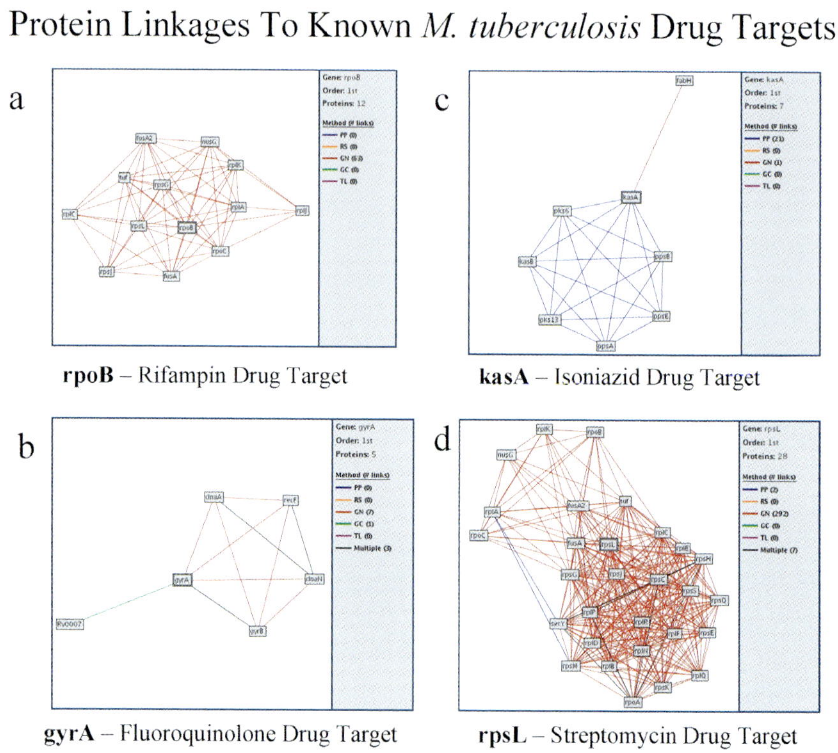

Figure 8.
Protein networks involving known *M. tuberculosis* drug targets. a) rpoB protein network (rifampin drug target), b) gyrA protein network (fluoroquinolone drug target), c) kasA protein network (isoniazid drug target), d) rpsL protein network (streptomycin drug target).

Linkage of known drug targets to uncharacterized proteins may not only suggest a potential function for these uncharacterized proteins, but may also suggest relevant leads for drug target discovery. Figures 8c and 8d show protein networks of the Isoniazid drug target, KasA, and the Streptomycin target, RpsL.

Protein networks in Figure 9 illustrate two *Streptococcus pneumoniae* drug targets, the penicillin binding proteins and the gyrase A subunit. Interestingly, the penicillin binding protein network also contains the vancomycin resistance operon member, VncR, as well as the Mur gene products, which are also involved in cell wall biosynthesis. Together, networks

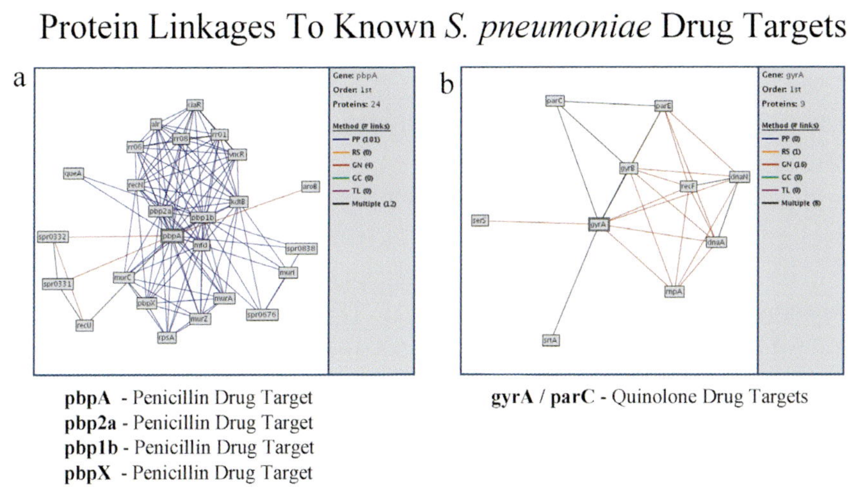

Figure 9.
Protein networks involving *S. pneumonia* drug targets. a) penicillin binding protein network, b) gyrA/parC protein network (quinolone drug targets). Protein networks such as these can be useful in identifying alternative drug targets.

such as these may suggest alternative drug targets as bacteria become resistant to current drugs.

In addition to suggesting alternative targets linked to current drug targets, protein networks can also help identify new drug targets that are associated with novel protein pathways, complexes, or cellular functions. Jeong et al. demonstrated that protein networks could be used to identify essential proteins, or proteins that are necessary for growth and survival. They found that proteins with higher connectivity in protein networks were more likely to be essential proteins, as compared to less connected proteins [58]. Essential proteins may provide useful drug targets, since the disruption of individual proteins may result in non-viable pathogens [59].

The methods described are not without noise, and methods such as the yeast two-hybrid assay are known to yield false positives in several cases. To address this situation, a number of methods have been developed to assess the reliability of various protein interaction datasets and methods for detecting protein interactions and protein linkages [60–62]. Such analyses are important, particularly when deciding which targets to pursue further.

From malaria to tuberculosis, protein networks have enabled researchers to identify and probe the global connectivity of proteins in relevant, disease-causing organisms [50, 63]. In some cases, such as in Plasmodium falciparum, protein connectivity differs from pathogenic to non-pathogenic organisms [64]. These networks enable researchers to better understand pathogens at the molecular level, and in turn can be used to identify novel drug targets. Such an approach facilitates a molecular approach to drug discovery, since drug targets are selected first at the molecular level, and then later tested at the cellular level. This is in contrast to the classical method of drug discovery, which identifies new drug compounds first at the cellular level, and later identifies the molecular target of the drug [65]. It is likely, that a combination of the two methods will yield the most promising results.

Some drugs, such as the breast cancer drug Herceptin, target the interactions between proteins. Specifically, Herceptin inhibits protein–protein interactions by binding to the extracellular domain of the human epidermal growth factor receptor, HER-2. Since protein networks often represent or suggest proteins that physically interact, protein networks may be useful for identifying relevant protein–protein interactions to target for disruption. Such a strategy is not without its challenges [66, 67], since interaction interfaces often lack amenable 'grooves' or 'binding sites' that are commonly targeted by small molecule drugs. As combinatorial drug screening advances, however, this may become an increasingly important area of focus in drug design and development.

6 Conclusion

Just as protein networks have helped us better understand the connectivity of proteins throughout the cell, protein networks also hold the promise to aid the identification of novel drug targets. As more pathogens become resistant to commonly used therapeutic agents, it will become increasingly important to pursue new strategies to combat disease. Specifically, protein networks can aid the identification of alternative protein drug targets that are linked to current drug targets, that are likely to be essential (based on network connectivity), and are linked to essential protein pathways or complexes. Protein networks also facilitate strategies that aim to target multiple proteins of the same pathway or complex. Analysis of gene expression within the context of protein networks can also help identify proteins and protein modules that may be important for virulence. Together, protein networks can help us better understand both normal and disease mechanisms at the protein level, and in turn may provide clues to identify more effective strategies to combat disease.

Acknowledgements

The authors thank the Howard Hughes Medical Institute, National Institutes of Health, and Department of Energy-Biological and Environmental Research (DOE-BER) for support.

References

1 Eisenberg D, Marcotte EM, Xenarios I, Yeates TO (2000) Protein function in the post-genomic era. *Nature* 405: 823–826
2 Uetz P, Giot L, Cagney G, Mansfield TA, Judson RS, Knight JR, Lockshon D, Narayan V, Srinivasan M, Pochart P et al (2000) A comprehensive analysis of protein–protein interactions in *Saccharomyces cerevisiae*. *Nature* 403: 623–627
3 Ito T, Chiba T, Ozawa R, Yoshida M, Hattori M, Sakaki Y (2001) A comprehensive two-hybrid analysis to explore the yeast protein interactome. *Proc Natl Acad Sci USA* 98: 4569–4574
4 Gavin AC, Bosche M, Krause R, Grandi P, Marzioch M, Bauer A, Schultz J, Rick JM, Michon AM, Cruciat CM et al (2002) Functional organization of the yeast proteome by systematic analysis of protein complexes. *Nature* 415: 141–147
5 Ho Y, Gruhler A, Heilbut A, Bader GD, Moore L, Adams SL, Millar A, Taylor P, Bennett K, Boutilier K et al (2002) Systematic identification of protein complexes in *Saccharomyces cerevisiae* by mass spectrometry. *Nature* 415: 180–183
6 Brown PO, Botstein D (1999) Exploring the new world of the genome with DNA microarrays. *Nat Genet* 21: 33–37
7 Eisen MB, Spellman PT, Brown PO, Botstein D (1998) Cluster analysis and display of genome-wide expression patterns. *Proc Natl Acad Sci USA* 95: 14863–14868
8 Marcotte EM, Pellegrini M, Ng HL, Rice DW, Yeates TO, Eisenberg D (1999) Detecting protein function and protein–protein interactions from genome sequences. *Science* 285: 751–753
9 Enright AJ, Iliopoulos I, Kyrpides NC, Ouzounis CA (1999) Protein interaction maps for complete genomes based on gene fusion events. *Nature* 402: 86–90

10 Moreno-Hagelsieb G, Collado-Vides J (2002) A powerful non-homology method for the prediction of operons in prokaryotes. *Bioinformatics* 18 Suppl 1: S329–336

11 Pellegrini M, Marcotte EM, Thompson MJ, Eisenberg D, Yeates TO (1999) Assigning protein functions by comparative genome analysis: protein phylogenetic profiles. *Proc Natl Acad Sci USA* 96: 4285–4288

12 Salgado H, Moreno-Hagelsieb G, Smith TF, Collado-Vides J (2000) Operons in *Escherichia coli*: genomic analyses and predictions. *Proc Natl Acad Sci USA* 97: 6652–6657

13 Strong M, Mallick P, Pellegrini M, Thompson MJ, Eisenberg D (2003) Inference of protein function and protein linkages in *Mycobacterium tuberculosis* based on prokaryotic genome organization: a combined computational approach. *Genome Biol* 4: R59

14 Overbeek R, Fonstein M, D'Souza M, Pusch GD, Maltsev N (1999) The use of gene clusters to infer functional coupling. *Proc Natl Acad Sci USA* 96: 2896–2901

15 Dandekar T, Snel B, Huynen M, Bork P (1998) Conservation of gene order: a fingerprint of proteins that physically interact. *Trends Biochem Sci* 23: 324–328

16 Wuchty S (2002) Interaction and domain networks of yeast. *Proteomics* 2: 1715–1723

17 Jeong H, Tombor B, Albert R, Oltvai ZN, Barabasi AL (2000) The large-scale organization of metabolic networks. *Nature* 407: 651–654

18 Marcotte EM, Pellegrini M, Thompson MJ, Yeates TO, Eisenberg D (1999) A combined algorithm for genome-wide prediction of protein function. *Nature* 402: 83–86

19 Ravasz E, Somera AL, Mongru DA, Oltvai ZN, Barabasi AL (2002) Hierarchical organization of modularity in metabolic networks. *Science* 297: 1551–1555

20 Rives AW, Galitski T (2003) Modular organization of cellular networks. *Proc Natl Acad Sci USA* 100: 1128–1133

21 Fields S, Song O (1989) A novel genetic system to detect protein–protein interactions. *Nature* 340: 245–246

22 Vidal M, Legrain P (1999) Yeast forward and reverse 'n'-hybrid systems. *Nucleic Acids Res* 27: 919–929

23 Li S, Armstrong CM, Bertin N, Ge H, Milstein S, Boxem M, Vidalain PO, Han JD, Chesneau A, Hao T et al (2004) A map of the interactome network of the metazoan *C. elegans*. *Science* 303: 540–543

24 Giot L, Bader JS, Brouwer C, Chaudhuri A, Kuang B, Li Y, Hao YL, Ooi CE, Godwin B, Vitols E et al (2003) A protein interaction map of *Drosophila melanogaster*. *Science* 302: 1727–1736

25 Rual JF, Venkatesan K, Hao T, Hirozane-ishikawa T, Dricot A, Li N, Berriz GF, Gibbons FD, Dreze M, Ayivi-Guedehoussou N et al (2005) Towards a proteome-scale map of the human interactome network. *Nature* 437: 1173–1178

26 Sambrook J, Russell DW (2005) Identification of associated proteins by coimmunoprecipitation. *Nature Methods* 2: 475–476

27 Database of Interacting Proteins: http://dip.doe-mbi.ucla.edu/

28 Salwinski L, Miller CS, Smith AJ, Pettit FK, Bowie JU, Eisenberg D (2004) The Database of Interacting Proteins: 2004 update. *Nucleic Acids Res* 32: D449–451

29 Gilbert D (2005) Biomolecular interaction network database. *Brief Bioinform* 6: 194–198

30 Zanzoni A, Montecchi-Palazzi L, Quondam M, Ausiello G, Helmer-Citterich M, Cesareni G (2002) MINT: a Molecular INTeraction database. *FEBS Lett* 513: 135–140

31 Kanehisa M, Goto S, Kawashima S, Nakaya A (2002) The KEGG databases at GenomeNet. *Nucleic Acids Res* 30: 42–46

32 Keseler IM, Collado-Vides J, Gama-Castro S, Ingraham J, Paley S, Paulsen IT, Peralta-Gil M, Karp PD (2005) EcoCyc: a comprehensive database resource for *Escherichia coli*. *Nucleic Acids Res* 33: D334–337

33 Mewes HW, Frishman D, Mayer KF, Munsterkotter M, Noubibou O, Pagel P, Rattei T, Oesterheld M, Ruepp A, Stumpflen V (2006) MIPS: analysis and annotation of proteins from whole genomes in 2005. *Nucleic Acids Res* 34: D169–172

34 Pellegrini M, Thompson M, Fierro J, Bowers P (2001) Computational method to assign microbial genes to pathways. *J Cell Biochem* 37: 106–109

35 GOLD – Genomes OnLine Database. http://www.genomesonline.org/

36 Bernal A, Ear U, Kyrpides N (2001) Genomes OnLine Database (GOLD): a monitor of genome projects world-wide. *Nucleic Acids Res* 29: 126–127

37 Cole ST, Brosch R, Parkhill J, Garnier T, Churcher C, Harris D, Gordon SV, Eiglmeier K, Gas S, Barry CE et al (1998) Deciphering the biology of *Mycobacterium tuberculosis* from the complete genome sequence. *Nature* 393: 537–544

38 Bowers PM, Pellegrini M, Thompson MJ, Fierro J, Yeates TO, Eisenberg D (2004) Prolinks: a database of protein functional linkages derived from coevolution. *Genome Biol* 5: R35

39 Salgado H, Santos-Zavaleta A, Gama-Castro S, Millan-Zarate D, Diaz-Peredo E, Sanchez-Solano F, Perez-Rueda E, Bonavides-Martinez C, Collado-Vides J (2001) RegulonDB (version 3.2): transcriptional regulation and operon organization in *Escherichia coli* K-12. *Nucleic Acids Res* 29: 72–74

40 ProLinks Database – http://www.doe-mbi.ucla.edu/

41 von Mering C, Huynen M, Jaeggi D, Schmidt S, Bork P, Snel B (2003) STRING: a database of predicted functional associations between proteins. *Nucleic Acids Res* 31: 258–261

42 Hollstein M, Sidransky D, Vogelstein B, Harris CC (1991) p53 mutations in human cancers. *Science* 253: 49–53

43 Vassilev LT, Vu BT, Graves B, Carvajal D, Podlaski F, Filipovic Z, Kong N, Kammlott U, Lukacs C, Klein C et al (2004) *In vivo* activation of the p53 pathway by small-molecule antagonists of MDM2. *Science* 303: 844–848

44 Patino MM, Liu JJ, Glover JR, Lindquist S (1996) Support for the prion hypothesis for inheritance of a phenotypic trait in yeast. *Science* 273: 622-626

45 Serio TR, Cashikar AG, Kowal AS, Sawicki GJ, Moslehi JJ, Serpell L, Arnsdorf MF, Lindquist SL (2000) Nucleated conformational conversion and the replication of conformational information by a prion determinant. *Science* 289: 1317-1321

46 DePace AH, Santoso A, Hillner P, Weissman JS (1998) A critical role for amino-terminal glutamine/asparagine repeats in the formation and propagation of a yeast prion. *Cell* 93: 1241-1252

47 Balbirnie M, Grothe R, Eisenberg DS (2001) An amyloid-forming peptide from the yeast prion Sup35 reveals a dehydrated β-sheet structure for amyloid. *Proc Natl Acad Sci USA* 98: 2375-2380

48 Nelson R, Sawaya MR, Balbirnie M, Madsen AO, Riekel C, Grothe R, Eisenberg D (2005) Structure of the cross-beta spine of amyloid-like fibrils. *Nature* 435: 747–749

49 Shorter J, Lindquist S (2004) Hsp104 catalyzes formation and elimination of self-replicating Sup35 prion conformers. *Science* 304: 1793–1797

50 Strong M, Graeber TG, Beeby M, Pellegrini M, Thompson MJ, Yeates TO, Eisenberg D (2003) Visualization and interpretation of protein networks in *Mycobacterium tuberculosis* based on hierarchical clustering of genome-wide functional linkage maps. *Nucleic Acids Res* 31: 7099–7109

51 Yeats C, Finn RD, Bateman A (2002) The PASTA domain: a beta-lactam-binding domain. *Trends Biochem Sci* 27: 438

52 Rachman H, Strong M, Schaible U, Schuchhardt J, Hagens K, Mollenkopf H, Eisenberg D, Kaufmann SHE (2006) *Mycobacterium tuberculosis* gene expression profiling within the context of protein networks. *Microbes and Infection* 8: 747–757

53 D'Costa VM, McGrann KM, Hughes DW, Wright GD (2006) Sampling the antibiotic resistome. *Science* 311: 342–343

54 Blower SM, Chou T (2004) Modeling the emergence of the 'hot zones': tuberculosis and the amplification dynamics of drug resistance. *Nature Medicine* 10: 1111–1116

55 Hecht FM, Grant RM, Petropoulos CJ, Dillon B, Chesney MA, Tian H, Hellmann NS, Bandrapalli NI, Digilio L, Branson B et al (1998) Sexual transmission of an HIV-1 variant resistant to multiple reverse-transcriptase and protease inhibitors. *N Engl J Med* 339: 307–311

56 Ohsaki Y, Tachibana M, Nakanishi K, Nakao S, Saito K, Toyoshima E, Sato M, Takahashi T, Osanai S, Itoh Y et al (2003) Alterations in penicillin binding protein gene of *Streptococcus pneumoniae* and their correlation with susceptibility patterns. *Int J Antimicrob Agents* 22: 140–146

57 Hatful G, Jacobs WR (eds) (2000) *Molecular Genetics of Mycobacteria*. American Society Microbiology Press, New York, USA

58 Jeong H, Mason SP, Barabasi AL, Oltvai ZN (2001) Lethality and centrality in protein networks. *Nature* 411: 41–42

59 Sassetti CM, Boyd DH, Rubin EJ (2003) Genes required for mycobacterial growth defined by high density mutagenesis. *Mol Microbiol* 48: 77–84

60 Deane CM, Salwinski L, Xenarios I, Eisenberg D (2002) Protein interactions: two methods for assessment of the reliability of high throughput observations. *Mol Cell Proteom* 1: 349–356

61 von Mering C, Krause R, Snel B, Cornell M, Oliver SG, Fields S, Bork P (2002) Comparative assessment of large-scale data sets of protein–protein interactions. *Nature* 417: 399–403

62 Sprinzak E, Sattath S, Margalit H (2003) How reliable are experimental protein–protein interaction data? *J Mol Biol* 327: 919–923

63 LaCount DJ, Vignali M, Chettier R, Phansalkar A, Bell R, Hesselberth JR, Schoenfeld LW, Ota I, Sahasrabudhe S, Kurschner C et al (2005) A protein interaction network of the malaria parasite *Plasmodium falciparum*. *Nature* 438: 103–107

64 Suthram S, Sittler T, Ideker T (2005) The Plasmodium protein network diverges from those of other eukaryotes. *Nature* 438: 108–112

65 Chaudhuri A, Chant J (2005) Protein-interaction mapping in search of effective drug targets. *Bioessays* 27: 958–969

66 Arkin MR, Wells JA (2004) Small-molecule inhibitors of protein–protein interactions: progressing towards the dream. *Nat Rev Drug Discov* 3: 301–317

67 Zhao L, Chmielewski J (2005) Inhibiting protein–protein interactions using designed molecules. *Curr Opin Struct Biol* 15: 31–34

Progress in Drug Research, Vol. 64
(Helena I. Boshoff and Clifton E. Barry III, Eds)

Toxicogenomics applied to predictive and exploratory toxicology for the safety assessment of new chemical entities: a long road with deep potholes

By François Pognan

AstraZeneca Pharmaceuticals,
Safety Assessment,
Macclesfield, Cheshire, UK
<francois.pognan@astrazeneca.com>

Abstract

Toxicology is the perturbation of metabolism by external factors such as xenobiotics, environmental factors or drugs. As such, toxicology covers a broad range of fields from studies of the whole organism responses to minute biochemical events. Mechanistic toxicogenomics is an attempt to harness genomic tools to understand the physiological basis for a toxic event based on an analysis of transcriptional, translational or metabolomic profiles. These studies are complicated by non-toxic adaptive responses in transcript, protein or metabolite expression levels that have to be distinguished from those that are proximally related to the toxic event. Substantial progress has been made on the identification of biomarkers and the establishment of screens derived from such toxicogenomics studies. The ultimate goal, of course, is predictive toxicogenomics, which is an attempt to infer the likelihood of occurrence of a toxic event with exposure to a new agent based upon comparative responses with large databases of gene, protein or metabolite expression data. Gene expression databases are currently limited by the fact that measurable toxic phenotypes generally precede or at best coincide with the earliest observable changes in transcriptional profiles. Unfortunately, predictive protein databases have been limited by technical difficulties. Metabonomics-based databases, which would probably have the highest predictive value, are limited in turn by the inability to perform high dose studies in humans. This chapter will conclude by reviewing those elements of toxicogenomics that apply specifically to the development of anti-infectives and the potential for accurately modelling the toxicity of future drugs.

1 Overview

Gene profiling, or more exactly mRNA transcript profiling, has relatively recently invaded all layers of biological sciences [1, 2], from fundamental research through to biomarker development and toxicology. This discipline, commonly called genomics or more precisely transcriptomics, allows the investigator to monitor the activity of a genome through measuring the relative abundance of thousands of mRNA or even a whole genome transcriptome, using so-called 'gene array' chips, nylon filters or glass slides [3, 4] (see Chapter 2). More recently, the term genomics has been used to embrace transcriptomics, proteomics and metabonomics, and systems biology approaches use the term genomics in its widest sense to include biostatistics and mathematical tools used in an attempt to integrate the huge amount of data generated into meaningful information [5]. Indeed, these 'omics terms immediately trigger in scientists minds gene arrays, 2D gels and nuclear magnetic resonance (NMR) spectroscopy techniques respectively, each of which can produce tens of thousands of data points. However, these 'omics also embrace many other complementary techniques, for example reverse transcription quantitative (RTQ)-polymerase chain reaction (PCR) for gene arrays ([6], see also Chapter 1). In this chapter, we use the term genomics in its broadest context; and transcriptomics for transcript profiling or 'gene expression profiling' (GEP) only. Likewise, the application of gene profiling to toxicology is usually called toxicogenomics; however toxicotranscriptomics is more accurate and will therefore be favoured in this article. Toxicogenomics will again be used in the meaning of the regrouping of the three disciplines applied to toxicology.

Being able to analyse a snapshot view of genome activity (mRNA, protein expression and metabolism) in one organ or even a cell subpopulation of one organ under specific conditions, allows in theory, a thorough understanding of biological events at a specific time point. This approach should allow a better understanding of fundamental biology at a molecular level, identify new pharmacological targets and biomarkers, and improve understanding of toxicology mechanisms [2, 7–10]. Technical issues linked to the monitoring and analyses of whole transcriptomes have been largely overcome and a variety of platforms are now available [11, 12]. However, there are still some technical limitations and every platform has advantages and disadvantages, but the choice is large enough to select or adapt appropriate, reliable technology from existing commercial or 'home made' kits [11, 12]. The very large amount of data generated by any genomics platform is simply too overwhelming for straightforward human analysis. Hence, bioinformatics solutions have been developed. There are numerous statistical tools to extract the relevant information or what is thought to be pertinent for the question under investigation. Here again no single method is absolute and a careful informed choice of analysis methods is a prerequisite to biological interpretation of the extracted data [2, 13]. Despite common assertions made in the pioneering times that GEP would be the ultimate tool and become the biological panacea, it has become very obvious that this was overoptimistic. More reasonably, it is now admitted that proteomics (see Chapter 4) and metabonomics (see Chapter 5) are exploratory tools that not only complement each other and gene profiling but also facilitate interpretation and confirm the biological meaning of the results [7, 14]. It should also be noted that intrinsic limitations of the 'omics' concept itself may be the most important aspect to consider before entering the path of genomics [15, 16]. It is therefore necessary to state that even well handled combined genomics will not solve all biological mysteries. However, these powerful tools have huge potentials that the scientific community is just starting to explore. The possibilities are open to all areas of biological science and toxicology is certainly one that may start to benefit from the strength of genomics.

The purpose of this chapter is not to detail these technologies, and excellent reviews dealing with either platforms and/or statistical analysis of data have been published [1, 2, 5, 7, 13], but to review toxicological applications in mechanistic and predictive mode applied to the safety assessment of new drugs, and to run a quick survey of its status regarding anti-infective drug-associated side effects.

2 Toxicogenomics

The field of toxicology is unique in that it engages almost all biological sciences. Indeed, toxicology can be seen as the disturbance of any aspect of life by external factors such as xenobiotics, environmental factors or drugs. Typically such aspects include main organ physiology, hormone communication, cellular functions, cell interactions, metabolism, central nervous system (CNS) function and behaviour, genetic integrity, and immunological regulation, etc. Information on the perturbation of one or more of these processes is combined with toxicology-related issues such as exposure to drug, routes of excretion or metabolism of a drug, pharmacokinetics, route of exposure, or risk assessment [17]. Due to the complexities of the interplay of these factors and the large variation in response observed between humans, toxicology like medicine is often perceived more as an art than a hard science. Toxicologists are faced with complex data derived from many different processes that need to be evaluated at many different levels, from molecules to broad physiological functions, for which a variety of *in vitro* and *in vivo* techniques and studies have been developed over the years. The latest additions to the toxicologist's toolbox are the toxicogenomics platforms. It is hoped that the systematic exploration of toxicological events at the molecular level by studying the entirety of mRNA, protein and metabolite perturbations in response to a xenobiotic challenge will yield a deeper understanding of the triggers of an adverse response. Hence, this knowledge should improve the understanding of animal models, and allow these models to be refined and optimised. It should also facilitate the design of improved informative *in vitro* assays and should even allow the prediction of toxicity, potentially including human idiosyncratic side effects. However, toxicotranscriptomics does not directly produce informative molecular toxicological insights on its own; neither will toxicogenomics if not integrated in the overall picture of a toxic event which often includes clinical pathology, histopathology, clinical examination, safety pharmacology and genetic toxicology observations. This rosy picture seems to be within our reach and toxicologists have embraced toxicogenomics into two different avenues that are quite contrary in their philosophies:

- A reactive approach consisting of exploring a toxicity event which has been previously characterised and well described by *in vivo* studies using classical approaches like histopathology. This is often referred to as 'mechanistic or investigative toxicogenomics'.
- A proactive approach which entails the building up of large databases of GEPs, protein profiles or metabolite profiles, derived from tissue samples or body fluids of drug-treated animals at sub-toxic and toxic doses, in order to identify the potential toxicity patterns of new chemical entities (NCE). This is often referred to as 'predictive toxicogenomics'.

Both approaches have their own distinct value but are anticipated to eventually converge to yield an identical outcome. However, each has very different drawbacks and pitfalls [16].

2.1 Mechanistic toxicogenomics

Small animal *in vivo* toxicology studies for the assessment of new chemical entities (NCEs) are classically designed with four different groups of animals: control vehicle treated, low-, medium- and high-dose treatment. The goal of early regulatory toxicity studies in the pharmaceutical industry is to define the main toxic liabilities. Until recently, describing those events and having a sufficient margin between the pharmacological or efficacious dose of a compound and the dose at which the very first adverse events are detectable, was seen as the best possible way to progress the development of a NCE to a usable marketable drug. However, the pharmaceutical industry together with regulatory authorities around the world is now increasingly inclined to try to understand toxicity events [18]. Traditionally, this involved the development of a hypothesis that was tested and possibly verified by all available techniques and disciplines. Having molecular clues, rather than just morphological, physiological and clinical observations, is obviously valuable for the generation of a more accurate and a more focussed mechanistic hypothesis. There are now more published data of classical chemical-, and to a lesser extent, drug-induced adverse events [19]. One of the best-studied cases is certainly the effect of acetaminophen toxicity in either mouse or rat liver [20–24]. These studies rapidly provided new insights into molecular events leading to acetaminophen-induced liver failure which had not previously been confirmed despite results generated by classical biochemical work over the three or four previous decades. However, the interpretation of this new knowledge was only possible due to the previous wealth of data regarding acetaminophen hepatotoxicity. There are very few examples of new mechanisms of toxicity unveiled by toxicogenomics that had not been previously hypothesised or which had not been partly previously explained based on classical biochemical and observational approaches [25]. Hence, the question arises if the genomics approach to unravel a unique toxicity event provides any real advantage over more classical approaches. Nonetheless, toxicogenomics is an important new tool allowing beneficial new angles of attack to a specific issue and will possibly become the workhorse of this field as the understanding and interpretation of the complex information generated by 'omic approaches improves.

Such studies have to be carefully designed. As is also the case for predictive toxicogenomics, non-toxic adaptive responses in transcript, protein or metabolite profiles have to be distinguished from those that are relevant to the toxic event. To achieve this, studies must have a low/medium dose of compound that would achieve a pharmacological effect without producing any observable adverse effect. Then, by subtracting the pharmacological profile from the toxicological profile, the amount of data that needs to be analysed is somewhat reduced. However, even this amount of data is usually too complex for simple manual comparisons and generally requires statistical informatics tools to extract the relevant information that can lead to an understanding of the studied event. Also, even in single dose studies, a time course of tissue sampling is intuitively necessary to obtain meaningful data [22–24]. Indeed, a single sampling time point will yield limited information compared to sequential observations after dosing. Likewise, the number of minutes or hours between a single high toxic dose and the time of necropsy will yield a potentially totally different panel of upregulated and downregulated effects, leading itself to potentially diametrically opposite interpretations. Indeed, early tissue collection after dosing will display many stress response proteins and genes that respond quickly, while very late collection will reveal gross pathology such as necrosis or attempts at tissue repair [16]. In other words, it is crucial for toxicogenomics data to collect tissues and samples during an appropriate time window, which should be more or less consistent with the dosing regimen, the dose level, the route of administration, the intrinsic clearance of the drug, the solubility of the drug, the vehicle used and inter-animal metabolic variations. All these parameters would ideally need to be pre-established for initiating a toxicogenomics study; however, this information is rarely available with only a few compounds such as acetaminophen being very well described from this perspective in the literature [20–24].

Equally important are the differences between toxicity-induced by a single high dose and that resulting from repeated lower doses. Repeat dose studies are far more complex and require such a plethora of sample analyses that as yet, there are very few such studies published. In toxicology it is a broadly accepted concept that the longer the treatment, the lower the dose necessary to obtain an adverse event. However, short high dose treatments do not necessarily induce similar pathology to longer duration lower dose treatment. Nevertheless, toxicologists still hope to find similar molecular features and clues in both cases. Thus, repeat dose regimen studies with much lower drug levels to induce toxicity than in single dose studies, are used to acquire better clues about long-term toxicity. In this case, the timing of early sampling time points after the last treatment is intuitively less important than that of single high dosing regimen. It is therefore common practice to collect less time point samples after the last treatment than in single dose-studies. In this regard, the hepatic gene profiling study induced by peroxisome proliferators published by Cornwell et al. [26] is a model of this type of approach. First of all, the use of peroxisome proliferator-activated receptor (PPARs) drugs was an astute choice, as the mechanism of tumour induction is known to be based on specific gene regulation [27]. Hence, such a study cannot fail in finding a whole wealth of gene deregulation directly responsible for the observed toxicity. Second, the design of the study itself was optimised for disentangling the mechanism of action of the drugs. In this study, six different but chemically and pharmacologically-related drugs were used at a toxic dose and an approximately ten-fold lower non-toxic dose, matching the previously described criteria for extracting relevant mechanistic data. Furthermore, animals were treated repeatedly for either 1, 3 or 7 days and the pathology which ensued as anticipated was recorded. This combined most of the parameters required to extract data allowing new insights into a toxicity event. However, as complete as this study was, only 1 sampling time after the last dose was used and arguably, maybe more fundamental knowledge could have been gained by analysing earlier samples than 24 h post-dosing. Undoubtedly, had the same liver samples been co-analysed using a proteomics platform, more insight would have been gained from this study and this would have provided proof that the observed gene expression changes translated into cellular changes at the protein level to bring about a biological impact. In any case, as for acetaminophen, this study did not unveil new mechanistic insights into the cellular basis of toxicity, but confirmed previous hypotheses about the toxic effects of these drugs.

Beside the search for mechanism of toxicity, one logical development is the identification of biomarkers and establishment of screens derived from this information [9]. Phospholipidosis (PLD) for example, is a disorder of lipid metabolism resulting in the accumulation of phospholipids and sphingomyelin in intracellular lysosomes, which can be induced in many organs by many drugs, including some antibiotics [28]. PLD can be modelled *in vitro* in different cells [29, 30]. Through the use of cell culture and about 30 reference phospholipidogenic and non-phospholipidogenic drugs, Sawada and collaborators [31] extracted a handful of genes common to inducers, most of them involved in pathways known to be involved in either the mechanism or in downstream consequences of PLD, which can be further used *in vitro* for screening for compounds that affect phospholipid metabolism and likely *in vivo* as potential markers of PLD induction. This is an example where the use of many structurally different drugs were used to investigate one cellular metabolic process (induction of PLD) leading to a better toxicological understanding of the mechanism. This approach falls between investigation of a specific toxicity and its prediction by analysing GEPs derived from using a variety of drugs with known effects on a specific cellular phenotype hereby producing sufficient data that can be statistically processed to start the building of a predictive database restricted to PLD.

2.2 Predictive toxicogenomics

Although understanding the molecular events underlying a toxic event is of scientific importance, avoidance of unacceptable toxicities in drug development would be more advantageous to the pharmaceutical industry. A lot of effort and money are currently devoted to predictive toxicogenomics, as the potential repercussion of avoiding toxic side effects would be enormous for the pharmaceutical industry [2, 6, 10]. Unlike mechanistic toxicogenomics which tries to unravel intimate mechanisms of toxicity, predictive toxicogenomics ignores the 'why' and tries to extrapolate the likelihood of the occurrence of a toxic event by using large databases of gene, protein or metabolite expression data. In principal, electronic databases consisting of gene, protein and/or metabolite profiles resulting from known toxicants with characterised pathology should allow relatively accurate toxicity predictions of new NCEs, by comparison of the unknown to the known ones [32, 33]. Different statistical tools have been developed and applied to this end [4, 13, 33, 34] and one of the most popular, but not necessarily the most informative, is the 3-D Principal Component Analysis (PCA) graph. Briefly, this approach consists of the collation of a large amount of data into three main features (or components), that have the most weight to discriminate one sample from another one [35]. Similar toxicants, i.e., producing identical or similar lesions in a specific organ, should produce a similar profile signature and cluster together in a relatively limited space portion of the PCA graph.

On the contrary, a different toxicant should have a combination of principle components placing it in a remote corner, away from other profiles. Control samples should cluster on their own, representing the non-toxic profile or fingerprint. Other statistical tools tend to use similar segregation approaches in a more or less visual way. Some pioneering studies have indeed demonstrated that it is possible to cluster a limited number of hepatotoxic chemicals and drugs according their induced pathologies in liver [36]. Based on this philosophy, the overall strategy to predict NCE toxicology becomes simple. Simple, but long and cumbersome in the initial stages, as the building of such databases is a huge task absolutely essential for the accuracy of the predictions. It is clear that the quality and the quantity of data available to evaluate a new fingerprint determine the accuracy of the prediction. Many databases, particularly those based on transcriptional profiles, are currently under construction in both the academic and industrial world [37, 38]. The aim in developing these databases is to attempt to gather as many fingerprints as possible from different organs from animals treated with known toxicants. Although these efforts are logical and straightforward, most efforts are limited to liver and to a much lesser extent to kidney and bone marrow. The largest databases so far are rat hepatotoxin-based and the best ones claim to bestow 85% accuracy of prediction [39]. The error in predictive value is produced by many limitations. For example, for the ability to discriminate genes that are regulated in response to a toxic insult, it is important that the database contains profiles derived from different families of toxicants with each compound family represented by as many representative members as possible to ascertain that compounds producing similar events do indeed produce similar fingerprints. In toxicology, broad categories of toxicities to simplify recording and interpretation of data have been defined (described in detail in [40]) which for liver include necrosis, phospholipidosis, steatosis, peroxisome proliferators or non-genotoxic carcinogens, cholestatics, tumour promoters. It is unclear how many distinct representatives of each class of toxic compounds are needed to gain a set of genes that accurately predict a certain type of toxic event. The precise delineation of a toxic event is impossible since any toxicity is the result of multiple events with multi-factorial consequences. Hence, building GEPs or other cellular profiles for one type of toxicity requires many samples, leading to a high cost of data generation per organ. Moreover, for every single compound, a meaningful number of independent replicates are required to attain the desired statistical power [13]. Intuitively, the data must be obtained from medicines and not from basic chemicals to be valuable for potential new drug toxicity prediction. This is introducing another layer of complexity, for those compounds will impact the fingerprints through their pharmacology, prior to and at lower doses, than the profiles of toxicological effects. At high doses, the pharmacological or adaptive non-toxicity related profiles will mix up with the one of interest. Hence, such databases must have a control dataset obtained from the vehicle treated animals, but also a low/pharmacological dose to be somehow subtracted from the high/toxic dose. This means larger studies and a larger number of samples to be processed and analysed. This is needed for every single organ for which a toxicity prediction is desired. However, there are different interpretations of what is meant by 'predictive toxicology'. Toxicologists in the pharmaceutical industry do not want to know if a compound will be toxic or not *per se*. Since Paracelsus (1493–1541), each and every one knows that all substances are toxic and only the dose differentiate the poison from the remedy. We also know that the duration of the treatment at low dose will have a great impact in the development of an undesired side effect or not. Hence, what interests the drug toxicologist is to be able to predict what dose will produce a toxic event, what kind of event, in what target organ(s) and which posology will trigger it. Consequently, databases must have more than one time point of sample collection and more than one dose for each compound. Here is the main caveat of predictive pattern recognition databases. It is hoped that transcript, protein, metabolite profiles or the combination of all, originating from single very high dose treatment will predict toxicities of short-term medium dose repeat studies, and that those of short-term repeat studies will be able to predict events of chronic studies at very low doses [33]. There is no strong demonstration of this using real case studies published in the literature at the present time. Also in our hands, it seems that toxic events defined as a histopathological finding or blood chemistry or haematology abnormalities, tends to precede or at best coincide with the very first observable gene changes. Indeed, another fundamental risky hypothesis is that most toxic events, if not all of them, will be preceded by gene modulation and even derive from them. This hypothesis is very often preached as a divine truth in literature reviews and congresses, but there are no hard facts so far to back up this belief. Actually, the opposite is likely to happen and that a single dose high enough to induce a toxic event will be too sudden and too overwhelming to allow any organism to have the time to signal and put in effect transcriptional modulations (Fig. 1) that will in turn induce a toxic event. It is more likely that post-translational protein modification such as (de)phosphorylation, (de)glycosylation, activation cleavage, or recruitment of stored enzymes could be of crucial significance in triggering a toxicity event. They also are likely to precede any transcript modulation that in fact may result from protein/transcription factors activation. Hence, protein databases would have more chances to be predictive than gene ones, but to date, protein data generation are impeded by the slow throughput of the cornerstone 2D gel analysis technique. Protein databases are unfortunately very slow to build up and are not commonly used for attempts of toxicity prediction. Until a technological breakthrough in protein technology, protein profiling will not be used to screen chemical series in the intention of elimination potential toxicants.

Supporters of predictive databases still point out that modifications deriving *from* a toxic event are still characteristic enough to fulfil their primary objective. Although a lot of gene modulation will be common to all injuries, such as heat shock proteins, early stress genes and many chaperones, as well as genes that are part of the cell housekeeping like the proteasome complex, there are still indeed transcript modulations specific enough to produce GEPs that will cluster in large families [32, 33]. However, the value of this tends to be lesser if detectable only after readily observable histopathology. Indeed, the very well established way of characterising toxicity by pathology is simpler, well validated and more cost effective [16].

There are many more trivial issues associated with predictive databases, like the fact that not all animals display the expected toxicology pattern when reproduced for gene transcript profiling studies, but those can be found elsewhere [16, 41]. All those caveats may be sorted out with time, but almost all those databases are derived from animal studies, when in the end, human adverse drug reactions are the real interest. There is however a certain concordance between animal studies and human clinical toxicity

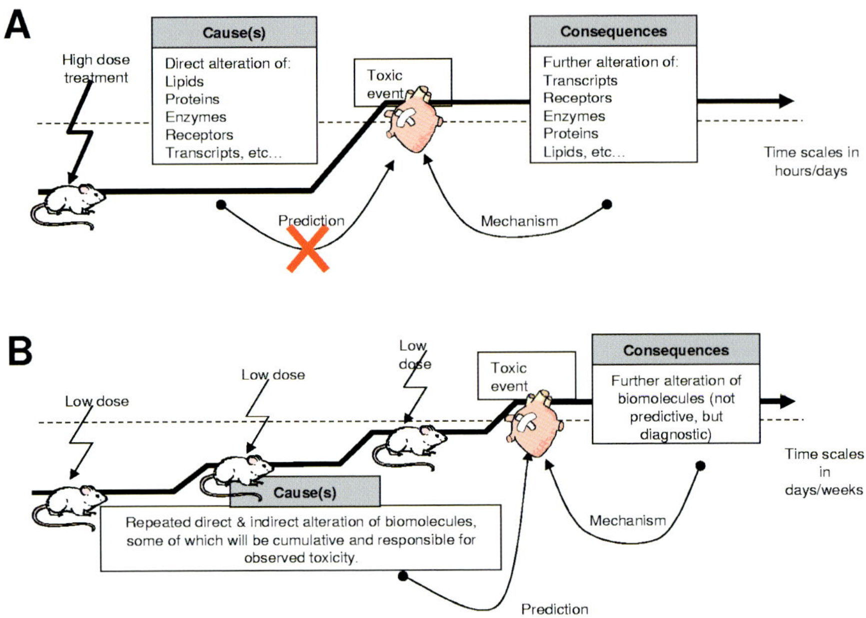

Figure 1.
A) A high dose of a toxic compound will induce a rapid onset of a pathology which will likely be a direct consequence of cell homeostasis disruption rather than gene deregulation. Hence, GEPs are unlikely to be of predictive value in this case. However, there are some hopes for protein profiles. Afterwards, GEPs can be used as diagnostics tools and gene upregulation and downregulation will be specific of the pathology, eventually allowing the understanding of its mechanism and the discovery of biomarkers.
B) Repeated compound administration at low doses will trigger toxic effects for which gene regulation and their products will have an impact on pathological events. These gene regulations may reflect either cellular defences or attempts of repair, as well as being part to the toxicity itself. In that case, toxicologists hope to find profiles that will predict the toxicity event.

[42] and if really of value to predict animal toxicity, those databases will eliminate a certain number of unwanted adverse events. However, they are very unlikely to provide clues about more specific and idiosyncratic human toxic side effects that are not even detected in classical animal studies. That is one of the reasons why non-invasive metabonomics studies may add so much value as they can be run from human samples. Metabonomics results present an exquisite challenge to the analysis as they reflect not only the toxic compound-induced changes, but also the basal metabolism of the

tested organism as determined by its genetics, the food intake, the diurnal variation and cycles, male and female hormonal differences and cycles, the very important microbial metabolism in quantity and quality, pre- or post-exercise samples and cross-interaction of all the above [43]. However, it is commonly hoped that pathological effects are overwhelmingly stronger than endogenous variations and hence relatively easily teased out from this messy background [44].

Metabonomics-based predictive databases may then be the best option for all of the above and because of its amenability to high-throughput platforms. However, it is not possible to deliberately dose humans with high doses of medicines; therefore metabonomics will never provide a thorough analysis of clinical samples relevant to toxicology. Hence, *in vitro* cell culture of human origin may also be used for building prediction databases [45, 46], but then the predictivity of *in vitro versus in vivo* as a whole needs first to be established, which is still very limited despite decades of multiple attempts by a variety of organisations such as the Interagency Coordinating Committee on the Validation of Alternative Methods (ICCVAM; http://iccvam.niehs.nih.gov) or the European Centre for the Validation of Alternative Methods (ECVAM; http://ecvam.jrc.cec.eu.int).

All this taken together may seem to paint a very grim picture, but the solution to the challenge may be in the realisation that the fundamental dogma one gene, one transcript, one protein, one function is an oversimplified concept and that in fact everything interacts with multiple partners at all levels, by association, inhibition, activation, translocation, amplification and so on. Despite the apparent additional complexity and thus a possible strengthening of the issue, analysis of those interactions by so-called pathway analysis and systems biology, may take us to a higher level of observation and hence enable us to see the true global picture of a toxic event [5]. Then, it would not be a specific subset of genes seemingly unrelated to each other, either up or down that would provide a predictive answer, but very well the activation or deactivation of one or several biological pathways, either partially or in total that would provide a real prediction of potential toxicity. There is little doubt that this approach is our best chance in matters of toxicity prediction, but there are so much more data to produce and collate into easily exploitable databases, that this avenue will not be in use before many years despite some efforts to gather data from many sources together [37, 38].

2.3 Specific considerations for toxicogenomics in anti-infectives

Toxicogenomics databanks are usually built from a patho-toxicological viewpoint rather than from a pharmacology perspective. For example, characteristics transcript profiles will be grouped by toxic event such as microvesicular steatosis, regardless of the nature of the inducer, which can range from psychiatric drugs to antivirals. Hence, as far as is known, there are no toxicogenomics databanks dedicated to anti-infective agents. However, many transcript-profiling databases include some antibiotics as organ specific toxicants. Toxicologists are grouping medicine-related side effects into two broad categories: 1) undesired effects linked to the pharmacology (exaggerated pharmacology), which may happen in any organ expressing the drug target, and 2) chemistry-related toxicities which can be either by direct toxicity (membrane lysis, uncoupling agent, etc...) or by interaction with another biomolecule other than that targeted (enzyme inhibitor, receptor modulator, etc...). Genomics has brought the possibility to develop a whole new range of microbe specific targets ([47, 48] and Chapter 2). This should decrease the incidence of pharmacology-related toxicities in preclinical investigations and ultimately in the clinic. However, this does not prevent chemistry-related toxicities from occurring.

Anti-infectives have not been thoroughly investigated in terms of toxicogenomics. In fact, bibliographical searches with numerous terms related to anti-infectives, antibiotics and antivirals in combination with genomics-related and toxicity-related items in a combination of databases like BIOSIS Previews, Current Contents, EMBASE, IPAB and MEDLINE does not yield a single article or review at the time this paper is written. This reflects the current pioneering status of toxicogenomics as a whole, but there is little doubt that anti-infective drugs will soon be included in such studies, as at least one abstract entitled "Toxicogenomics and anti-infective agents" has been deposited in the *Abstract of Interscience Conference on Antimicrobial Agents and Chemotherapy* in 2001.

For example, chloramphenicol and the oxazolidinone antibiotics class represented by Zyvox^{TM}(linezolid) have a relatively close pharmacology. They both specifically inhibit bacterial protein synthesis, though through different mechanisms [49, 50]. Their chemical structures are very different but their toxic effects on the bone marrow are remarkably similar as they both specifically induce red cell anaemia [51, 52]. A thorough mechanistic study comparing the transcript profiling in bone marrow red cell lineage only would likely bring clues of the mechanism of toxicity of these two antibiotics, which so far remains unknown. Although of different chemistry and similar but not identical pharmacology, molecular clues would help to dissociate or associate chloramphenicol and oxazolidinones in an antibiotics specific class of toxicity. In our hands, oxazolidinone compounds also induced blood reticulocyte reduction and bone marrow erythroblast diminution. We used a potent erythropenia-inducer oxazolidinone to study the total bone marrow transcript profile of mice treated for 5 days at 100 mg/kg/day, by means of the Affymetrix platform and U74Av2 chip which displays about 12,500 genes and Expressed Sequence Tags (ESTs). We found a total of 328 transcripts significantly upregulated by two-fold or more and 301 transcripts significantly downregulated by two-fold or more. Without going into details, many red cell specific mRNAs were found to be decreased which may or not just reveal the decline of the targeted population. Interestingly, upregulated transcripts were largely belonging to granulocytic, myeloid and lymphoid lineages, some of which like the granulocyte colony-stimulating factor receptor (G-CSF, accession number: 93198_at) was increased by 14-fold compared to controls. Despite the number of modulated genes in this short study, it has not been possible to establish a firm conclusion about the mode of toxicity, but rather to postulate a number of hypotheses, which all would require many more biochemical investigations to refine a likely mechanism. This demonstrates that in absence of previous knowledge, a simple but thorough transcriptomics study is not enough to provide deep insight into toxicity mechanisms.

Mammals have a whole range of specific 'visiting' and syncytial bacteria and fungi not just colonising the gastrointestinal (GI) tract, but in and on almost any possible area like skin, mouth or nasal cavity to mention only a few [53]. They maintain a complex and intimate relationship with the host, and GI microbial genomes taken altogether may surpass their human host genetic diversity by a factor 100 [53]. It is also well known that one of the main side effects of antibiotics is precisely to disturb this gut flora leading to displeasing digestive malfunctions. These intestinal hosts have a very active metabolic life, including cytochrome P450s that are interacting with host drug metabolism, producing active and inactive metabolites, as well as toxic metabolites, which in turn can display a whole range of remote toxicity, i.e., away from the intestinal tract [54]. Studying all the possible interactions between host, endogenous bacteria and antibiotics appears impossible, even using an 'omics approach. First, it is unlikely that we will soon determine the complete genome and the subsequent biology of the thousand odd species populating our guts, as some are even not known yet [53]. Second, the level of co-metabolism and metabolic exchanges are such that only a global approach, ignoring the intermediate steps could provide some insight [54]. And third, the gut flora is highly variable from one individual to the next for all the possible reasons of life style, food variety, environment and so on [54]. Those differences are even more pronounced between humans and the species that we use for safety preclinical studies. It is after all possible that the poor concordance of toxicity between species may reside in large part into the vast differences of our respective 'microbiomes' [54].

Hence, because of all of the above, prediction of anti-infective toxicity is treated in the same way as for any other drug. However, toxicogenomics applied to anti-infectives could be centred on their most common target organs for toxicity like the GI tract, bone marrow, liver and kidney.

3 Conclusion

Toxicogenomics as a tool grouping transcriptomics, proteomics and metabonomics, is in an even more pioneering stage than genomics applied to other biological sciences. Investigative toxicogenomics has already made some respectable advances in the exploration of mechanisms of drug side effects whereas predictive toxicogenomics still faces many hurdles. The construction of meaningful databases sufficiently populated with profiles deriving from medicines administered at toxic level to animal models is currently benefiting from a significant effort from the scientific community. It is unfortunately too early to decide if the reward will live up to the hopes and promises. Toxicogenomics applied specifically to anti-infective drugs is so far absent from the literature. However, antibiotics are being used as model toxicants to populate predictive databases with respect to the specific toxicities they trigger. By increasing the number of entries in predictive databanks, it may be possible that anti-infectives will generate some specific sub-classes of toxicity, which could be further exploited for accurate toxicity modelling of future drugs. However, the complexities of the interactions between endogenous bacteria, pathogenic bacteria, hosts and antibiotics appear so multifaceted that these drugs are currently dealt with in the same way as any other drug.

Acknowledgements

Drs H. Powell and P. Greaves are sincerely thanked for their most valuable help in reviewing this chapter.

References

1 Colebatch G, Trevaskis B, Udvardi M (2002) Functional genomics: Tools of the trade. *New Phytol* 153: 27–36

2 Mahler SM, Chin DY, Van Dyk DD (2003) The application of emerging technologies in genomics and proteomics to drug development. *J Pharm Pract Res* 33: 7–11

3 van Hall NL, Vorst O, van Houwelingen AM, Kok EJ, Peijnenburg A, Aharoni A, van Tunen AJ, Keijer J (2000) The application of DNA microarray in gene expression analysis. *J Biotechnol* 78: 271–280

4 Butte A (2002) The use and analysis of microarray data. *Nat Rev Drug Disc* 1: 951–960

5 Nicholson JK, Wilson ID (2003) Understanding 'global' systems biology: metabonomics and the continuum of metabolism. *Nat Rev Drug Discov* 2: 668–676

6 De Longueville F, Bertholet V, Remacle J (2004) DNA microarrays as a tool in toxicogenomics. *Comb Chem High Throughput Screening* 7: 207–211

7 Witkampt RF (2005) Genomics and system biology – how relevant are the developments to veterinary pharmacology, toxicology and therapeutics? *J Vet Pharmacol Therap* 28: 235–245

8 Loferer H, Jacobi A, Posch A, Gauss C, Meier-Ewert S, Seizinger B (2000) Integrated bacterial genomics for the discovery of novel antimicrobials. *Drug Discovery Today* 5: 107–114
9 Tugwood JD, Hollins LE, Cockerill MJ (2003) Genomics and the search for novel biomarkers in toxicology. *Biomarkers* 8: 79–92
10 Kramer JA, Kolaja K (2002) Toxicogenomics: an opportunity to optimise drug development and safety evaluation. *Expert Opin Drug Saf* 1: 275–286
11 Wildsmith S, Spence F (2003) Preparation and utilisation of microarrays. In: ME Burczynski (ed): *An introduction to toxicogenomics*. CRC Press, Boca Raton, USA, pp 3–16
12 Li J, Johnson JA (2003) Comparative studies using cDNA vs. oligonucleotide arrays. In: ME Burczynski (ed): *An introduction to toxicogenomics*. CRC Press, Boca Raton, USA. pp 17–27
13 Sebastiani P, Gussoni E, Kohane IS, Ramoni MF (2003) Statistical challenges in functional genomics. *Stat Sci* 18: 33–60
14 Ge H, Walhout AJ, Vidal M (2003) Integrating 'omic' information: a bridge between genomics and systems biology. *Trends Genet* 19: 551–560
15 Guerreiro N, Staedtler F, Grenet O, Kehren J, Chibout S-D (2003) Toxicogenomics in drug development. *Toxicol Pathol* 31: 471–479
16 Pognan F (2004) Genomics, proteomics and metabonomics in toxicology: Hopefully not 'fashionomics'. *Pharmacogenomics* 5: 879–893
17 Muckter H (2003) What is toxicology and how does it occur? *Baillieres Best Pract Res Clin Anaes* 17: 5–27
18 Chan VSW, Theilade MD (2005) The use of toxicogenomic data in risk assessment: A regulatory perspective. *Clin Toxicol* 43: 121–126
19 Scheel J, von Brevern M-C, Storck T (2003) An overview of mechanistic toxicogenomics studies. In: ME Burczynski (ed): *An introduction to toxicogenomics*. CRC Press, Boca Raton, USA. pp 183–209
20 Fountoulakis M, Berndt P, Boelsterli UA, Crameri F, Winter M, Albertini S, Suter L (2000) Two-dimensional database of mouse liver proteins: Changes in hepatic protein levels following treatment with acetaminophen or its nontoxic regioisomer 3-acetamidophenol. *Electrophoresis* 21: 2148–2161
21 Reilly TP, Bourdi M, Brady JN, Pise-Masison CA, Radonovich MF, George JW, Pohl LR (2001) Expression profiling of acetaminophen liver toxicity in mice using microarray technology. *Biochem Biophys Res Com* 282: 321–328
22 Ruepp SU, Tonge RP, Shaw J, Wallis N, Pognan F (2002) Genomics and proteomics analysis of acetaminophen toxicity in mouse liver. *Toxicol Sci* 65: 135–150
23 Coen M, Lenz EM, Nicholson JK, Wilson ID, Pognan F, Lindon JC (2003). An integrated metabonomic investigation of acetaminophen toxicity in the mouse using NMR spectroscopy. *Chem Res Tox* 16: 295–303
24 Coen M, Ruepp SU, Lindon JC, Nicholson JK, Pognan F, Lenz EM, Wilson ID (2004) Application of transcriptomics and metabonomics yields new insight into the toxicity due to paracetamol in the mouse. *J Pharm Biomed Anal* 35: 93–105
25 Milano J, McKay J, Dagenais C, Foster-Brown L, Pognan F, Gadient R, Jacobs RT, Zacco A, Greenberg B, Ciaccio PJ (2004) Modulation of notch processing by

gamma-secretase inhibitors causes intestinal goblet cell metaplasia and induction of genes known to specify gut secretory lineage differentiation. *Toxicol Sci* 82: 341–358
26 Cornwell PD, de Souza AT, Ulrich RG (2004) Profiling of hepatic gene expression in rats treated with fibric acid analogs. *Mut Res* 549: 131–145
27 Peters JM, Cattley RC, Gonzalez FJ (1997) Role of PPAR alpha in the mechanism of action of the nongenotoxic carcinogen and peroxisome proliferator Wy-14,643. *Carcinogenesis* 18: 2029–2033
28 Montenez JP, Van Bambeke F, Piret J, Brasseur R, Tulkens PM, Mingeot-Leclercq MP (1999) Interactions of macrolide antibiotics (Erythromycin A, roxithromycin, erythromycylamine [Dirithromycin], and azithromycin) with phospholipids: computer-aided conformational analysis and studies on acellular and cell culture models. *Toxicol Appl Pharmacol* 156: 129–140
29 Casartelli A, Bonato M, Cristofori P, Crivellente F, Dal Negro G, Masotto I, Mutinelli C, Valko K, Bonfante V (2003) A cell-based approach for the early assessment of the phospholipidogenic potential in pharmaceutical research and drug development. *Cell Biol Toxicol* 19: 161–176
30 Morelli JK, Buehrle M, Pognan F, Barone L, Fieles W, Ciaccio PJ (2006) Validation of an *in vitro* screen for phopholipidosis using a high content biology platform. *Cell Biol Toxicol* 22: 15–27
31 Sawada H, Takami K, Asahi SA (2005) Toxicogenomic approach to drug-induced phospholipidosis: Analysis of its induction mechanism and establishment of a novel *in vitro* screening system. *Tox Sci* 83: 282–292
32 Suter L, Babiss LE, Wheeldon EB (2004) Toxicogenomics in predictive toxicology drug development. *Chem Biol* 11: 161–171
33 Porter MW, Castle AL, Orr MS, Mendrick DL (2003) Predictive toxicogenomics. In: ME Burczynski (ed): *An introduction to toxicogenomics*. CRC Press, Boca Raton, USA. pp 183–209
34 Sherlock G (2000) Analysis of large-scale gene expression data. *Curr Opin Immunol* 12: 201–205
35 Joliffe IT, Morgan BJ (1992) Principal component analysis and exploratory factor analysis. *Stat Methods Med Res* 1: 69–95
36 Waring JF, Jolly RA, Ciurlionis R, Lum PY, Praestgaard JT, Morfitt DC, Buratto B, Roberts C, Schadt E, Ulrich RG (2001) Clustering of hepatotoxins based on mechanism of toxicity using gene expression profiles. *Toxicol Appl Pharmacol* 175: 28–42
37 Mattes WB, Pettit SD, Sansone S-A, Bushel PR, Waters MD (2004) Database development in toxicogenomics: Issues and efforts. *Environ Health Perspect* 112: 495–505
38 Hayes KR, Vollrath AL, Zastrow GM, McMillan BJ, Craven M, Jovanovich S, Rank DR, Penn S, Walisser JA, Reddy JK et al (2005) EDGE: A centralized resource for the comparison, analysis, and distribution of toxicogenomic information. *Mol Pharmacol* 67: 1360–1368
39 Huby R, Tugwood JD (2005) Gene expression profiling for pharmaceutical safety assessment. *Expert Opin Drug Metab Toxicol* 1: 247–260

40 Klaassen CD (ed) (2001) *Casarett and Doull's toxicology: the basic science of poisons.* Sixth Edition. McGraw-Hill, New York, USA

41 Luhe A, Suter L, Ruepp S, Singer T, Weiser T, Albertini S (2005) Toxicogenomics in the pharmaceutical industry: Hollow promises or real benefit? *Mut Res* 575: 102–115

42 Olson H, Betton G, Robinson D, Thomas K, Monro A, Kolaja G, Lilly P, Sanders J, Sipes G, Bracken W et al (2000) Concordance of the toxicity of pharmaceuticals in humans and in animals. *Regul Toxicol Pharmacol* 32: 56–67

43 Bollard ME, Holmes E, Lindon JC, Mitchell SC, Branstetter D, Zhang W, Nicholson JK (2001) Investigations into biochemical changes due to diurnal variation and estrus cycle in female rats using high-resolution (1)H NMR spectroscopy of urine and pattern recognition. *Anal Biochem* 295: 194–202

44 Wang Y, Tang H, Nicholson JK, Hylands PJ, Sampson J, Holmes E (2005) A metabonomic strategy for the detection of the metabolic effects of chamomile (Matricaria recutita L.) ingestion. *J Agric Food Chem* 53: 191–196

45 Boess F, Kamber M, Romer S, Gasser R, Muller D, Albertini S, Suter L (2003) Gene expression in two hepatic cell lines, cultured primary hepatocytes, and liver slices compared to the *in vivo* liver gene expression in rats: possible implications for toxicogenomics use of *in vitro* systems. *Toxicol Sci* 73: 386–402

46 Kier LD, Neft R, Tang L, Suizu R, Cook T, Onsurez K, Tiegler K, Sakai Y, Ortiz M, Nolan T et al (2004) Applications of microarrays with toxicologically relevant genes (tox genes) for the evaluation of chemical toxicants in Sprague Dawley rats *in vivo* and human hepatocytes *in vitro*. *Mutat Res* 549: 101–113

47 de Backer MD, van Dijck P (2003) Progress in functional genomics approaches to antifungal drug target discovery. *Trends in Microbiol* 11: 470–478

48 Parkinson T (2002) The impact of genomics on anti-infectives drugs discovery and development. *Trends in Microbiol* 10: S22–26

49 Contreras A, Barbacid M, Vazquez D (1974) Binding to ribosomes and mode of action of chloramphenicol analogues. *Biochim Biophys Acta* 349: 376–388

50 Matassova NB, Rodnina MV, Endermann R, Kroll HP, Pleiss U, Wild H, Wintermeyer W (1999) Ribosomal RNA is the target for oxazolidinones, a novel class of translational inhibitors. *RNA* 5: 939–946

51 Turton JA, Yallop D, Andrews CM, Fagg R, York M, Williams TC (1999) Haemotoxicity of chloramphenicol succinate in the CD-1 mouse and Wistar Hanover rat. *Hum Exp Toxicol* 18: 566–576

52 Gerson SL, Kaplan SL, Bruss JB, Le V, Arellano FM, Hafkin B, Kuter DJ. (2002) Hematologic effects of linezolid: summary of clinical experience. *Antimicrob Agents Chemother* 46: 2723–2726

53 Xu J, Gordon JI (2003) Honor thy symbionts. *Proc Natl Acad Sci USA* 100: 10452–10459

54 Nicholson JK, Holmes E, Wilson ID (2005) Gut microorganisms, mammalian metabolism and personalized health care. *Nat Rev Microbiol* 3: 431–438

Progress in Drug Research, Vol. 64
(Helena I. Boshoff and Clifton E. Barry III, Eds)

Biological robustness in complex host-pathogen systems

By Hiroaki Kitano[1,2]

[1]The Systems Biology Institute,
Suite 6A,
M31 6-31-15 Jingumae,
Shibuya, Tokyo 150-0001, Japan

[2]Sony Computer Science Laboratories, Inc.,
3-14-13 Higashi-Gotanda,
Shinagawa, Tokyo 141-0022, Japan

Abstract

Infectious diseases are still the number one killer of human beings. Even in developed countries, infectious diseases continue to be a major health threat. This article explores a conceptual framework for understanding infectious diseases in the context of the complex dynamics between microbe and host, and explores theoretical strategies for anti-infectives. The central pillar of this conceptual framework is that biological robustness is a fundamental property of systems that is closely interlinked with the evolution of symbiotic host-pathogen systems. There are specific architectural features of such robust yet evolvable systems and interpretable trade-offs between robustness, fragility, resource demands, and performance. This concept applies equally to both microbes and host. Pathogens have evolved to exploit the host using various strategies as well as effective escape mechanisms. Modular pathogenicity islands (PAI) derived from horizontal gene transfer, highly variable surface molecules, and a range of other countermeasures enhance the robustness of a pathogen against attacks from the host immune system. The host has likewise evolved complex defensive mechanisms to protect itself against pathogenic threats, but the host immune system includes several trade-offs that can be exploited by pathogens and induces undesirable inflammatory reactions. Due to the complexity of the dynamics emerging from the interactions of multiple microbes and a host, effective counter-measures require an in-depth understanding of system dynamics as well as detailed molecular mechanisms of the processes that are involved.

1 Robustness is a fundamental organizational principle of biological systems

Robustness is the property of systems to maintain a certain function despite external and internal perturbations. This property is ubiquitously observed in various aspects of biological systems as reviewed extensively [1, 2]. It is distinctively a system-level property that cannot be observed simply by looking at isolated components. The specific components of a system and their interactions, the system functions that are required to be maintained, and the types of perturbations that the system shows robustness against must be well defined in order to understand the biological significance of the particular system and its behavior. For example, modern airplanes (system) have complex instrumentation allowing them to maintain a flight path (function) against atmospheric turbulence (perturbation). Bacterial chemotaxis is a well documented example of system robustness. Chemotaxis of a bacterial cell along a ligand concentration gradient is maintained against perturbations such as dramatic changes in ligand concentration and different rate constants for the interactions involved [3–5]. The network for segmental polarity formation during embryogenesis of *Drosophila* robustly produces repetitive stripes of differential gene expressions despite variations in the initial concentration of substances involved, as well as variation in the kinetic parameters of these interactions [6, 7].

Why is robustness so important? First, it is a feature that is observed ubiquitously in biological systems; from such fundamental processes as phage fate decision switching [8] and bacterial chemotaxis [3–5] to developmental plasticity [6] and even at the level of whole ecosystems [9]. This implies that robustness may be a basic universal principle of biological systems.

Second, robustness against environmental and genetic perturbations is essential for evolvability [10–12]. Evolvability requires the generation of a variety of non-lethal phenotypes and genetic buffering [13, 14]. Mechanisms that attain robustness against environmental perturbations may also be used for attaining robustness against mutations, developmental stability, and other features that facilitate evolvability [1, 10–12].

Third, various human diseases can be usefully considered as perturbations that threaten a robust host, or as a separate robust system emerging with the host as perturbant. For example, cancer can be considered as a robust system and approaches to interfere with the robustness of tumors have been argued as essential [15, 16]. Type 2 diabetes may be a result of robustness mechanisms acquired through human evolution during long periods of malnutrition, with selection for specific pathogen resistance, and other hostile environmental conditions that now leave us maladapted for modern living conditions [17]. This perspective is particularly relevant in infectious diseases as these are essentially a dynamic interaction between host and pathogen systems which both have their own robustness and fragility properties.

2 Four underlying general mechanisms for robustness

2.1 System control

Extensive system control is typically encountered in robust systems, particularly negative feedback loops, to make the system dynamically stable around a specific state. Integral feedback used in bacterial chemotaxis is a typical example [3–5]. Due to integral feedback, bacteria can sense changes of chemoattractant and chemorepellant independent of absolute concentration so that proper chemotaxis behavior is maintained over a wide range of ligand concentration. In addition, the same mechanism makes the bacteria insensitive to changes in rate constants involved in the circuit. Positive feedback is often used to create bi-stability in signal transduction and cell cycle systems, to make them tolerant against minor perturbations in stimuli and rate constants [18–20].

2.2 Alternative (fail-safe)

Alternative (or fail-safe) mechanisms increase tolerance against component failure and environmental changes by providing alternative components or methods to ultimately maintain system functions. Sometimes, there are multiple components that are similar to each other that are redundant. In other cases, different means are used to cope with perturbations that cannot be handled by other means. This is often called phenotypic plasticity [21, 22] or diversity. Redundancy and phenotypic plasticity are often considered as opposites, but it is more consistent to view them as different ways to provide alternative fail-safe mechanisms.

2.3 Modularity

Modularity provides isolation of perturbations from the rest of the system. The cell is the most significant example. More subtle and less obvious examples are modules of biochemical and gene regulatory networks. Modules also play an important role during developmental processes by buffering perturbations so that proper pattern formation can be accomplished [6, 23, 24]. The definition of modules and how to detect such modules are still controversial, but the general consensus is that modules do exist and play an important role [25].

2.4 Decoupling

Decoupling isolates low-level noise and fluctuations from functional level structures and dynamics. For example Hsp90 provides genetic buffering in which misfolding of proteins due to environmental stresses is fixed, and thus the effects of such perturbations are isolated from the functions of circuits. This mechanism applies also to genetic variations where genetic changes in a coding region that may affect protein structures are masked because protein folding is fixed by Hsp90 unless such masking is removed by extreme stress [11, 26, 27]. Emergent behaviors of complex networks also exhibit such buffering property [28]. These effects may constitute canalization proposed by Waddington [29]. The recent discovery by Uri Alon's group on oscillatory expression of p53 upon DNA damage may exemplify decoupling at the signal encoding level [30], because stimuli invoked pulses of p53 activation level, instead of gradual changes, effectively converting analog signals into digital signals. Digital pulse encoding may indicate robust information transmission, although further investigations are required before any conclusions can be drawn.

An example of a sophisticated engineering system clearly illustrates how these mechanisms work as a whole system. An airplane maintains its flight path by following the commands of the pilot against atmospheric perturbations and various internal perturbations including changes in the center of gravity due to fuel consumption and movement of passengers, as well as mechanical inaccuracies. This function is carried out by controlling flight control surfaces (rudder, flaps, elevators, etc.) and the propulsion system (engines) by an automatic flight control system (AFCS). Extensive negative feedback control is used to correct deviations of flight path. The reliability of the AFCS is critically important for a stable flight. To increase reliability, the AFCS is composed of three independently implemented modules (a triple redundancy system) that all meet the same functional specifications. Most of the AFCS is digitalized, so that low-level noise of voltage fluctuations is effectively decoupled from the digital signals that define the functions of the system. Due to these mechanisms, modern airplanes are highly robust against various perturbations.

3 Intrinsic features of robust systems: Evolvability and trade-offs

Robustness is a basis of evolvability, and evolution tends to select individuals with robust traits [1]. For the system to be evolvable, it must be able to produce a variety of non-lethal phenotypes [14]. At the same time, genetic variations need to be accumulated as a neutral network, so that pools of genetic variants are exposed when the environment changes suddenly. Systems that are robust against environmental perturbations employ mechanisms such as system control, fail-safe alternatives, modularity, and decoupling. These mechanisms also support the generation of non-lethal phenotypes and genetic buffering. In addition, the capability to generate flexible phenotypes and robustness require the emergence of a bow-tie structure as an architectural motif [31]. One of the reasons why robustness in biological systems is so ubiquitous is because it facilitates evolution, and evolution tends to select traits that are robust against environmental perturbations. This leads to successive addition of system controls.

Systems that have acquired robustness against certain perturbations through design or evolution have intrinsic trade-offs between robustness, fragility, performance, and resource demands. Carlson and Doyle argued, using simple examples from physics and forest fires, that systems that are optimized for specific perturbations are extremely fragile against unexpected perturbations [32, 33]. Systems that have been designed, or have evolved, optimally (either global optimal or sub-optimal) against certain perturbations are called High Optimized Tolerance (HOT) systems. Csete and Doyle further argued that robustness is a conserved quantity [34]. This means that when robustness is enhanced against a range of perturbations, then there must be a trade-off by fragility elsewhere as well as compromised performance and increased resource demands.

A robust yet fragile trade-off can be understood intuitively using the airplane example again. Comparing modern commercial airplanes and the Wright Flyer, modern commercial airplanes are several orders of magnitude more robust against atmospheric perturbations than the Wright Flyer, owing to sophisticated flight control systems. However, such flight control systems rely entirely on electricity. In the inconceivable event of a total power failure in which all electrical power is lost in the airplane, the airplane can no longer be controlled at all. Obviously, airplane manufacturers are well aware of this issue, and take every possible countermeasure to minimize such a risk. On the other hand, despite its vulnerability against atmospheric perturbations, the Wright Flyer could never have been affected by a power failure because there was no reliance on electricity. This extreme example illustrates that systems that are optimized for certain perturbations could be extremely fragile against unusual perturbations.

Highly Optimized Tolerance (HOT) model systems are successively optimized and designed (although not necessarily globally optimized) against perturbations, whereas Self-Organized Criticality (SOC) [35] or Scale-Free Networks [36] are the unconstrained stochastic addition of components without design or optimization. Such differences affect the failure patterns of the systems, and so have direct implications for understanding the nature of disease and therapy design.

Unlike Scale-Free Networks, HOT systems are robust against perturbations such as the removal of hubs provided the systems are optimized against such perturbations. However, systems are generally fragile against 'fail-on' type failures in which a component failure results in a continuous malfunction, instead of ceasing to function ('fail-off'), so that incorrect signals keep being transmitted. This type of failure is known in engineering as the Byzantine Generals Problem [37], named after a problem in the Byzantine army that arose when there were multiple generals dispersed in the field, some of whom were traitors who sent incorrect messages to confuse the army.

Disease often reflects systemic failure triggered by a fragility of the system. Diabetes mellitus is an excellent example of how systems that are optimized for near-starving, intermittent food supply, high energy utilization lifestyle, and highly infectious conditions, are fragile against unusual perturbations such as high energy content foods and low energy utilization lifestyle [17]. Due to optimization to the near-starving condition, extensive control to maintain minimum blood glucose level has been acquired so that activities of the central nervous system and innate immunity are maintained. However, no effective regulatory loop has been developed against excessive energy intake, and feedback regulation serves to reduce glucose uptake by adipocyte and skeletal muscle cells because it may reduce plasma glucose level below the acceptable level. These mechanisms lead to the state that blood glucose level is chronically maintained at higher than the desired level and for a longer time than it has been optimized for, leading to cardiovascular complications.

4 Robustness attributes of pathogens

Pathogens exploit host systems for their survival and proliferation. Often, they exploit host immune reactions to achieve this goal. There are several means that pathogens employ to attain a certain level of robustness against host immunity including countermeasures to neutralize the effects of host immunity, evade host recognition through countermeasures and genetic variations, and mechanisms to hijack host immune reactions seen in some of pathogens. *Shigella* avoids autophage by secreting IcsB effector [38]. In the initial phase of *Salmonella* infection of a macrophage, it triggers apoptosis by the SipB protein coded on SPI1 that activates caspase-1 [39]. Soon after the infection, SPI1 transcribed SipB is inhibited, and *Salmonella* replicate within *Salmonella*-containing vacuole (SCV) in which SPI2 encoded genes triggers a series of events for replication and further proliferation [40]. *Listeria monocytogenes* escapes the hazards of the phagosome by creating pores on its membrane with listeriolysin O (LLO) that is encoded by the *hly* gene on the *Listeria* pathogenicity island-1 (LIPI-1) [41]. It is interesting to note that these counter measures depend on the function of a single gene on a modular DNA region called Pathogenicity Island (PAI) of each pathogen, and have been acquired through evolution [42, 43]. Knockout of such gene disables escape capability of pathogens. Thus, in a sense each pathogen's capacity to maintain pathogenicity against mutation is not robust, but the system can be robust in terms of the global pathogen population as a whole because genes accountable for pathogenicity may be horizontally transferred. For example, *Vibrio cholerae* is a pathogen that periodically causes epidemics in many developing countries through contamination of food and water supplies. It produces a toxin that interacts with G-protein, and causes diarrhea. Cholerae-toxin is encoded by a PAI, which is considered to have been acquired through horizontal gene transfer (HGT) [44]. Likewise, some pathogenic attributes of enteroinvasive *E. coli*, such as O157, have been demonstrated to have resulted from the acquisition of toxic genes in its PAI by HGT. Emergence of drug resistant bacteria sometimes involves emergence of one or more bacteria that acquired the drug resistance followed by horizontal transfer of genes that encoded genes responsible to resistant phenotype. The modular structure of PAI enhances HGT-based acquisition of pathogenicity, thus contributing to robust maintenance of pathogenicity of the pathogen population, rather than individual.

It should be noted that within pathogens there are also trade-offs between robustness, fragility, resource demands, and performance of specific functions. It is clear that each individual pathogen is not so robust against host immunity and mutation is the mechanism through evolution to foster faster replication under minimum resource requirements. Assuming that each pathogen is built to be more robust against mutation and host immune responses it must incorporate a range of complex mechanisms that requires more resources to survive and more time to replicate. Such trade-off is certainly not desirable for pathogens. This is particularly the case for a class of pathogens that carry out ‘frontal attack’ strategies, according to Merrell and Falkow. They classified host attack strategies of pathogens into two types: frontal attack and stealth attack [45]. Frontal attack is to infect the host and quickly replicate itself and possibly overwhelm the host defense before the host adaptive immune system counteracts. This is the strategy taken by many pathogens including *V. cholerae*, and exploits the problem of time-lag to activate adaptive immunity. Thus, one general strategy of some pathogens chosen through evolution is to sacrifice individual robustness, in favor of population robustness.

Although robustness at pathogen-wide level is an interesting feature that is unique to microbial populations, each individual often exhibits robustness against host immune responses by providing variations of surface molecules to escape from the host immune recognition, and by being totally invisible to the host system. The strategy of evading immune recognition by changing biologic markers that appear on the membrane surface is illustrated by Trypanosomes that can generate highly variable surface molecules known as variant surface glycoprotein (VSG) coat to evade B cell response [46]. While the strategy of switching surface molecules to involves some level of host recognition of the pathogen, another strategy is to be totally invisible from the host immune system. For example, *Helicobacter pylori*, which infects the human stomach and is associated with stomach cancer [47], has flagellins that are not detectable by the host's TLR5. It also inhibits proliferation of T cells and B cell by vacuolating cytotoxin (VacA) and CagA that blocks T cell receptor and B cell's JAK-STAT signaling, respectively [48]. Thus, these pathogens effectively blind the host immune system. While these strategies generally enhance survivability of pathogens, it does not enhance robustness of pathogens against host immune response once it is triggered. The strategy exploits the fragility of the host immune system to allow the pathogen to escape from the response.

Hijackers invade the host immune system without being noticed, or induce the host immune cells to take up such microbes, and proliferate as well as attack the host using the host immune reactions. The most significant example of the hijacker is human immunodeficiency virus (HIV). Acquired immune deficiency syndrome (AIDS) is a syndrome in which HIV specifically invades and attacks the core of the innate immune response, CD4+ T cells [49]. HIV infection depletes CD4+ T cells as the disease progresses, causing the immune system to be gradually disabled and become prone to opportunistic pathogens [49]. HIV infection is robust against the immune response and against various therapies to which drug-resistant escape mutants readily appear [50]. Thus, HIV can be viewed as a hijacker of the immune system as actions to remove the virus infection in general triggers further spread of the HIV virus itself. One countermeasure for the genetic diversity of HIV is to use combinations of drugs that do not give cross resistance in their target. A specific mutation that gave resistance to one drug would leave sensitivity to the other, and *vice versa*. AZT-3TC combination therapy illustrates a successful case where resistance mechanisms for two drugs used are independent of each other. The HIV-1 virus can acquire resistance to 3'-azidothymidine (AZT, zidovudine) by a stepwise accumulation of four out of five mutations in reverse transcriptase (RT) at codons 41, 67, 70, 215, or 219 [51]. For HIV-1 to be resistant against

(-)2′-deoxy-3′-thiacytidine (3TC), it must substitute Val or Leu for Met at codon 184 in RT [52]. Therefore, AZT-resistant virus is 3TC-sensitive, while 3TC-resistant virus is AZT-sensitive [53].

While chemotherapy can suppress disease progress, the underlying robustness of this epidemic remains intact. One interesting countermeasure that has been proposed is to take over mechanisms that provide the robustness of HIV infection. The idea is to design a decoy, a conditionally replicating HIV-1 vector (crHIV-1) [54, 55]. It is designed to contain cis, but does not contain a trans-element that is required for producing virus packaging proteins. It also carries antivirus genes that inhibit wild type HIV replication [56]. This is an interesting 'Trojan Horse' strategy, because it sends in decoys with specific agents that exploit essential mechanisms that ensure the robustness of HIV-1 infection in order to force AIDS into the latent stage, instead of eliminating the HIV-1 virus itself.

5 Limits of a robust system: Pathogen-triggered diseases

A major issue for the host immune system is the trade-off between the ability to cope with a broad range of pathogens without risking misrecognition and possibly harmful inflammation owing to its architectural features as well as inherent fragility of the signaling network that entail non-redundant core in the bow-tie structure in both innate and adaptive immunity [57]. Although the immune system evolved to be very robust to host organisms, there are trade-offs inherent in the system. The fragilities of the immune system arise directly from the inherent properties that have been optimized on an evolutionary time scale. There are five major weak links: (1) reliance on MyD88 in TLR signaling, (2) MHC presentation and recognition, (3) reliance on CD4+ T cells as the cornerstone for adaptive immunity, (4) a cytokine network that has been tuned to be highly proinflammatory and which may cause damage to the host organism when hyper-activated, and (5) the time lag between detection of pathogens and activation of adaptive immunity. While no report has been made on infectious disease that actively neutralizes MyD88 functions, all other four weaknesses have been critical in certain infectious diseases. HIV infects

CD4+ T cell – the core of adaptive immunity and gradually destroy adaptive immunity. 'Frontal attack' type pathogens make use of the time lag between detection of pathogens and activation of adaptive immunity.

5.1 Proinflammatory architecture of the host immune system

Analysis of molecular interaction networks of the host immune system indicates that it is fundamentally proinflammatory [58], and requires active control to reduce inflammatory reactions once started [59–61]. There are many positive feedback loops that escalate secretion of cytokines and promote further inflammation. Hyper-activation of a cytokine network, often called 'cytokine storm', is one of the major factors that aggravates patient health and may results in death. For example, influenza infection causes a range of cytokine release as its acute response [62, 63]. However, the infection is generally localized to epithelial cells yet extensive cytokine release often takes place systemically. This systemic release of cytokines particularly IL-1α and IFN-γ aggravates inflammation leading to fever and lung inflammation, and sometimes leads to fatality. Mice infected with influenza virus in which IL-1α and IFN-γ are suppressed show substantial mitigation of such risks [64, 65]. Similarly, infection with herpes simplex virus (HSV) triggers elevated production of IL-4 from CD4+ T cells and aggravates encephalitis [66]. The use of a certain types of drugs, such as vesarinone, for encephalomyocarditis (EMC) virus induced heart failure remarkably improved the survival rate of patients by reducing production of IL-1, IL-6, TNF-α, and IFN-γ [67]. As vesarione is not an antiviral agent, it was concluded that the improvement in outcome heart failure reduction was due to suppression of TNF-α production that may be induced by lipopolysaccharide (LPS) stimulation [68]. Perhaps the most dramatic example of such cytokine overproduction is fulminant hepatitis where significant elevation of TNF-α and IL-1 has been reported [69].

A series of experimental and clinical observations naturally leads to the conclusion that control of cytokine production may effectively prevent escalation of infection-triggered organ dysfunctions, and more generally systemic inflammatory response syndrome (SIRS). While various mouse experiments confirmed mitigation of SIRS [70], clinical experiments reported so far have had mixed outcomes. System-level studies that involve individual variations of cytokine production and resulting dynamics may be warranted for proper development of cytokine modulation therapies.

5.2 Autoimmune disorders

The immune system enhances robustness of the host system against broad range of pathogenic perturbations. It has to be able to react against a greater variety of pathogens within the resource limitations of the host system. The major constraint in immune system is resource limitation. Host immune systems must cope with an infinite variety of pathogens using finite number of T cells. Antigen processing and trimming is an effective mechanism that enables recognition of a broader range of pathogens using limited numbers of T cells. The trade-off is increased risk of misrecognition of a pathogen associated signature with the host's tissues. At the same time, resource limitation forces the system to take activation-triggered maturation of adaptive immune cells, rather than making themselves ready to be dispatched immediately. It is conceivable that this requirement has imposed selective pressures that have shaped the global structure of the immune system. A typical architecture of a bow-tie, or hour-glass, comprises conserved and efficient core processes with diverse and redundant input and output processes [1, 71]. The host immune system encompasses a nested tandem bow-tie architecture which can be observed in TLR signaling in innate immunity [58], processing and recognition of MHC-peptides between APC and T cells, and convergence of signaling from various cells into CD4+ T cells to foster polarized proliferation involving a complex cytokine network [57].

The most relevant issue in the current context is the bow tie structure of antigen presentation and recognition. In this process, various exogenous materials are captured by antigen presenting cells (APCs) through phagocytosis, macropinocytosis, and fluid phase endocytosis; also it expresses a broad range of receptors that induce receptor-mediated endocytosis. Exogenous materials captured undergo peptide processing to be loaded onto MHC II followed by trimming. The size of loaded peptides on MHC II ranges between 13–17 [72], and only a core of short peptides of 9–10 amino acids epitope binds to a receptor on CD4+ helper T cells [73]. A proper binding of TCR to MHC II activates signal transduction pathways, triggering cytokine secretion and polarization. MHC Class I is yet another bow-tie structure where a huge variety of peptides of endogenous origin are processed for loading and trimming on MHC I with the length of 8–10 amino acids and recognized by CD8+ T cells [74]. While this mechanism enabled robust host adaptive immune response to a broad range of pathogens, it is fragile against misrecognition so that, in some cases, molecular signature for pathogens and that of host tissue systems can be misrecognized that may trigger autoimmune reactions.

Some autoimmune diseases are now identified as infection-triggered, such as Crohn's disease (CD), which is an intestine autoimmune disease that causes chronic inflammation. Recently, it was shown that inflammation induced by bacterial infection triggers chronic inflammation, and mutation of NOD2 increases disease susceptibility [75, 76]. Extensive concentration of bacteria such as *Mycobacterium paratuberculosis* and *Listeria monocytogenes* has been observed by biopsy of CD patients using 16S rDNA PCR and DNA hybridization analysis [77]. Such infection-triggered autoimmune disorders are not specific to Crohn's disease reflecting the inherent fragility of the immune system where antigen patterns presented for immune reaction are sufficiently similar to the host's own signature, causing the immune system to react against the self [78]. The MHC antigen presentation and receptor system is the core of the bow-tie architecture, and so a breach in this system seriously affects its functionality. Dilated cardiomyopathy is associated with cardiotropic virus infection triggering dendritic cell-induced autoimmune heart failure [79]. It has been argued that the broad range of autoimmune disorders discussed above as well as rheumatoid arthritis (RA), systemic lupus erythematosus (SLE), and others, are due to multiple exposures to pathogenic bacteria and virus [80]. This class of autoimmune diseases can be attributed to breaches of the immune response against pathogens, by which invaded pathogens trigger a sustained immune response by molecular mimicry [78], possibly with TCR-dependent bystander activation [80].

Chlamydia pneumoniae has been found to associate with atherosclerosis [81, 82]. *Chlamydia* was found to infect lymphocytes and monocytes to escape host immune reactions and to proliferate [83]. Promotions of atherosclerosis due to *Chlamydia* may be due to its ability to transform macrophage into foam cells as well as possible autoimmune reactions [84] as similarity between *Chlamydia* external membrane protein and human cardio-muscle myosin has been identified [85].

6 Does microbial flora affect vulnerability against pathogenic infections?

The immune system is not the only mechanism for the host defense. Mammalian species host a range of symbionts, mostly bacterial, which often provide essential functions for the organism. In human beings, the intestinal microbiota contains 500–1,000 species of diverse microorganisms, and about 10^{14} bacteria totaling about 1.5 kg of biomass [86]. As a result, a typical human being considered as a symbiotic system would consist of approximately 90% prokaryotes and 10% eukaryotes [87]. A random shotgun sequencing of an individual person would result in predominantly bacterial genome readouts of about 2 million genes with sporadic mammalian genes [88]. Bacterial flora play essential roles in host physiology by helping to develop the mucosal immune system, rejecting pathogens, and providing metabolic functions for synthesizing certain vitamins that cannot be synthesized by the host alone [88].

Germ-free mice that have no commensal bacterial flora have an undeveloped mucosal immune system that has hypoplastic Peyer's patches, as well as significantly reduced numbers of IgA-producing plasma cells and lamina propria CD4+ T cells [89, 90]. A recent study on one commensal bacteria species, *Bacteroides thetaiotaomicron*, revealed that it stimulates angiogenesis during postnatal intestine development to enhance nutrient absorbing capability [91]. Due to the intricate relationship between bacterial flora and the host, some believe that flora should be considered as an 'organ', rather than unwanted guests [88]. It should also be noted that evolutionary history indicates that living systems increased robustness by acquiring 'non-self' into 'self' through evolution, which the author termed Self-Extending Symbiosis [92]. Bacterial flora is one of recent additions to this strategy to enhance robustness.

The central interest in the context of this article is whether commensal bacteria reduce the risk of infection. The bacterial flora functions antagonistically against pathogenic bacteria through a phenomenon known as colonization resistance. Continuous flow experiments using a smaller subset of commensal bacteria revealed that this effect is due to the anti-pathogen function of commensal bacteria including *E. coli* and competition for nutrients and spaces that are sustained by the dynamics of an inter-microbial metabolic network [93, 94]. In order for commensal bacterial flora to function to protect the host from pathogen invasion, maintenance of biodiversity of the flora seems to be a critical issue as it may enhance intestinal epithelial barrier functions [95] and suppress proliferation and attachment of pathogenic bacteria to the intestine [96]. It is well recognized that loss of diversity of flora due to extensive use of antibiotics allows pathogenic bacteria such as *Clostridium difficile* to proliferate and cause antibiotic associated diarrhea (AAD) [97]. While a general mechanistic explanation of how high biodiversity flora can reject pathogens has yet to be proven, it is clear that loss of diversity in an ecosystem leads to reduced stability and resistance against invasion [98]. A similar conclusion was reached by researchers at the NASA Kennedy Space Center who investigated the stability of advanced life support systems using a bacteria ecosystem [99].

In addition, it has been found that loss of biodiversity of the bacterial flora of the intestine is associated with inflammatory bowel diseases (IBD) [100], perhaps due to excessive growth of specific bacteria species [101] triggered by the loss of diversity [102]. Association between loss of diversity in bacterial flora and autoimmune disorders is documented even in cases of CD and ulcerative colitis. A recent study revealed that diversity of bacterial flora in Crohn's disease (CD) patients and ulcerative colitis was reduced by 50% and 30% compared to the healthy control group, respectively, and such reduction of diversity was attributed to the loss of normal anaerobic bacteria including *Bacteroides* species, *Eubacterium* species, and *Lactobacillus* species [100]. These bacteria that are significantly lost in the population are consistent with specific species that are observed to have high intra-division biodiversity [103] such as Cytophage-Flavobacterium-Bacteroides (CFB) and the Firmicutes. Extensive concentration of bacteria such as *Mycobacterium paratuberculosis* and *Listeria monocytogenes* has been observed by biopsy of CD patients using 16S rDNA PCR and DNA hybridization analysis [77]. Combined with the genetic susceptibility of the subpopulation of CD patients with NOD2 mutation [75, 76], perturbations of bacteria flora might have lost the capability to suppress such pathogenic bacteria and allowed them to grow and invade. However, due to the highly interactive nature of bacteria flora and the mucosal immune system, it is unclear whether such reduction in biodiversity of flora is a part of the cause, or the result of disease.

7 Future directions

This paper discussed possible issues related to robustness and trade-offs particular to the pathogen and host interaction in the context of infectious diseases. There have been a great many molecular details revealed in recent studies from both pathogen and host systems, and their complex interactions are starting to be revealed. As living systems have evolved to acquire robustness against a certain set of perturbations, it results in intrinsic trade-offs. Pathogens and the host system are no exception. Pathogens acquire robustness against host immune response by a variety of counter measures, variable surface molecule presentation, as well as by being invisible from immune recognition. Some of them are consistent with mechanisms for robustness observed in more complex living organisms. However, pathogens have generally evolved to be less robust against mutations, perhaps opting for efficient and faster replication. The modular PAI structure enables some pathogens to exchange pathogenicity genes. Effective drugs for such pathogens that specifically target the weaker aspects of pathogenesis systems stand the best chance of being meaningful interventions.

The host immune system is a complex and characteristic structure that has evolved to defend the host from a broad range of pathogenic threats. It has, however, several fragile points which are effectively exploited by a variety of pathogens. At the same time, the proinflammatory nature of cytokine network and risk of misrecognition by molecular mimicry make the host system prone to infection-triggered organ dysfunctions, such as ECM-induced heart failure, fulminent hepatitis, and a series of autoimmune disorders such as Crohn's disease.

Prevention and treatment of infectious diseases has to take into account the complex nature of the host–pathogen interaction. Bacterial flora has been featured as one possible risk factor for a variety of diseases and autoimmune disorders by preventing pathogen invasion from mucosal surfaces. A comprehensive understanding of the whole host system and pathogen interactions needs to be made to design effective therapeutic and preventive options. 'Biological robustness' provides viable conceptual framework for coherent understanding of infectious diseases and infection-triggered autoimmune disorders to guide future research and therapeutic efforts.

Acknowledgements

This research was supported in part by the ERATO-SORST Program (Japan Science and Technology Agency), the Systems Biology Institute, the Center of Excellence program, the special coordination funds (Ministry of Education, Culture, Sports, Science, and Technology) to Keio University.

References

1 Kitano H (2004) Biological robustness. *Nat Rev Genet* 5(11): 826–837
2 Stelling J, Sauer U, Szallasi Z, Doyle FJ 3rd, Doyle J (2004) Robustness of cellular functions. *Cell* 118(6): 675–685
3 Alon U, Surette MG, Barkai N, Leibler S (1999) Robustness in bacterial chemotaxis. *Nature* 397(6715): 168–171
4 Barkai N, Leibler S (1997) Robustness in simple biochemical networks. *Nature* 387(6636): 913–917
5 Yi TM, Huang Y, Simon MI, Doyle J (2000) Robust perfect adaptation in bacterial chemotaxis through integral feedback control. *Proc Natl Acad Sci USA* 97(9): 4649–4653
6 von Dassow G, Meir E, Munro EM, Odell GM (2000) The segment polarity network is a robust developmental module. *Nature* 406(6792): 188–192
7 Ingolia NT (2004) Topology and robustness in the *Drosophila* segment polarity network. *PLoS Biol* 2(6): E123
8 Little JW, Shepley DP, Wert DW (1999) Robustness of a gene regulatory circuit. *Embo J* 18(15): 4299–4307
9 Yachi S, Loreau M (1999) Biodiversity and ecosystem productivity in a fluctuating environment: the insurance hypothesis. *Proc Natl Acad Sci USA* 96(4): 1463–1468
10 Wagner GP, Altenberg L (1996) Complex adaptations and the evolution of evolvability. *Evolution* 50(3): 967–976
11 Rutherford SL (2003) Between genotype and phenotype: protein chaperones and evolvability. *Nat Rev Genet* 4(4): 263–274

12 de Visser J, Hermission J, Wagner GP, Meyers L, Bagheri-Chaichian H, Blanchard J, Chao L, Cheverud J, Elena S, Fontana W et al (2003) Evolution and detection of genetics robustness. *Evolution* 57(9): 1959–1972
13 Gerhart J, Kirschner M (1997) *Cells, embryos, and evolution: toward a cellular and developmental understanding of phenotypic variation and evolutionary adaptability.* Blackwell Science, Malden, Massachusetts, USA
14 Kirschner M, Gerhart J (1998) Evolvability. *Proc Natl Acad Sci USA* 95(15): 8420–8427
15 Kitano H (2004) Cancer as a robust system: implications for anticancer therapy. *Nat Rev Cancer* 4(3): 227–235
16 Kitano H (2003) Cancer robustness: tumour tactics. *Nature* 426(6963): 125
17 Kitano H, Oda K, Kimura T, Matsuoka Y, Csete M, Doyle J, Muramatsu M (2004) Metabolic syndrome and robustness tradeoffs. *Diabetes* 53 Suppl 3: S6–S15
18 Tyson JJ, Chen K, Novak B (2001) Network dynamics and cell physiology. *Nat Rev Mol Cell Biol* 2(12): 908–916
19 Ferrell JE Jr (2002) Self-perpetuating states in signal transduction: positive feedback, double-negative feedback and bistability. *Curr Opin Cell Biol* 14(2): 140–148
20 Chen KC, Calzone L, Csikasz-Nagy A, Cross FR, Novak B, Tyson JJ (2004) Integrative analysis of cell cycle control in budding yeast. *Mol Biol Cell* 15(8): 3841–3862
21 Agrawal AA (2001) Phenotypic plasticity in the interactions and evolution of species. *Science* 294(5541): 321–326
22 Schlichting C, Pigliucci M (1998) *Phenotypic evolution: a reaction norm perspective.* Sinauer Associates, Inc., Sunderland, MA, USA
23 Eldar A, Dorfman R, Weiss D, Ashe H, Shilo BZ, Barkai N (2002) Robustness of the BMP morphogen gradient in *Drosophila* embryonic patterning. *Nature* 419(6904): 304–308
24 Meir E, von Dassow G, Munro E, Odell GM (2002) Robustness, flexibility, and the role of lateral inhibition in the neurogenic network. *Curr Biol* 12(10): 778–786
25 Schlosser G, Wagner G (eds) (2004) *Modularity in development and evolution.* The University of Chicago Press, Chicago, USA
26 Rutherford SL, Lindquist S (1998) Hsp90 as a capacitor for morphological evolution. *Nature* 396(6709): 336–342
27 Queitsch C, Sangster TA, Lindquist S (2002) Hsp90 as a capacitor of phenotypic variation. *Nature* 417(6889): 618–624
28 Siegal ML, Bergman A (2002) Waddington's canalization revisited: developmental stability and evolution. *Proc Natl Acad Sci USA* 99(16): 10528–10532
29 Waddington CH (1957) *The strategy of the genes: a discussion of some aspects of theoretical biology.* Macmillan, New York, USA
30 Lahav G, Rosenfeld N, Sigal A, Geva-Zatorsky N, Levine AJ, Elowitz MB, Alon U (2004) Dynamics of the p53-Mdm2 feedback loop in individual cells. *Nat Genet* 36(2): 147–150
31 Csete ME, Doyle J (2004) Bow ties, metabolism and disease. *Trends Biotechnol* 22(9): 446–450

32 Carlson JM, Doyle J (1999) Highly optimized tolerance: a mechanism for power laws in designed systems. *Phys Rev E Stat Phys Plasmas Fluids Relat Interdiscip Topics* 60(2 Pt A): 1412–1427
33 Carlson JM, Doyle J (2002) Complexity and robustness. *Proc Natl Acad Sci USA* 99 Suppl 1: 2538–2545
34 Csete ME, Doyle JC (2002) Reverse engineering of biological complexity. *Science* 295(5560): 1664–1669
35 Bak P, Tang C, Wiesenfeld K (1988) Self-organized criticality. *Physical Review A* 38(1): 364–374
36 Barabasi AL, Oltvai ZN (2004) Network biology: understanding the cell's functional organization. *Nat Rev Genet* 5(2): 101–113
37 Lamport L, Shostak R, Pease M (1982) The Byzantine generals problem. *ACM Transactions on Programming Language and Systems* 4(3): 382–401
38 Ogawa M, Yoshimori T, Suzuki T, Sagara H, Mizushima N, Sasakawa C (2005) Escape of intracellular *Shigella* from autophagy. *Science* 307(5710): 727–731
39 Hersh D, Monack DM, Smith MR, Ghori N, Falkow S, Zychlinsky A (1999) The *Salmonella* invasin SipB induces macrophage apoptosis by binding to caspase-1. *Proc Natl Acad Sci USA* 96(5): 2396–2401
40 Waterman SR, Holden DW (2003) Functions and effectors of the *Salmonella* pathogenicity island 2 type III secretion system. *Cell Microbiol* 5(8): 501–511
41 Cossart P, Pizarro-Cerda J, Lecuit M (2003) Invasion of mammalian cells by *Listeria* monocytogenes: functional mimicry to subvert cellular functions. *Trends Cell Biol* 13(1): 23–31
42 Hacker J, Kaper JB (2000) Pathogenicity islands and the evolution of microbes. *Annu Rev Microbiol* 54: 641–679
43 Groisman EA, Ochman H (1996) Pathogenicity islands: bacterial evolution in quantum leaps. *Cell* 87(5): 791–794
44 Waldor MK, Mekalanos JJ (1996) Lysogenic conversion by a filamentous phage encoding cholera toxin. *Science* 272(5270): 1910–1914
45 Merrell DS, Falkow S (2004) Frontal and stealth attack strategies in microbial pathogenesis. *Nature* 430(6996): 250–256
46 Dubois ME, Demick KP, Mansfield JM (2005) Trypanosomes expressing a mosaic variant surface glycoprotein coat escape early detection by the immune system. *Infect Immun* 73(5): 2690–2697
47 Blaser MJ (2005) An endangered species in the stomach. *Sci Am* 292(2): 38–45
48 Umehara S, Higashi H, Ohnishi N, Asaka M, Hatakeyama M (2003) Effects of *Helicobacter pylori* CagA protein on the growth and survival of B lymphocytes, the origin of MALT lymphoma. *Oncogene* 22(51): 8337–8342
49 McCune JM (2001) The dynamics of CD4+ T-cell depletion in HIV disease. *Nature* 410(6831): 974–979
50 McMichael AJ, Rowland-Jones SL (2001) Cellular immune responses to HIV. *Nature* 410(6831): 980–987
51 Larder BA, Kemp SD (1989) Multiple mutations in HIV-1 reverse transcriptase confer high-level resistance to zidovudine (AZT). *Science* 246(4934): 1155–1158

52 Tisdale M, Kemp SD, Parry NR, Larder BA (1993) Rapid *in vitro* selection of human immunodeficiency virus type 1 resistant to 3′-thiacytidine inhibitors due to a mutation in the YMDD region of reverse transcriptase. *Proc Natl Acad Sci USA* 90(12): 5653–5656
53 Larder BA, Kemp SD, Harrigan PR (1995) Potential mechanism for sustained antiretroviral efficacy of AZT-3TC combination therapy. *Science* 269(5224): 696–699
54 Dropulic B, Hermankova M, Pitha PM (1996) A conditionally replicating HIV-1 vector interferes with wild-type HIV-1 replication and spread. *Proc Natl Acad Sci USA* 93(20): 11103–11108
55 Weinberger LS, Schaffer DV, Arkin AP (2003) Theoretical design of a gene therapy to prevent AIDS but not human immunodeficiency virus type 1 infection. *J Virol* 77(18): 10028–10036
56 Mautino MR, Morgan RA (2002) Gene therapy of HIV-1 infection using lentiviral vectors expressing anti-HIV-1 genes. *AIDS Patient Care STDS* 16(1): 11–26
57 Kitano H, Oda K (2006) Robustness trade-offs and host-microbial symbiosis in the immune system. *Mol Sys Biol* msb4100039-E1
58 Oda K, Kitano H (2006) A comprehensive molecular interaction map of Toll-like receptor signaling network. *Mol Sys Biol* msb4100057
59 Gilroy DW, Lawrence T, Perretti M, Rossi AG (2004) Inflammatory resolution: new opportunities for drug discovery. *Nat Rev Drug Discov* 3(5): 401–416
60 Nathan C (2002) Points of control in inflammation. *Nature* 420(6917): 846–852
61 O'Shea JJ, Ma A, Lipsky P (2002) Cytokines and autoimmunity. *Nat Rev Immunol* 2(1): 37–45
62 Conn CA, McClellan JL, Maassab HF, Smitka CW, Majde JA, Kluger MJ (1995) Cytokines and the acute phase response to influenza virus in mice. *Am J Physiol* 268(1 Pt 2): R78–84
63 Hennet T, Ziltener HJ, Frei K, Peterhans E (1992) A kinetic study of immune mediators in the lungs of mice infected with influenza A virus. *J Immunol* 149(3): 932–939
64 Wyde PR, Wilson MR, Cate TR (1982) Interferon production by leukocytes infiltrating the lungs of mice during primary influenza virus infection. *Infect Immun* 38(3): 1249–1255
65 Oda T, Akaike T, Hamamoto T, Suzuki F, Hirano T, Maeda H (1989) Oxygen radicals in influenza-induced pathogenesis and treatment with pyran polymer-conjugated SOD. *Science* 244(4907): 974–976
66 Ikemoto K, Pollard RB, Fukumoto T, Morimatsu M, Suzuki F (1995) Small amounts of exogenous IL-4 increase the severity of encephalitis induced in mice by the intranasal infection of herpes simplex virus type 1. *J Immunol* 155(3): 1326–1333
67 Matsumori A, Shioi T, Yamada T, Matsui S, Sasayama S (1994) Vesnarinone, a new inotropic agent, inhibits cytokine production by stimulated human blood from patients with heart failure. *Circulation* 89(3): 955–958
68 Matsui S, Matsumori A, Matoba Y, Uchida A, Sasayama S (1994) Treatment of virus-induced myocardial injury with a novel immunomodulating agent, ves-

narinone. Suppression of natural killer cell activity and tumor necrosis factor-alpha production. *J Clin Invest* 94(3): 1212–1217

69 Muto Y, Nouri-Aria KT, Meager A, Alexander GJ, Eddleston AL, Williams R (1988) Enhanced tumour necrosis factor and interleukin-1 in fulminant hepatic failure. *Lancet* 2(8602): 72–74

70 Wakabayashi G, Gelfand JA, Burke JF, Thompson RC, Dinarello CA (1991) A specific receptor antagonist for interleukin 1 prevents *Escherichia coli*-induced shock in rabbits. *Faseb J* 5(3): 338–343

71 Csete M, Doyle J (2004) Bow ties, metabolism and disease. *Trends Biotechnol* 22(9): 446–450

72 Rudensky A, Preston-Hurlburt P, Hong SC, Barlow A, Janeway CA Jr (1991) Sequence analysis of peptides bound to MHC class II molecules. *Nature* 353(6345): 622–627

73 Brown JH, Jardetzky TS, Gorga JC, Stern LJ, Urban RG, Strominger JL, Wiley DC (1993) Three-dimensional structure of the human class II histocompatibility antigen HLA-DR1. *Nature* 364(6432): 33–39

74 Yewdell JW, Bennink JR (2001) Cut and trim: generating MHC class I peptide ligands. *Curr Opin Immunol* 13(1): 13–18

75 Maeda S, Hsu LC, Liu H, Bankston LA, Iimura M, Kagnoff MF, Eckmann L, Karin M (2005) Nod2 mutation in Crohn's disease potentiates NF-kappaB activity and IL-1beta processing. *Science* 307(5710): 734–738

76 Kobayashi KS, Chamaillard M, Ogura Y, Henegariu O, Inohara N, Nunez G, Flavell RA (2005) Nod2-dependent regulation of innate and adaptive immunity in the intestinal tract. *Science* 307(5710): 731–734

77 Tiveljung A, Soderholm JD, Olaison G, Jonasson J, Monstein HJ (1999) Presence of eubacteria in biopsies from Crohn's disease inflammatory lesions as determined by 16S rRNA gene-based PCR. *J Med Microbiol* 48(3): 263–268

78 Baum H, Davies H, Peakman M (1996) Molecular mimicry in the MHC: hidden clues to autoimmunity? *Immunol Today* 17(2): 64–70

79 Eriksson U, Ricci R, Hunziker L, Kurrer MO, Oudit GY, Watts TH, Sonderegger I, Bachmaier K, Kopf M, Penninger JM (2003) Dendritic cell-induced autoimmune heart failure requires cooperation between adaptive and innate immunity. *Nat Med* 9(12): 1484–1490

80 von Herrath MG, Fujinami RS, Whitton JL (2003) Microorganisms and autoimmunity: making the barren field fertile? *Nat Rev Microbiol* 1(2): 151–157

81 Saikku P, Leinonen M, Mattila K, Ekman MR, Nieminen MS, Makela PH, Huttunen JK, Valtonen V (1988) Serological evidence of an association of a novel Chlamydia, TWAR, with chronic coronary heart disease and acute myocardial infarction. *Lancet* 2(8618): 983–986

82 Campbell LA, Kuo CC (2004) *Chlamydia pneumoniae* – an infectious risk factor for atherosclerosis? *Nat Rev Microbiol* 2(1): 23–32

83 Haranaga S, Yamaguchi H, Friedman H, Izumi S, Yamamoto Y (2001) *Chlamydia pneumoniae* infects and multiplies in lymphocytes *in vitro*. *Infect Immun* 69(12): 7753–7759

84 Wick G, Perschinka H, Xu Q (1999) Autoimmunity and atherosclerosis. *Am Heart J* 138(5 Pt 2): S444–449
85 Bachmaier K, Neu N, de la Maza LM, Pal S, Hessel A, Penninger JM (1999) Chlamydia infections and heart disease linked through antigenic mimicry. *Science* 283(5406): 1335–1339
86 Xu J, Gordon JI (2003) Inaugural article: Honor thy symbionts. *Proc Natl Acad Sci USA* 100(18): 10452–10459
87 Savage DC (1977) Microbial ecology of the gastrointestinal tract. *Annu Rev Microbiol* 31: 107–133
88 Hooper LV, Midtvedt T, Gordon JI (2002) How host-microbial interactions shape the nutrient environment of the mammalian intestine. *Annu Rev Nutr* 22: 283–307
89 Macpherson AJ, Hunziker L, McCoy K, Lamarre A (2001) IgA responses in the intestinal mucosa against pathogenic and non-pathogenic microorganisms. *Microbes Infect* 3(12): 1021–1035
90 Macpherson AJ, Martinic MM, Harris N (2002) The functions of mucosal T cells in containing the indigenous commensal flora of the intestine. *Cell Mol Life Sci* 59(12): 2088–2096
91 Stappenbeck TS, Hooper LV, Gordon JI (2002) Developmental regulation of intestinal angiogenesis by indigenous microbes via Paneth cells. *Proc Natl Acad Sci USA* 99(24): 15451–15455
92 Kitano H, Oda K (2006) Self-extending symbiosis: a mechanism for increasing robustness through evolution. *Biological Theory* 1(1): 61–66
93 Ushijima T, Ozaki Y (1988) Factors influencing potent antagonistic effects of *Escherichia coli* and *Bacteroides ovatus* on *Staphylococcus aureus* in anaerobic continuous flow cultures. *Can J Microbiol* 34(5): 645–650
94 Ushijima T, Ozaki Y (1986) Potent antagonism of *Escherichia coli*, *Bacteroides ovatus*, *Fusobacterium varium*, and *Enterococcus faecalis*, alone or in combination, for enteropathogens in anaerobic continuous flow cultures. *J Med Microbiol* 22(2): 157–163
95 Madsen K, Cornish A, Soper P, McKaigney C, Jijon H, Yachimec C, Doyle J, Jewell L, De Simone C (2001) Probiotic bacteria enhance murine and human intestinal epithelial barrier function. *Gastroenterology* 121(3): 580–591
96 Sartor RB (2005) Probiotic therapy of intestinal inflammation and infections. *Curr Opin Gastroenterol* 21(1): 44–50
97 Bergogne-Berezin E (2000) Treatment and prevention of antibiotic associated diarrhea. *Int J Antimicrob Agents* 16(4): 521–526
98 Cardinale BJ, Palmer MA, Collins SL (2002) Species diversity enhances ecosystem functioning through interspecific facilitation. *Nature* 415(6870): 426–429
99 Roberts MS, Garland JL, Mills AL (2004) Microbial astronauts: assembling microbial communities for advanced life support systems. *Microb Ecol* 47(2): 137–149
100 Ott SJ, Musfeldt M, Wenderoth DF, Hampe J, Brant O, Folsch UR, Timmis KN, Schreiber S (2004) Reduction in diversity of the colonic mucosa associated bacterial microflora in patients with active inflammatory bowel disease. *Gut* 53(5): 685–693

101 Sartor RB (2003) Targeting enteric bacteria in treatment of inflammatory bowel diseases: why, how, and when. *Curr Opin Gastroenterol* 19(4): 358–365
102 Swidsinski A, Ladhoff A, Pernthaler A, Swidsinski S, Loening-Baucke V, Ortner M, Weber J, Hoffmann U, Schreiber S, Dietel M et al (2002) Mucosal flora in inflammatory bowel disease. *Gastroenterology* 122(1): 44–54
103 Backhed F, Ley R, Sonnenburg J, Peterson D, Gordon JI (2005) Host-bacterial mutualism in the human intestine. *Science* 307: 1915–1920

Progress in Drug Research, Vol. 64
(Helena I. Boshoff and Clifton E. Barry III, Eds)

Toward whole cell modeling and simulation: Comprehensive functional genomics through the constraint-based approach

By Andrew R. Joyce[1]
and Bernhard Ø. Palsson[2]

[1]Bioinformatics Program,
University of California, San Diego,
La Jolla, California, USA
<ajoyce@ucsd.edu>

[2]Department of Bioengineering,
University of California, San Diego,
La Jolla, California, USA
<bpalsson@bioeng.ucsd.edu>

Abstract

The increasing availability of various system-level, or so-called 'omics', datasets, in concert with existing data from the primary research literature, is facilitating the development of genome-scale metabolic models for many organisms. By incorporating the metabolic reaction stoichiometry as well as other physicochemical properties into systemic network reconstructions, these models account for the constraints that restrict an organism's phenotypic behavior. Accordingly, unlike many contemporary modeling strategies, this constraint-based modeling approach does not attempt to predict network behavior exactly; rather, it seeks to clearly distinguish those network states that a system can achieve from those that it cannot. A variety of analytical tools have been designed and developed to probe these models, thus enabling studies that investigate the metabolic capabilities of a number of organisms, that generate and test experimental hypotheses, and that predict accurately metabolic phenotypes and evolutionary outcomes. This chapter introduces the concepts that underlie the constraint-based modeling approach, and describes several of its applications with an emphasis on those potentially relevant to the drug development field. In addition, while this chapter focuses on the primary application of the constraint-based approach to date, namely in modeling metabolic networks, the latter sections of the chapter discuss its relatively recent application to modeling other cellular systems. Finally, the chapter concludes with an assessment of future directions focusing on the efforts that will be required to utilize the constraint-based approach in generating a holistic model of a viable organism.

Keywords: systems biology, Flux Balance Analysis (FBA), mathematical modeling of biological systems, constraint-based reconstruction and analysis, extreme pathway analysis

1 Introduction to modeling using the constraint-based approach

The development of high-throughput experimental techniques in recent years has led to an explosion of genome-scale datasets for a variety of organisms. Considerable efforts have yielded complete genomic sequences for hundreds of organisms [1], from which gene annotation provides a list of individual cellular components. Microarray technology affords researchers the ability to probe gene expression patterns of cells and tissues on a genome scale thus providing insight into components available to the system at a given time and condition. Furthermore, advances in the fields of proteomics, as well as significant high-throughput gene product localization and high-throughput phenotyping efforts further add to the vast quantity of data currently available to researchers. Integration of these datasets to extract the most relevant information in formulating a comprehensive view of biological systems is a major challenge currently facing the biological research community [2]. Achieving this task will require comprehensive models of cellular processes.

A prudent approach to gain biological understanding from these complex datasets involves the development of mathematical modeling, simulation, and analysis techniques [3]. For many years, researchers have developed and analyzed models of biological systems via simulation, but these efforts often have been hampered by lack of complete or reliable data. Some examples of the modeling philosophies and approaches that have been pursued include deterministic kinetic modeling [4, 5], stochastic modeling [6, 7], and Boolean modeling [8]. Many of these approaches are implicitly limited in that they require knowledge of unknown parameters that are difficult to experimentally determine or approximate. Furthermore, the above approaches typically require substantial computational power, thus limiting the scale of the models that can be developed.

In recent years, however, great strides have been made in developing and using genome-scale metabolic models of a number of organisms using another modeling technique that is not subject to the above limitations. This approach, known as constraint-based reconstruction and analysis [9–13], has been employed to generate genome-scale models for organisms from all three major branches of the tree of life. While bacterial models dominate this growing collection, a model from archaea has recently appeared, and several eukaryotic models are also available (see Fig. 1 and Tab. 1 for an overview of existing constraint-based metabolic models).

In complimentary efforts, many analytical tools have been developed to use these models in computational investigations of model organisms (reviewed in [10]), some of which have the potential to aid drug development efforts. For example, Flux Balance Analysis (FBA) [14, 15], is a powerful mathematical approach that uses optimization by linear programming to study the properties of metabolic networks under various conditions. Additionally, uniform random sampling of the steady-state flux space defined in these models can be used to assess network structure and capabilities, and has been used to examine enzymopathies [16, 17].

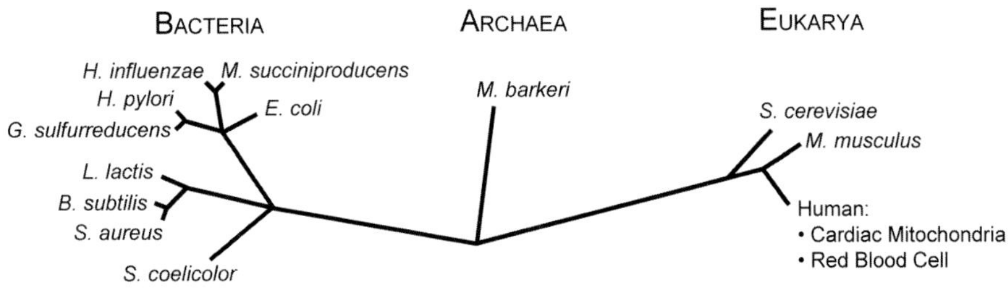

Figure 1.
Distribution of constraint-based metabolic models across the tree of life. This approximation of the tree of life, which is derived from the Taxonomy Browser available through NCBI [101], lists all currently available genome-scale, constraint-based models of metabolism. Table 1 summarizes model details and lists references for each respective model.

Table 1.
Currently available constraint-based models. This table summarizes content statistics for the models developed and published to date. *This number is based on the protein species identified in a proteomics study of the human cardiac mitochondria from which the components of the reconstruction were derived [106]. NA – Not applicable.

Organism	Total Genes	Model Genes	Model Metabolites	Model Reactions	Reference
Bacteria					
Bacillus subtilis	4,225	614	637	754	[102]
Escherichia coli	4,405	904	625	931	[58]
		720	438	627	[60]
Geobacter sulfurreducens	3,530	588	541	523	[64]
Haemophilus influenzae	1,775	296	343	488	[76]
		400	451	461	[103]
Heliobacter pylori	1,632	341	485	476	[62]
		291	340	388	[61]
Lactococcus lactis	2,310	358	422	621	[104]
Mannheimia succinciproducens	2,463	335	352	373	[105]
Staphylococcus aureus	2,702	619	571	641	[63]
		551	712	682	[80]
Streptomyces coelicolor	8,042	700	500	700	[65]
Archaea					
Methanosarcina barkeri	5,072	692	558	619	[66]
Eukarya					
Mus musculus	28,287	1156	872	1220	[72]
Saccharomyces cerevisiae	6,183	750	646	1149	[68]
		672	636	1038	[69]
		708	584	1175	[67]
Human Cardiac Mitochondria	615*	298	230	189	[55]
Human Red Blood Cell	NA	NA	39	32	[73]

In this chapter, we provide an introduction to the principles that underlie constraint-based reconstruction and analysis with an emphasis on modeling metabolic networks. Furthermore, we show directly how FBA can be used to analyze these models and interrogate their properties. We also review several published studies that utilize FBA and uniform random sampling to illustrate their potential utility in drug development applications. Finally, we introduce the application of the constraint-based approach to modeling other cellular systems aside from metabolism and discuss the steps that remain in generating a holistic model of a viable organism.

2 Building a constraint-based model

This section outlines the general procedure (Fig. 2) followed in constructing a constraint-based model with a slant towards metabolic network. Furthermore, we introduce FBA as an example of a useful analytical method that can be used in conjunction with these models. This model building and analysis approach can be divided approximately into four successive steps:

1. Network reconstruction
2. Stoichiometric (S) matrix compilation
3. Identification and assignment of appropriate constraints to molecular components
4. Network analysis (in the presented case using FBA).

2.1 Network reconstruction

The first step in constraint-based modeling, known as network reconstruction, involves generating a model that describes the system of interest. This process can be decomposed into three parts typically performed simultaneously during model construction. First, data collection is conducted to define the network of interest; second, a corresponding metabolic reaction list is generated; and third gene-protein-reaction (GPR) relationships are determined.

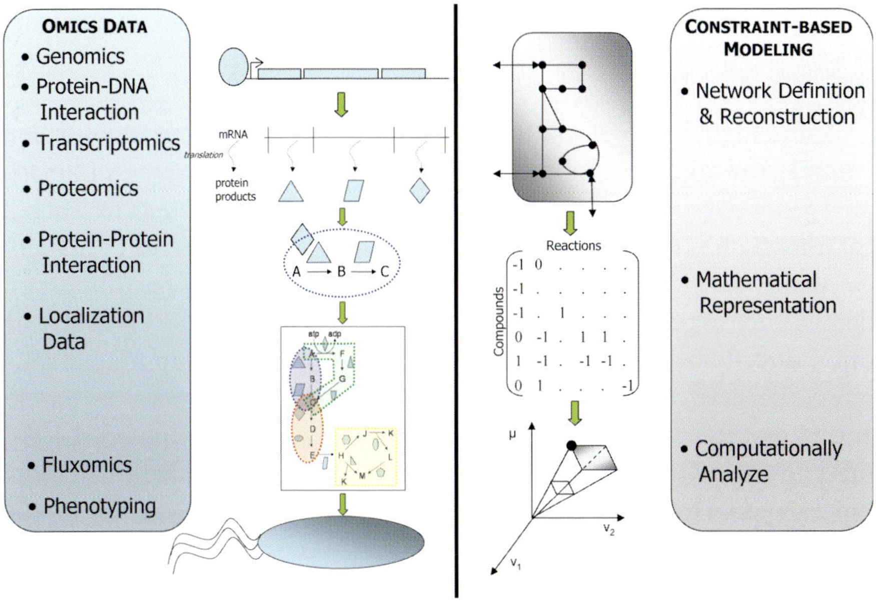

Figure 2.
From 'omics' data to constraint-based models. Omics datasets are appearing that describe the levels, subcellular localization, and interactions between many of the biomolecules within the cell. These data are facilitating the construction and analysis of genome-scale, constraint-based models of biological systems. For example, genomics, transcriptomics, and proteomics yield information regarding the cellular components to be included in the network to be reconstructed (*left panel*). Protein–protein interaction data helps identify the enzyme complexes to be included in the network reconstruction, and protein–DNA interactions are useful when integrating transcriptional regulatory information into the model. Finally, localization data, when available, is extremely useful for multi-compartmental models in which components must be properly assigned to their respective subcellular compartments. Having defined and reconstructed the system based on these and older data from the literature, the model can be represented in mathematical form as a matrix (*right panel*). Finally, computational analyses using this matrix can be performed and compared to fluxomics and phenotyping data for model validation and refinement purposes.

2.1.1 Data collection

Perhaps the most critical component of the constraint-based modeling approach involves data collection relevant to the system of interest. Not long ago, this was among the most challenging steps as researchers had access to very limited amounts of biochemical data. However, the success of recent genome sequencing and annotation projects, advances in high-throughput technologies, as well as the development of detailed and extensive online database resources, has improved matters dramatically.

Many high quality data resources exist to help researchers identify and compile the appropriate metabolites, biochemical reactions, and associated genes to be included in the network reconstruction. Direct biochemical information found in the primary literature usually contains the highest quality data for use in reconstructing biochemical networks. Important details, such as precise reaction stoichiometry and reaction reversibility, are often directly available. Given that scrutinizing each study individually is an excessively time-consuming and tedious task, biochemical textbooks and review articles should be utilized when available, relying on the primary literature to resolve conflicts as necessary. Furthermore, many volumes devoted to individual organisms and organelles, such as *E. coli* [18], and the mitochondria [19], are increasingly becoming available and are typically excellent resources.

High-throughput datasets are also generally excellent resources, particularly for less-studied, non-model organisms. In recent years, the complete genome sequence of hundreds of organisms has been determined, and many more sequencing projects are underway [20]. This collection is dominated by microbial and viral sequences, but several highly publicized higher eukaryotic sequences are also available [21–24]. Furthermore, extensive bioinformatics-based annotation efforts continue to make great strides toward automatically identifying all coding regions contained within the sequence [25–27]. Interestingly, efforts are underway to automatically reconstruct networks based on annotated sequence information alone [28]. However, these automated approaches are limited in that they can only be as good as the genome annotation from which they are derived. Therefore, considerable quality control efforts should be conducted prior to extensive use of these networks.

The proteome of a biological system defines the full complement, localization, and abundance of proteins. Although these data are generally difficult to obtain, data for some subcellular components and bacteria are available [29, 30]. Proteomic data are of particular importance in eukaryotic systems modeling, in which care must be taken to assign reactions to their appropriate subcellular compartment or organelle. Similarly, when modeling a system under a single condition, these data are important in identifying active components.

In recent years, significant efforts also have been devoted to developing comprehensive databases that integrate many information sources, including those data types previously described. Of particular interest for metabolic modeling efforts are resources that have incorporated these disparate data sources into metabolic pathway maps. Kyoto Encyclopedia of Genes and Genomes (KEGG) [31] is perhaps the most extensive and well known among these resource types, providing pathway maps for numerous metabolic processes and information regarding gene orthology across many organisms.

Additional organism-specific database resources are also available. EcoCyc [32] incorporates gene and regulatory information, as well as enzyme reaction pathways particular to *E. coli*. The Comprehensive Yeast Genome Database (CYGD) [33] and *Saccharomyces* Genome Database (SGD) [34] are other examples of *S. cerevisiae*-specific comprehensive resources. Finally, the BioCyc resource [35, 36] contains automated annotation-derived pathway/genome databases for 205 individual organisms.

An additional important wealth of information can be found in resources that provide functional information for individual genes and gene products. These ontology-based tools strive to describe how gene products behave in a cellular context. The most well-known resource is Gene Ontology Consortium (GO) [37, 38], which contains information for a variety of organisms. In recent years, organism-specific ontologies, such as GenProtEC [39] for *E. coli*, also have appeared. Table 2 lists some popular online high-throughput data resources as well as integrative organism-specific and ontological resources.

2.1.2 Metabolic reaction list generation

The next step in putting together a constraint-based model requires clearly specifying the reactions to be included based on the metabolite and enzyme information collected in the previous step. A metabolic reaction can be viewed simply as substrate(s) conversion to product(s), often by enzyme-mediated catalysis. In light of this notion, each reaction in a metabolic network must adhere to the fundamental laws of physics and chemistry; therefore, reactions must be balanced in terms of charge and

Table 2.
Online data resources. This table details some of the databases that store and distribute genome-scale data, gene ontological information, and organism specific data. It should also be noted that this table is by no means comprehensive in its content, but rather provides a reasonably broad sample of the data and resources that are readily accessible to researchers today. 2D-PAGE – two-dimensional polyacrylamide-gel electrophoresis; *E. coli* – *Escherichia coli*; GFP – green fluorescent protein; *S. cerevisiae* – *Saccharomyces cerevisiae*; SAGE – serial analysis of gene expression.

Data Type	Resource	Description	URL
Genomic	Genomes OnLine Database (GOLD)	Repository of completed and ongoing genome projects	http://www.genomesonline.org
	The Institute for Genomic Research (TIGR)	Curated databases for microbial, plant, and human genome projects	http://www.tigr.org
	National Center for Biotechnology Information (NCBI)	Curated databases of DNA sequences as well as other data	http://www.ncbi.nlm.nih.gov
	The SEED	Database resource for genome annotations using the subsystem approach	http://www.theseed.org
Transcriptomic	Gene Expression Omnibus (GEO)	Microarray and SAGE-based genome-wide expression profiles	http://www.ncbi.nlm.nih.gov/geo
	Stanford Microarray Database (SMD)	Microarray-based genome-wide expression data	http://genome-www5.stanford.edu/
Proteomic	Expert Protein Analysis System (ExPASy)	Protein sequence, structure, and 2-D PAGE data.	http://au.expasy.org
	BRENDA	Enzyme functional data.	http://www.brenda.uni-koeln.de/
	Open Proteomics Database (OPD)	Mass-spectrometry-based proteomics data	http://bioinformatics.icmb.utexas.edu/OPD
Protein–DNA Interaction	Biomolecular Network Database (BIND)	Published protein–DNA interactions	http://www.bind.ca/Action/
	Encyclopedia of DNA Elements (ENCODE)	Database of functional elements in human DNA	http://genome.ucsc.edu/encode/

Table 2 (continued)

Data Type	Resource	Description	URL
Protein–protein Interaction	Munich Information Center for Protein Sequences (MIPS)	Links to protein–protein interaction data and resources	http://mips.gsf.de/proj/ppi
	Database of Interacting Proteins (DIP)	Published protein–protein interactions	http://dip.doe-mbi.ucla.edu
Subcellular Localization	Yeast GFP-fusion Localization Database	Genome-scale protein localization data for yeast	http://yeastgfp.ucsf.edu
Phenotype	A Systematic Annotation Package For Community Analysis of Genomes (ASAP)	Single-gene-deletion phenotype microarray data for *E. coli*	http://www.genome.wisc.edu/tools/asap.htm
	General Repository for Interaction Datasets (GRID)	Synthetic lethal interactions in yeast	http://biodata.mshri.on.ca/grid
Pathway	Kyoto Encyclopedia of Genes and Genomes (KEGG)	Pathway maps for many biological processes	http://www.genome.ad.jp/kegg/
	BioCarta	Interactive graphic models of molecular and cellular pathways	http://www.biocarta.com/genes/index.asp
Organism Specific	EcoCyc	Encyclopedia of *E. coli* K12 genes and metabolism	http://www.ecocyc.org
	Saccharomyces Genome Database (SGD)	Scientific database of the molecular biology and genetics of *S. cerevisiae*	http://www.yeastgenome.org
	BioCyc	A collection of 205 pathway/genome databases for individual organisms.	http://www.biocyc.org

elemental composition. For example, the biochemical reaction that represents the first step of glycolysis, in which hexokinase phosphorylates glucose yielding glucose-6-phosphate, can be depicted as:

$$C_6H_{12}O_6 + ATP^{3-} \xrightarrow{Hexokinase} C_6H_{11}O_6PO_3^{2-} + ADP^{2-}.$$

However, this equation is neither elementally nor charge balanced. However, inclusion of hydrogen, as shown below:

$$C_6H_{12}O_6 + ATP^{3-} \xrightarrow{Hexokinase} C_6H_{11}O_6PO_3^{2-} + ADP^{2-} + H^+$$

...balances the reaction in both regards. This level of detail, however minor it seems, is very important when building chemically consistent constraint-based models.

Biological boundaries also must be considered when defining reaction lists. Metabolic networks are comprised of both intracellular and extracellular reactions. For example, in bacteria the reactions of glycolysis and the tricarboxylic acid cycle (TCA) generally take place intracellularly in the cytosol. However, glucose must be transported into the cell via an extracellular reaction in which a glucose transporter takes up extracellular glucose. An additional boundary consideration must be recognized particularly when modeling eukaryotic cells. Given that certain metabolic reactions take place in the cytosol and others take place in various organelles, reactions must be compartmentalized properly. Data is now being generated in which proteins are tagged, with green fluorescent protein (GFP) for example, or recognized by antibodies and localized to subcellular compartments or organelles [40–42]. Furthermore, computational tools have also been developed to predict subcellular location of proteins in eukaryotes [43].

Finally, reaction reversibility must be defined. Certain metabolic reactions can proceed in both directions. Thermodynamically, this permits reaction fluxes to take on both positive and negative values. The KEGG and BRENDA online resources (Tab. 2) are two useful resources that catalog enzyme reversibility.

2.1.3 Determining gene-protein-reaction (GPR) relationships

Upon completing the reaction list, the protein, or protein complexes that facilitate each metabolite substrate to product conversion must be determined. Each subunit protein from a complex must be assigned to the same reaction. Additionally, certain individual reactions can be catalyzed by different distinct enzymes. Collectively, each enzyme that fits this criterion is known as an isozyme for a particular reaction. Accordingly, isozymes must all be assigned to the same appropriate reaction. Biochemical textbooks often provide the general name of the enzyme(s) responsible; however, the precise gene and associated gene product specific for the model organism of interest must be identified. The database resources detailed in Section 2.1.1 and Table 2 assist this process. In particular, KEGG and GO provide considerable enzyme-reaction information for a variety of organisms. Furthermore, protein–protein interaction datasets, derived from yeast two-hybrid experiments [44], for example, may be useful resources for defining enzymatic complexes in less defined situations. One must take care in using these data, however, given their generally high false positive rate and questionable reproducibility [45, 46].

2.2 Defining the stoichiometric (S) matrix

Having reconstructed the network of interest, the compiled reaction list can be represented mathematically in the form of a stoichiometric (S) matrix. The S matrix for metabolic networks is formed from the stoichiometric coefficients of the reactions that participate in the defined reaction network. It has $m \times n$ dimensions, where m is the number of metabolites and n is the number of reactions. Therefore, the S matrix is organized such that every column corresponds to a reaction, and every row corresponds to a metabolite. The S matrix describes how many reactions a compound participates in, and thus, how reactions are interconnected and thus effectively represents a two dimensional annotation of the genome [9, 47].

Figure 3 shows how a simple two reaction system can be represented as an S matrix. In this example, v_1 and $v_2$denote reaction fluxes and are associated with individual proteins or protein complexes that catalyze the reactions. Element S_{ij} represents the coefficient of metabolite i in reaction j.

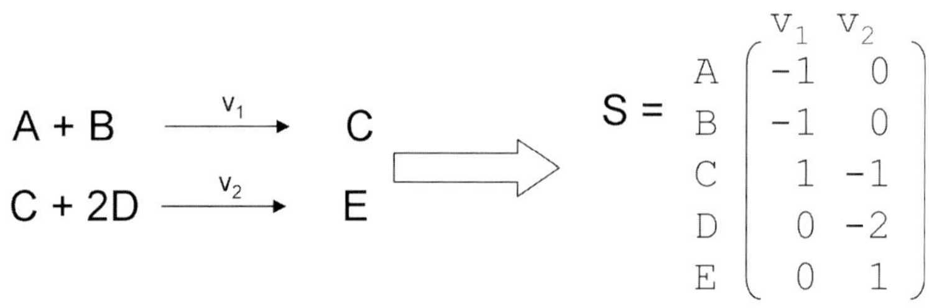

Figure 3.
Generating the stoichiometric (S) matrix. The reaction list on the left is mathematically represented by the S matrix on the right. As a convention, each row represents a metabolite and each column represents a reaction in the network. Additionally, input or reactant metabolites have negative coefficients and outputs or products have positive coefficients. Metabolites that do not participate in a given reaction are assigned a zero value.

Furthermore, notice that substrates are assigned negative coefficients and products are given positive coefficients. Also, for those reactions in which a metabolite does not participate, the corresponding element is assigned a zero value.

2.3 Identifying and applying constraints

Having developed a mathematical representation of a metabolic network in the form of the S matrix, the next step requires that any constraints be identified and imposed on the system. Cells are subject to a variety of constraints from environmental, physiochemical, evolutionary, and regulatory sources [10, 12]. In and of itself, the S matrix is a constraint in that it defines the mass and charge balance requirements for all possible metabolic reactions available to the cell. These stoichiometric constraints establish a geometric solution space that in principle contains all possible metabolic behaviors.

Additional constraints can be identified and imposed on the model, which has the effect of further limiting the metabolic solution space. Maximum enzyme capacity (V_{max}), which can be determined experimentally for some reactions, is one example, and can be imposed by limiting the flux through any associated reactions to that maximum value. Furthermore, the uptake rates of certain metabolites can be determined experimentally and used to restrict metabolite uptake to the appropriate levels when mathematically analyzing the metabolic model. Additional types of constraints have also been applied, including thermodynamic limitations [48], internal metabolic flux determinations [11], and transcriptional regulation [49–52].

2.4 Network analysis: Assessing the model using Flux Balance Analysis

With a mathematical representation of the network in hand, a variety of analytical techniques can be utilized to assess its properties. Flux Balance Analysis (FBA) is a powerful computational method that relies on linear programming-based optimization [53] to investigate the production capabilities and systemic properties of a metabolic network. By defining an objective, such as biomass production, ATP production, or byproduct secretion, linear optimization may be used to find an optimal flux distribution for the network model that maximizes the stated objective. This section briefly introduces some main concepts that underlie FBA, with an emphasis on how FBA can be utilized to assess gene essentiality in a metabolic network.

2.4.1 Linear optimization

As previously stated, the solution space defined by constraint-based models can be explored via optimization by linear programming (LP). The LP problem corresponding to the search for the optimal flux distribution through a metabolic network can be formulated as follows:

$$\begin{aligned} &\text{Maximize } \mathbf{Z} = c^{\mathrm{T}} v \\ &\text{Subject to } \mathbf{S} \cdot v = 0 \\ &\qquad \alpha_i \leq v_i \leq \beta_i \text{ for all reactions i} \end{aligned}$$

In the above representation, **Z** represents the objective function, and c is a vector of weights on the fluxes v. The weights are used to define the properties of the particular solution that is sought. The latter statements represent the flux constraints for the metabolic network. S is the matrix defined in the previous section and contains the mass and charge balanced representation of the system. Furthermore, each reaction flux v_i in the system is subject to lower and upper bound constraints, represented in α_i and β_i respectively.

The solution to this problem yields not only a value for Z but also results in an optimal flux distribution (v) that allows the highest flux through the chosen objective function, Z. Furthermore, computational assessment of gene essentiality is performed easily within this framework. By setting the upper and lower flux bound constraints to zero for the reaction(s) corresponding to the gene(s) of interest, a simulated gene deletion strain may be created. An examination of the results of simulations run before and after knocking out a gene leads directly to gene essentiality predictions.

Problems of this type can be readily formulated and solved by a variety of commercial software packages. Box 1 presents a simple, hypothetical example solved with Matlab for three cases using the system depicted in Figure 4. It should also be noted that these types of analyses yield a single flux distribution; however, it is possible that multiple equivalent flux distributions exist that yield a maximal biomass function value for a given network and simulation conditions. This topic has been explored using mixed integer linear programming (MILP) techniques with genome-scale metabolic models [54, 55], but is beyond the scope of this chapter and will not be further discussed.

2.4.2 Constraints

As previously stated, the S matrix constrains the system by defining the mass and charge balances for all possible metabolic reactions within the system. In mathematical terms, the stoichiometric (S) matrix is a linear transformation of the reaction flux vector,

$$\mathbf{v} = (\mathrm{v}_1, \mathrm{v}_2, \ldots, \mathrm{v}_\mathrm{n})$$

to a vector of time derivatives of metabolic concentrations

$$\mathbf{x} = (\mathrm{x}_1, \mathrm{x}_2, \ldots, \mathrm{x}_\mathrm{n})$$

Box 1: FBA using Matlab

Here we use Matlab to solve an FBA problem for 3 cases using the system in **Figure 4**. The **linprog()** function accepts six arguments and returns two values in the following form:

$$[v, Z] = \text{linprog}(c, Aeq, beq, S, b, \alpha, \beta).$$

This solves the following LP problem:

$$\begin{aligned} &\text{Minimize} && Z = c^T \cdot v \\ &\text{Subject to} && Aeq \cdot v \le beq \\ &&& S \cdot v = b \\ &&& \alpha \le v \le \beta \end{aligned}$$

Since the system does not have inequality constraints other than flux vector bounds, Aeq is set equal to the identity matrix and beq to β, so that

$$Aeq \cdot v \le beq$$

is equivalent to

$$v \le \beta.$$

The code to solve the wild type problem (Case 1) of interest in Matlab's framework follows, using α and β as defined in the text :

```
>> S = [-1 -1 0 0 0 0 1 0;
        1 0 -1 1 -1 0 0 0;
        0 1 1 -1 0 -1 0 0;
        0 0 0 0 1 1 0 -1];
>> b = [0 0 0 0]';
>> alpha = [0 0 0 0 0 0 0 0]';
>> beta = [2 10 4 6 10 8 100 100]';
>> c = [0 0 0 0 0 0 0 1];
>> Aeq = eye(8);
>> [v,Z] = linprog(-c,Aeq,beta,S,b,alpha,beta)
Optimization terminated successfully.

v = 2.0000   10.0000   0.1822   3.9137   5.7315   6.2685
    12.0000  12.0000
Z =  -12.0000
```

Note that since Matlab defaults to solving a minimization problem we use the negative of the optimization vector. The resulting flux distributions for three cases (1: Wild-type; 2: Impaired Single Deletion Strain; and 3: Lethal Double Deletion Strain) are displayed on network maps to the right.

Case 1: Wild Type

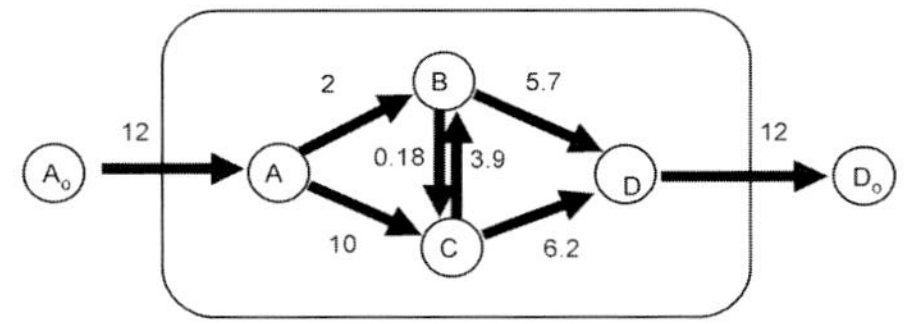

Case 2 solves the same problem, but this time after knocking out reaction v5 by modifying the β vector:

```
>> beta = [2 10 4 6 10 0 100 100]';
```

Case 2: v6 Knockout

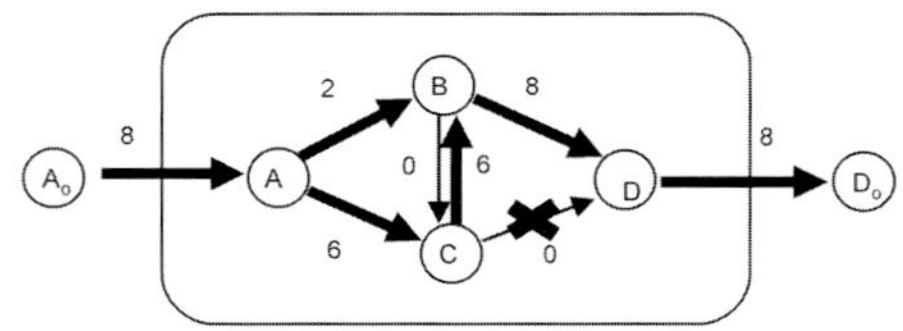

Finally, Case 3 simulates a "lethal" deletion strain by knocking out both v5 and v6:

```
>> beta = [2 10 4 6 0 0 100 100]';
```

Case 3: v5 & v6 Double Knockout

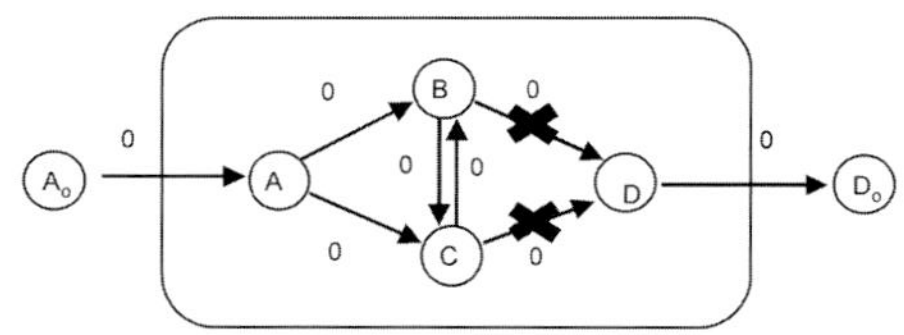

a

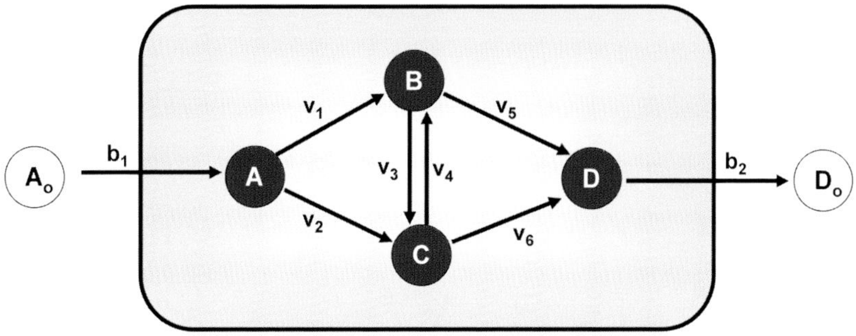

b

```
b1:     → A
v1: A → B
v2: A → C
v3: B → C
v4: C → B
v5: B → D
v6: C → D
b2: D →
```

c

S=

Metabolites \ Reactions	v1	v2	v3	v4	v5	v6	b1	b2
A	-1	-1	0	0	0	0	1	0
B	1	0	-1	1	-1	0	0	0
C	0	1	1	-1	0	-1	0	0
D	0	0	0	0	1	1	0	-1

Figure 4.
An example system. (**a**) A four metabolite, eight reaction system is first decomposed into individual reactions in (**b**), and then represented mathematically in the S matrix depicted in (**c**). By convention, internal reactions are denoted by v_1, and reactions that span the system boundary are denoted by b_1. External metabolites A_0 and D_0 need not be explicitly represented explicitly within this framework as they are outside the system under consideration. This system is used in the calculations shown in Box 1.

such that

$$\frac{d\mathbf{x}}{dt} = \mathbf{S} \cdot \mathbf{v}$$

Therefore, a particular flux distribution **v** represents the flux levels through each reaction in the network. Since the time constants that describe metabolic transients are fast (on the order of tens of seconds or less), whereas the time constants for cell growth are comparatively long (on the order of hours to days) the behavior of cellular components can be considered as existing in a quasi-steady state. This assumption leads to the reduction of the previous equation to:

$$\mathbf{S} \cdot \mathbf{v} = 0.$$

By focusing only on the steady-state condition, assumptions regarding reaction kinetics are not needed. Furthermore, based on this premise it is possible to determine all chemically balanced metabolic routes through the metabolic network.

The second constraint set is imposed on the individual reaction flux values. The constraints defined by

$$\alpha_i \leq v_i \leq \beta_i \quad \text{for all reactions i}$$

specify lower and upper flux bounds for each reaction. If all model reactions are irreversible, α equals 0. Similarly, if the enzyme capacity, or V_{max}, is experimentally defined, setting β to the known experimental value limits the allowable reaction flux through the enzyme. In contrast, a gene knockout is simulated by setting both α_i and $\beta_i = 0$ for gene i (see Box 1). If no constraints on flux values through reaction v_i can be identified, then α_i and β_i are set to $-\infty$ and $+\infty$, respectively, to allow for all possible flux values. In practice, ∞ is typically represented as an arbitrarily large number that will exceed any feasible internal flux.

A brief consideration should also be given to specifying input and output constraints on the system. When analyzing metabolic models in the context of assessing cellular growth capabilities, input constraints effectively define the environmental conditions being considered. For example, organisms have various elemental requirements that must be provided in the environment in order to support growth. Some organisms that lack certain biosynthetic processes are auxotrophic for certain biomolecules, such as amino acids, and these compounds must also be provided in the environment. From an FBA standpoint, these issues mean that input sources must be specified in the form of input flux constraints specified in v. For example, if one desires to simulate rich medium conditions, flux constraints are specified such that all biomolecules that can be inputs to the system, in other words all compounds that are available extracellularly, are left unconstrained and can flow freely into the system. In contrast, when modeling minimal medium conditions (see [56] for an example of a large-scale analysis performed of *E. coli* growth simulations on minimal media) only those inputs required for cell growth, or biomass formation in the formalism being considered here, are allowed to flow into the system with all other input fluxes constrained to zero. It should also be noted that certain output flux constraints may need to be set appropriately in order to allow for the simulated secretion of biomolecules that may 'accumulate' in the process of forming biomass.

2.4.3 The objective function

Given that multiple possible flux distributions exist for any given network, linear optimization is used to identify a particular solution that maximizes or minimizes a defined objective function. Commonly used objective functions include production of ATP, or production of a secreted byproduct. When assessing the growth capabilities of a microbe using its associated metabolic model, growth rate, as defined by the weighted consumption of metabolites needed to make biomass, is maximized. The general analysis strategy asks the question "is the metabolic reaction network able to support growth under the specified growth conditions?" Therefore, biomass generation in this modeling framework is represented as a reaction flux that drains intermediate metabolites, such as ATP, NADPH, pyruvate, and amino acids, in appropriate ratios (defined in the vector c of the biomass function Z) to support growth. As a convention, the biomass function is typically written to reflect the needs of the cell in order to make one gram of cellular dry weight, and has been experimentally determined for *E. coli* [57]. In sum, the choice of biomass as an objective function means that cell growth, depicted as a non-zero value for Z, will only occur if all the components in the biomass function can be provided for by the network in the correct relative amounts.

3 Metabolic model applications and computational challenges

The previous sections provided the basic concepts of constraint-based reconstruction and analysis. We will now turn to the current state of the field by first touching on some of the computational challenges that are commonly encountered when scaling up to genome-scale network reconstruction and analysis. We will also introduce many of the metabolic models that have appeared in the literature and that are being utilized in many follow-up analytical studies. We will then discuss FBA-based analysis of gene essentiality and uniform random sampling analysis, two applications that use constraint-based models and have potential utility for drug development purposes. Model validation and improvement opportunities will be discussed in the context of the former application as well.

3.1 The current state of affairs

This chapter presents the basic steps required to build and conduct analyses of constraint-based cellular models with an emphasis on modeling metabolic networks. These model systems quickly grow in size and scale, introducing computational challenges that need to be addressed. With large-scale models it becomes necessary to use a robust computational platform designed specifically for sophisticated optimization problems, such as those developed by LINDO Systems, Inc (Chicago, Ill) and available through GAMS (GAMS Development Corporation, Washington, DC).

Furthermore, data management becomes difficult as models scale up in size. For example, the most current published *E. coli* model contains 904 genes and 931 unique biochemical reactions [58]. Constructing and analyzing a genome-scale model within the framework proposed in Section 2 is possible, but would be slow, unwieldy, and error prone. In recent years, an integrative data management and analysis software platform called SimPheny (Genomatica, San Diego, CA) has been developed specifically to address the data management and computational challenges inherent in building large-scale cellular models. This versatile platform provides network visualization, database, and various analytical tools that greatly facilitate the construction and study of genome-scale cellular models.

Currently, more than a dozen genome-scale metabolic models have been published and are available (Fig. 1 and Tab. 1) for further research and analysis. Most of these models represent bacteria and range from the important model organism *E. coli* [58–60] to pathogenic microbes such as *H. pylori* [61, 62] and *S. aureus* [63]. Furthermore, recently developed models of *G. sulfurreducens* [64] and *S. coelicolor* [65] are potentially important for their facilitation of studies that probe these organisms' respective potential bioenergetic and therapeutics-producing properties.

Representative constraint-based models have also appeared from the other two major branches of the tree of life. The recently developed metabolic reconstruction of *M. barkeri* [66], an interesting methanogen with bioenergetic potential, represents the first constraint-based model of an archaea that has been used to aid in the analysis of experimental data from this relatively obscure group of organisms. Furthermore, several eukaryotic models also have been developed. The metabolic models of the baker's or brewer's yeast *S. cerevisiae* [67–69] are second only to the *E. coli* models in terms of relative maturity and have been used in a variety of studies designed to assess network properties (for recent examples, see [70, 71]). Metabolic models of higher order systems are also becoming available, such as a model of mouse (*Mus muculus* [72]) as well as human cardiac mitochondria [55] and red blood cell [73].

As more of these genome-scale models are developed, the issue of making their contents available to the broader research community is of primary concern. Given their inherent complexity there is a need for a standardized format in which their contents can be consistently represented in order to circumvent potential problems associated with the current typical means of distribution via non-standard flat file or spreadsheet format. In an effort to address this concern, the Systems Biology Markup Language (SBML) [74], for example, has been developed to provide a uniform framework in which models can be represented, and the recently initiated MIRIAM ('minimum information requested in the annotation of biochemical models') project [75] and affiliated databases have appeared to provide greater transparency as to the contents, and potential deficiencies in models made publicly available. The adoption of these or similar standards will be important to the advancement of the field and in promoting its general utility in biological research.

3.2 Predicting gene essentiality

One application of constraint based modeling in conjunction with FBA that has been particularly successful in computationally assessing metabolic networks is in studies of gene essentiality. Recent studies have used genome-scale constraint-based models to assess gene essentiality for several organisms under various growth conditions, in particular using models of *E. coli* [52, 60], *H. influenzae* [76], *H. pylori* [61], *M. barkeri* [66] and *S. cerevisiae* [68, 77], under various growth conditions. Each study simulated gene deletions by constraining the flux through the associated reaction(s) to zero, as described in Section 2.4.2 and Box 1. Interestingly, relatively few central metabolic genes are predicted to be lethal. This observation likely reflects the inherent redundancy and high degree of interconnectivity that is characteristic of central metabolism. In addition, *H. influenzae* seems to be less robust than *E. coli* against single gene deletions as a higher percentage of central metabolic genes are predicted to be essential. Furthermore, given that metabolic networks appear generally robust against single gene deletions, perhaps future studies should focus on lethal double mutants, known as synthetic lethal mutants, which are commonly studied in *S. cerevisiae* [78, 79]. Results from such studies are beginning to appear [62, 69] and may provide additional insight into gene and reaction essentiality, as well as metabolic network robustness.

Beyond being useful for basic research purposes, these gene essentiality studies may also have significant importance for drug development projects. For example, each essential gene identified in these assessments represents a potential drug target as any therapy directed at these genes or associated gene products should significantly impact the organism's viability. A recent gene essentiality analysis using a genome-scale metabolic model of *Staphylococcus aureus* N315 revealed that glycan and lipid biosynthetic pathways in particular were sensitive to gene deletions [80]. Given this organism's frequent involvement in antibiotic-resistant, hospital-acquired infection, the genes involved in these processes may prove to be fruitful avenues for novel antibiotic development.

3.2.1 Model performance assessment

Validating model predictions is a critical component in constraint-based model analysis, and these gene essentiality assessments provide an ideal testing ground for this purpose. Growth phenotype data, available for a number of knockout strains and organisms, can be acquired from biochemical literature [81] and online databases, including ASAP [82] for *E. coli*, as well as CYGD and SGD for *S. cerevisiae*. Experimental growth phenotype data is available to assess directly the predictive power of the model for four of the five organisms listed previously, and shows that correct predictions were made in ~60%, 86%, 83%, and 92% of cases for *H. pylori* [61], *E. coli* [52], *S. cerevisiae* [68], and *M. barkeri* [66], respectively. These comparisons serve two important functions: validation of the general predictive potential of the model, and identification of areas that require refinement. In this sense, constraint-based models are particularly useful in experimental design by directing research to the most or least poorly understood biological components. The next section details how to interpret incorrect model predictions and their likely causes.

3.2.2 Troubleshooting incorrect predictions

In the studies discussed in Section 3.2, the model predictions, when compared to experimental findings, failed most often by falsely predicting growth when the gene deletion leads to a lethal phenotype *in vivo*. This trend indicates that the most common cause of false predictions is due to lack of information included in the network. For example, certain important pathways not related to metabolism in which the deleted gene participates may not be represented. In addition, the objective function may not be defined properly by failing to include the production of a compound required for growth. This case was shown to account for many false predictions when using a yeast metabolic model to account for strain lethality [69] when a few relatively minor changes to the biomass function dramatically improved the model's predictive capability. Alternatively, the gene deletion may lead to the production of a toxic byproduct that ultimately kills the cell, a result for which this approach cannot account. Furthermore, certain isozymes are known to be dominant, whereas metabolic models typically assign equal ability to each isozyme. The model would predict viable growth for the dominant isozyme deletion, whereas *in vivo*, the minor isozyme(s) would not sufficiently rescue the strain from the lethal phenotype perhaps due to lower gene expression or enzymatic activity.

An additional major error source stems from the lack of regulatory information incorporated into the previously described models. Including transcription factor–metabolic gene interactions, using a Boolean logic approach, enhances the accuracy of constraint-based model predictions [52]. Regulatory information is available in the primary literature, in addition to online resources such as EcoCyc and RegulonDB [83]. Furthermore, these interactions can be derived from ChIP-chip analysis of transcription factors and corresponding gene expression microarray data [49]. A more detailed treatment of this latter topic is presented in Section 4.3.

Incorrect predictions are less often due to false predictions of lethality. These uncommon cases often suggest the presence of previously unidentified enzyme activities, which, if added to the model, would lead to accurate predictions. They may also reflect improper biomass function definition, but in a different sense from the situation described above. For example, rather than failing to include compounds required for growth, it is also possible that certain compounds are included in the biomass function erroneously, and may actually not be essential to support biological growth. In any case, inaccurate [10, 84] predictions are most often attributed to a paucity of information available for inclusion in the model and not simply a failure of the technique, thus validating the general strategy of constraint-based modeling.

3.3 Uniform random sampling

Uniform random sampling of points throughout a metabolic network's solution space (see Fig. 5 for a conceptual representation of the solution space) can be used to characterize the range of metabolic functions available to the organism [70, 85, 86]. The basic strategy for using this technique with genome-scale metabolic models involves choosing an initial point, defined by a high dimensional network flux distribution vector within the solution space, by using FBA on a slightly more constrained space than normal [17]. The second step in the process involves randomly choosing another point within the space by perturbing one or more dimensions of the original flux distribution vector. This basic process, which can be thought of as a random walk within the solution space, is repeated many times, on the order of 10^5 points with every 500 points or so recorded, ultimately converging to a uniform distribution of points within the solution space.

This technique can be used to identify network modules by examining the correlation of elements within each flux distribution vector and also to readily assess the impact on functional properties of the network with the addition of new constraints to the system [10]. Interestingly, this latter

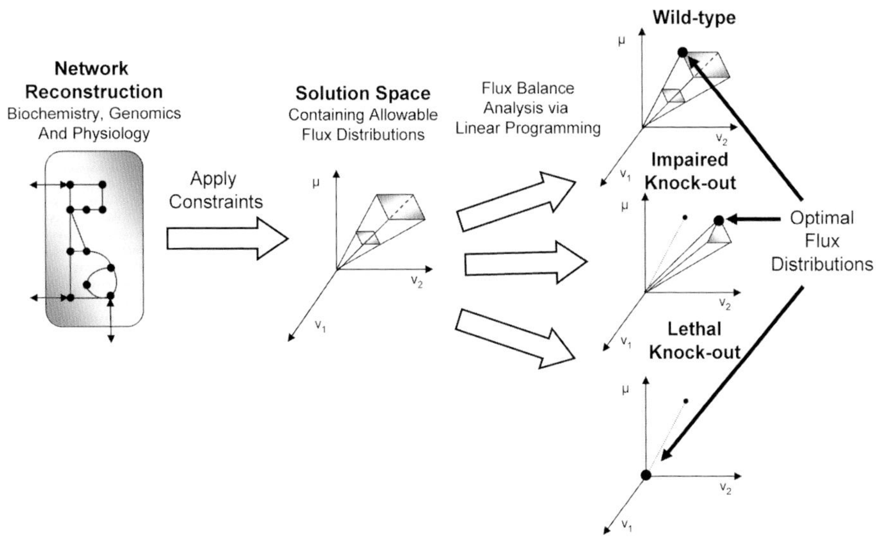

Figure 5.
Constraint-based modeling and analysis. Application of constraints to a reconstructed metabolic network (left) leads to a defined solution space that specifies a cell's allowable metabolic phenotypes (middle). Flux Balance Analysis uses linear programming to find solutions in the space that maximize or minimize a given objective (right). In the graphical representation on the right, the optimal flux distributions that maximize μ, which represents growth/biomass production for this example, are highlighted. The effects of gene knockouts on the solution space and resulting metabolic capabilities can be assessed by simulating a gene knockout and comparing its ability to grow *in silico* relative to wild type. Impaired knockout strains are those which have a lower maximum value for the objective function than wild-type, and lethal knockout strains are those which have a zero value for the objective function, indicating no growth capability when the strain harbors that particular gene deletion. As a reference the wild-type flux distribution vector is also depicted by the dashed line on the impaired and lethal knockout plots.

application has been used to study enzymopathies in the human red blood cell [16]. By imposing additional V_{max} constraints on one or more enzymes, one can simulate the adverse effect of single nucleotide polymorphisms (SNPs), for example, on the overall metabolic capabilities of the cell. This strategy showed that altering the activity level of pyruvate kinase, which is the most common enzyme deficiency to be reported in the glycolytic pathway, can have profound impacts on distant network components, thus having a broad impact on the network as a whole. A further study using this approach with the human cardiac mitochondria revealed that network perturbations designed to mimic diabetic, ischemic, and dietetic conditions can have broad, system-wide impacts, sometimes quite distant from the point of specific network insult [17]. Both of these examples highlight the potential utility of this approach in identifying potential therapeutic targets (in the case of modeling of diseased or disordered states) and for assessing potential pleiotropic effects that might be expected from certain therapeutics (in the case of modeling network impacts associated with targeted treatments).

4 Future directions for constraint-based modeling

Thus far, constraint-based models have had their primary success in assessing the metabolic capabilities of cells. However, current models generally fail to account for many other important aspects of cellular biology. In the past several years, however, several efforts have been initiated to apply the constraint-based modeling and analysis techniques to other cellular processes. Below we briefly describe relatively recent work that is setting the stage for including RNA and protein synthesis [87] as well as other processes governed by cell signaling [88] and transcriptional regulatory networks into genome-scale, constraint-based models of the cell.

4.1 Modeling of RNA and protein synthesis

RNA and protein synthesis represent two of the primary energy drains on the cell [57] and are of obvious vital importance in that these processes give rise to many of the active components responsible for cellular activities. Existing constraint-based genome-scale metabolic models do not explicitly account for these processes; rather they are included as abstract, lumped sum quantities of monomeric amino acid and nucleotide triphosphate demands required to support cellular growth [89]. The specific values for these quantities are determined from measurements of biomass constituents [57] and are independent of the genome sequence. In order to alleviate this deficiency, a scalable, constraint-based framework was developed to capture the metabolic requirements for gene expression and protein synthesis directly from the genome sequence itself [87].

a

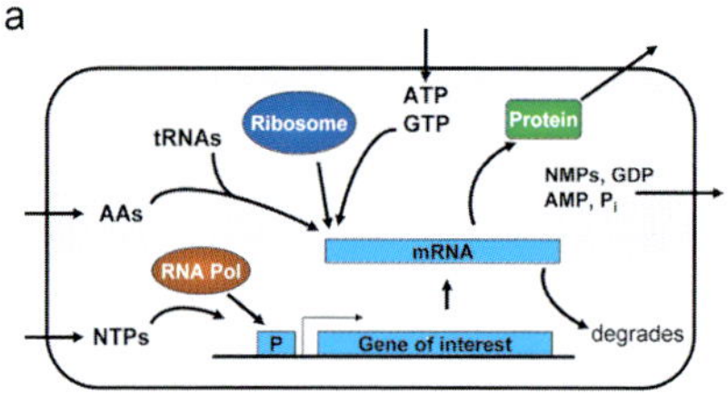

b

Transcription Initiation:	Gene + RNA Pol	→	Gene*
Transcription:	Gene* + n NTP	→	mRNA + Gene + RNA Pol + $2n$ P_i
mRNA decay:	mRNA	→	n NMP
Translation Initiation:	mRNA + Ribosome	→	Ribosome*
Translation:	Ribosome* + a AAtRNA +$2a$ GTP	→	a tRNA +$2a$ GDP + $2a$ P_i + Ribosome + mRNA + Protein
tRNA Charging:	AA + tRNA + ATP	→	AMP + $2P_i$ + AAtRNA
Exchange Reactions:	AA_{ext}	→	AA
	NTP_{ext}	→	NTP
	ATP_{ext}	→	ATP
	GTP_{ext}	→	GTP
	Protein	→	$Protein_{ext}$
	NMP	→	NMP_{ext}
	AMP	→	AMP_{ext}
	GDP	→	GDP_{ext}
	Pi	→	$P_{i\,ext}$

c

	Transcription Init.	Transcription	mRNA decay	Translation Init.	Translation	tRNA Charging	AA influx	NTP influx	ATP influx	GTP influx	Protein efflux	NMP efflux	AMP efflux	GDP efflux	P_i efflux
Gene	-1	1	0	0	0	0	0	0	0	0	0	0	0	0	0
Gene*	1	-1	0	0	0	0	0	0	0	0	0	0	0	0	0
RNA Pol	-1	1	0	0	0	0	0	0	0	0	0	0	0	0	0
NTP	0	-n	0	0	0	0	0	0	0	0	0	0	0	0	0
mRNA	0	1	-1	-1	1	0	0	0	0	0	0	0	0	0	0
P_i	0	2n	0	0	2a	2	0	0	0	0	0	0	0	0	1
NMP	0	0	n	0	0	0	0	0	0	0	0	0	0	0	0
Ribosome	0	0	0	-1	1	0	0	-1	0	0	0	0	0	0	0
Ribosome*	0	0	0	1	-1	0	0	0	0	0	0	0	0	0	0
AAtRNA	0	0	0	0	-a	1	0	0	0	0	0	0	0	0	0
Protein	0	0	0	0	1	0	0	0	0	0	1	0	0	0	0
GTP	0	0	0	0	-2a	0	0	0	0	-1	0	1	0	0	0
GDP	0	0	0	0	2a	0	0	0	0	0	0	0	0	1	0
AA	0	0	0	0	0	-1	-1	0	0	0	0	0	0	0	0
tRNA	0	0	0	0	a	-1	0	0	0	0	0	0	0	0	0
ATP	0	0	0	0	0	-1	0	0	-1	0	0	0	0	0	0
AMP	0	0	0	0	0	1	0	0	0	0	0	0	1	0	0

Figure 6.
Constraint-based modeling of RNA and protein synthesis. (**a**) A hypothetical system that represents the RNA and protein synthesis network associated with the transcription and translation of a single gene is depicted. The processes of transcription initiation, transcription, mRNA decay, translation initiation, translation, and tRNA charging are depicted. Also shown are some of the exchange fluxes required to balance the system. (**b**) A biochemical reaction list for the included processes and appropriate exchange reactions can be compiled. Note that the precise stoichiometry can and should be included in each reaction definition. In this system the gene and associated protein length can vary. Accordingly, variables for the number of bases (n) and number of amino acids (a) are included in the reaction stoichiometry. (**c**) The stoichiometric (S) matrix can then be formulated based on the reaction list. System components are represented in respective rows and each column denotes individual system reactions. AA, amino acid; AAtRNA, charged tRNA; Gene*, gene undergoing transcription; NMP, nucleotide monophosphate; P, Promoter; Pi, inorganic phosphate; Ribosome*, actively translating ribosome; RNA Pol, RNA polymerase.

The general strategy stems from the observation that RNA and protein synthesis can be broken down into constitutive biochemical reactions that underlie the processing of these polymers. As illustrated in Figure 6, the expression of a given gene and the synthesis of the protein which it encodes can be modeled by six essential biochemical reactions. These reactions include transcription initiation, transcription elongation, mRNA degradation, translation initiation, translation elongation, and tRNA charging. Biochemical equations representing each of these processes can be compiled (Fig. 6b), and used to formulate an associated stoichiometric (S) matrix (Fig. 6c).

Many of the previously introduced analytical tools can then be used to computationally assess the properties of the S matrix. For example, by choosing protein production as the objective, FBA can be used to determine how much protein the RNA and protein synthesis machinery within the cell can produce for a given set of environmental conditions and resources [87]. One can also incorporate promoter strength, transcription elongation, and translational initiation constraints on the system if such information is known or can be approximated. Extreme pathway analysis can also be used to assess the capabilities of these systems and their characteristic states [87]. Thus far, however, this framework and analysis methods have only been applied to small biological systems, namely the malate dehydrogenase (*mdh*) gene and the *lac* operon [87]. Accordingly, the limitations associated with studying large-scale systems in this manner remain to be assessed, although an ongoing study of the *E. coli* RNA and protein synthesis network (I. Thiele and B. Palsson, personal communication) is certain to be illuminating.

4.2 Modeling cell signaling networks

The signal transduction pathways that comprise cell signaling networks are responsible for many critical processes. Signaling events operate both on relatively quick time-scales, such as those that cause post-translational protein changes, and long time-scales, such as cell-cycle control, cell proliferation and migration, as well as apoptosis. Cell signaling networks are generally highly connected, complex, and involve many molecular players. In an effort to quantitatively characterize their properties, researchers are beginning to reconstruct these networks and apply mathematical methods to analyze them.

One approach to computationally analyzing cell signaling networks relies on many of the same constraint-based modeling principles discussed earlier in this chapter for metabolic networks [88, 90]. The key insight is to treat signaling pathways as a series of biochemical transformations starting with an input (the signal) and resulting in an output (post-translational protein modification, apoptosis, etc.). Accordingly, just as in modeling metabolic networks the first steps of this process focus on network reconstruction. One must first identify the components in the signaling network of interest and the interactions that occur between them. In contrast to modeling of metabolic networks where enzymes and metabolites are the primary players, signaling networks typically include receptors and their corresponding receptor ligands, metabolites such as ATP and ADP, as well as intracellular signal-transducing proteins. These networks also often include transcription factors, transcription factor binding sites, and the resulting target genes.

The data from which components and their interactions are derived have been traditionally difficult to obtain due to the often laborious effort involved in mapping signaling pathways using standard molecular biology techniques. Recently developed high-throughput, genome-scale techniques are mitigating this issue, however. For example, whole genome sequencing and annotation identifies the possible network components, ChIP-chip assays identify protein–DNA interactions, and yeast two-hybrid assays identify protein–protein interactions. As previously noted, Table 2 summarizes many useful online resources that contain publicly accessible data. Several strategies for mapping signaling pathways and networks have been developed in recent years by integrating these and other high-throughput data [2]. These methods have been employed to map DNA damage response as well as developmental pathways [2] among others.

Having identified the components and interactions that occur between them, a list of biochemical reactions that describes the cell signaling network can be listed. A stoichiometric matrix is then derived from this list (Fig. 7) in very much the same manner as previously described for metabolic as well as RNA and protein synthesis networks. It is important to note that each state of a component must be explicitly accounted for in the network. For example, a protein must be differentially represented in separate phosphorylated and unphosphorylated forms [90, 91].

This stoichiometric framework explicitly defines the underlying network reactions in a chemically consistent form. Accordingly, network properties can be readily and quantitatively assessed using previously in-

a

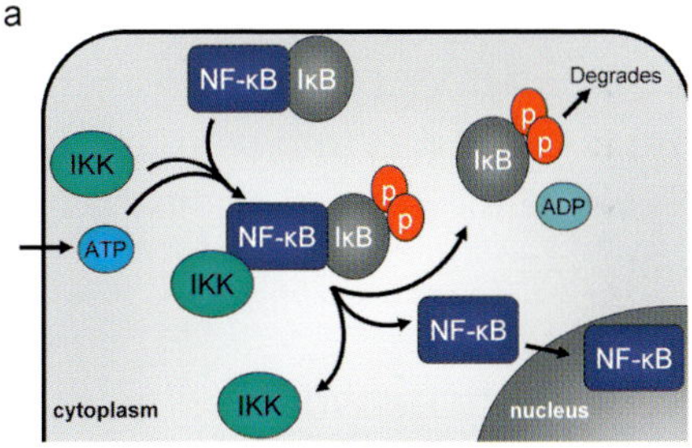

b

IKK complex formation:	IKK + IκB-NF-κB + 2ATP	→	IKK-IκB-NF-κB-ATP
IKK complex dissociation	IKK-IκB-NF-κB-ATP	→	IKK + IκBpp-NF-κB + 2ADP
NF-κB release:	IκBpp-NF-κB	→	IκBpp + NF-κB (cytoplasm)
NF-κB nuclear translocation:	NF-κB (cytoplasm)	→	NF-κB (nucleus)
IκBpp decay:	IκBpp	→	
Exchange Fluxes:	ATP (external)	→	ATP
	ADP	→	ADP (external)

c

	IKK complex form.	IKK complex dissoc.	NF-κB release	NF-κB nuclear transloc.	IκBpp decay	ATP influx	ADP efflux
IKK	-1	1	0	0	0	0	
IKK-IκB-NF-κB-ATP	1	-1	0	0	0	0	0
IκB-NF-κB	-1	0	0	0	0	0	0
IκBpp-NF-κB	0	1	-1	0	0	0	0
IκBpp	0	0	1	0	-1	0	0
NF-κB (cytoplasm)	0	0	1	-1	0	0	0
NF-κB (nucleus)	0	0	0	1	0	0	0
ATP	-2	0	0	0	0	-1	0
ADP	0	2	0	0	0	0	1

Figure 7.
Constraint-based modeling of cell signaling networks. (**a**) A schematic that includes a portion of the nuclear factor (NF)-κB signaling-related network is depicted. (**b**) A reaction list that corresponds to the schematic in (**a**) is detailed. Reactions are included for the interaction of IκB kinase (IKK) with the inhibitor of NF-κB (IκB)-NF-κB complex. The subsequent phosphorylation of IκB and release of NF-κB are also shown in addition to the degradation of phosphorylated IκB (IκBpp) and NF-κB translocation to the nucleus, and exchange fluxes required for the system. (**c**) The associated stoichiometric (S) matrix is compiled based on the reaction list. System components are depicted in each respective row, and reactions are represented in each column.

troduced analytical tools. Extreme pathway analysis, in particular, is an immensely useful tool for characterizing cell signaling networks. Using existing software [92, 93], one can enumerate the extreme pathways using the stoichiometric matrix from the reconstructed cell signaling network. Further processing of these extreme pathways allows one to derive many interesting network properties such as crosstalk, signaling redundancy, correlated reaction sets, and reaction participation [90].

Thus far, this constraint-based approach to modeling signaling networks has only been applied to a prototypic network [90] and the human B cell JAK (Janus activated kinase)-STAT (signal transducer and activator of transcription) signaling network [91]. While the prototypic network study served simply as proof of concept, the work on the JAK-STAT network showed that the constraint-based approach can be used to analyze real biological systems and yield quantitative insights into its properties. Accordingly, as more signaling networks are delineated and reconstructed, this approach will likely be of great utility.

4.3 Modeling of transcriptional regulatory networks

With the huge success of whole genome sequencing efforts and the appearance of hundreds of genome sequences [20], there is an increased interest in understanding how the genes within a given genome are regulated through complex transcriptional regulatory networks (TRNs). Consequently, efforts are underway to define and catalog the set of regulatory rules for model organisms [49]. Due to the large number of regulated genes and associated regulatory proteins as well as their extensive interconnectivity, there is a significant need for a structured framework to integrate regulatory rules and interrogate TRN functions in a systematic fashion.

Previous work has integrated models of regulatory networks with constraint-based models of metabolism to analyze and predict the effect of transcriptional regulation on cellular metabolism at the genome-scale [49, 51, 52, 94]. These studies developed and utilized a framework in which regulatory rules are represented as Boolean logic rules that control the expression of enzyme encoding genes that ultimately facilitate metabolic reactions within a constraint-based metabolic model of the type described previously within this chapter. The regulatory rules are defined such that metabolic enzyme genes are determined to be present or absent based on the presence or absence of extracellular and intracellular metabolites. If an enzyme encoding gene is determined to be absent then the flux through that enzyme is set to zero in the metabolic model, which adds a temporary constraint on the system. In effect, this is equivalent to carrying out FBA on the network following a gene deletion.

This iterative computational scheme in which Boolean rules are evaluated and FBA simulations are conducted on the appropriately constrained system has been used in analyses of small prototypic systems [51], and in genome-scale models of both *E. coli* [49] and yeast [94]. In the study of *E. coli* this analysis was performed in conjunction with dual perturbation growth experiments coupled with genome-wide expression analysis [49]. This systematic approach to reconstructing and interrogating the integrated network of *E. coli* led to the identification of many novel regulatory rules, and an expanded characterization of the genome-scale TRN, based on a model-driven analysis of multiple high-throughput datasets. Furthermore, a recent study has also used the integrated *E. coli* model in a large-scale simulation project to study all potential network states and found them to be organized primarily based upon terminal electron acceptor availability [56]. However, one shortcoming of this framework is that it does not facilitate a detailed analysis of transcriptional regulatory network properties.

In an effort to address this limitation, a structured and self-contained representation of TRNs that can be quantitatively interrogated has been developed relying on the principles of the constraint-based approach [95]. This strategy, which effectively connects environmental cues to transcriptional responses, is conceptually similar to the previously described constraint-based approach to modeling cell signaling networks. The first step in the process involves defining the components of the system and interactions between them based on legacy data from traditional molecular biology studies or from recently generated high-throughput data, such as ChIP-chip data which defines network connectivity, and microarray gene expression data which helps define upregulation and downregulation of genes.

Having gathered this type of information that describes the regulatory system of interest, the next step is to write quasi-stoichiometric, biochemical equations that describe the regulatory logic for each interaction in the network (Fig. 8b). To illustrate directly some of these concepts, we briefly consider the *lac* operon in *E. coli*. For the purpose of this investigation, the system is defined to include the *lac* operon (*lacZYA*) and the proteins each gene encodes, the inhibitor of the operon (*lacI*), an activator of the operon (Crp), and the intracellular inducer molecule allolactose, which inhibits the LacI inhibitor thus activating *lacZYA* transcription (Fig. 8a) by way of de-repression.

Having defined the system (Fig. 8a) and Boolean rules that specify the regulatory logic of this small transcriptional regulatory network (Fig. 8b), the system can be formulated and the associated **R** matrix constructed

a

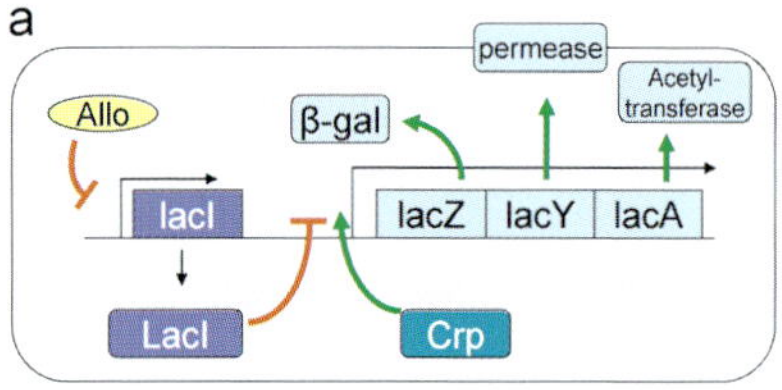

b

Genes	Rules
LacI	NOT(Allo)
LacZ	Crp AND NOT(LacI)
LacY	Crp AND NOT(LacI)
LacA	Crp AND NOT(LacI)

c

	vlacI	vLacI	vNOTLacI	vlacOperon	vLacOperon	Allo	Crp	LacI	LacA	LacZ	LacY
lacI	-1	1	0	0	0	0	0	0	0	0	0
*lacI**	1	-1	0	0	0	0	0	0	0	0	0
LacI	0	1	-1	0	0	0	0	-1	0	0	0
Allo	0	0	-1	0	0	-1	0	0	0	0	0
NOT_LacI	0	0	1	-1	0	0	0	0	0	0	0
Crp	0	0	0	-1	0	0	-1	0	0	0	0
lacZYA	0	0	0	-1	1	0	0	0	0	0	0
*lacZYA**	0	0	0	1	-1	0	0	0	0	0	0
LacZ	0	0	0	0	1	0	0	0	0	-1	0
LacY	0	0	0	0	1	0	0	0	0	0	-1
LacA	0	0	0	0	1	0	0	0	-1	0	0

d

$\mathbf{r}^T =$

vlacI	vLacI	vNOTLacI	vlacOperon	vLacOperon	Allo	Crp	LacI	LacZ	LacY	LacA
1	1	0	0	0	0	0	1	0	0	0
1	1	1	1	1	-1	-1	0	1	1	1

e f

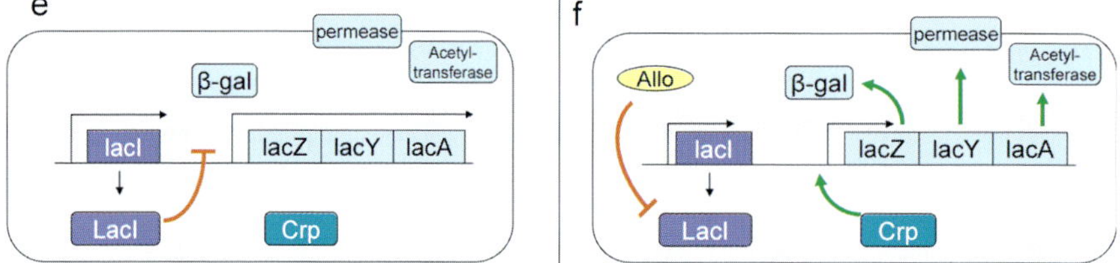

Extreme Pathway $\mathbf{r_1}$:
lac operon not expressed

Extreme Pathway $\mathbf{r_2}$:
lac operon expressed

Figure 8.
Constraint-based modeling and analysis of transcriptional regulatory networks. (**a**) The *lac* operon regulatory system is depicted and defined to include the *lac* operon genes (*lacZ*, *lacY*, *lacA*), the inhibitor gene *lacI*, the activator *Crp*, and the inducer allolactose (*Allo*). (**b**) A reaction list that summarizes the Boolean rules that capture the regulatory logic of the system is shown. (**c**) The R matrix that corresponds to the regulatory rule list from (**b**) is depicted with each row corresponding to system components and each column specifying regulatory reactions in a quasi-stoichiometric formalism. Accordingly, a '−1' represents a 'consumed' component, whereas a '+1' represents a 'produced' component. (**d**) The two extreme pathways for this system are listed in **r** with the corresponding reaction labels listed as well for reference. A non-zero value indicates that the corresponding reaction is active. The negative coefficients in the second extreme pathway reflect that *Allo* and *Crp* can be thought of as conceptually flowing into the system. (**e**) Pathway 1 is graphically illustrated and reflects the conditions for the LacI-mediated inhibition of the *lac* operon. (**f**) The graphical depiction of Pathway 2 shows the activation of the *lac* operon (i.e., inhibition of LacI by allolactose, thus allowing for de-repression and Crp-activated expression of *lacZYA*). $\mathbf{r}^T$, the transpose of the extreme pathway vectors reported in r (depicted in this way simply out of space considerations).

(Fig. 8c) in which each row represents a system component and each column represents a regulatory interaction or transport reaction. For the purposes of this analysis, each gene/operon is depicted within the matrix twice: *lacI* and *lacI**, as well as *lacZYA* and *lacZYA**. The former entity represents the open form, whereas the latter, asterisk-marked entity represents the actively transcribed form of the gene. This level of detail is not required in formulating **R** as the actively transcribed form of the gene is only a transient entity between transcription and translation. Rather, this is meant to show concretely that such mechanistic detail about ORFs and other network relationships can be readily incorporated into the current formalism as the data becomes available.

It should be noted that one peculiarity of this methodology is that it requires the inclusion of the converse of regulatory rules in addition to the regulatory rules themselves. The *converse* of the regulatory rules – i.e., the regulatory reactions that lead to the inhibition of gene transcription in our sample system – is necessary to reflect the lack of protein production for a given set of environmental cues. Many regulatory rules are inhibitory, such that the expression of a protein depends on the absence of a given metabolite or protein product. Additional reactions that include the converse of the regulatory rules and the absence of metabolites and protein products where appropriate must be included in the system. Also, note that regulatory rules of the Boolean type 'OR' require two separate reactions to indicate that there are two independent ways in which the target gene can be transcribed.

The **R** matrix can be analyzed using many of the tools previously described for analysis of the metabolic **S** matrix. For example, extreme pathway analysis on this system yields two vectors, denoted in *r*, (Fig. 8d) that represent the two possible expression states for the *lac* system. Each entry in the *r* vectors represents the activity of a reaction in the expression state, or pathway. For reaction names prefaced with a 'v', a 1 indicates that the reaction is active, and a 0 indicates that it is inactive. In the remaining reactions that specify flow across the system boundary, a 1 indicates flow out of the system (for example, a protein is produced), a -1 indicates flow into the system, and a 0 indicates that the associated component is neither produced nor consumed. Note that the entries are not quantitative but denote an active connection, and further, that a series of connections leads to a 'causal path'. As depicted graphically in Figure 8e and 8f respectively, vector r_1 represents the LacI-mediated inhibition of the *lac* operon and r_2 defines the inhibition of LacI by allolactose, thus resulting in de-repression and Crp-activated expression of *lacZYA*.

Thus far this approach has only been applied to the small *lac* operon system described above and a larger 25 gene prototypic network [95]. While this proof of concept study validates the utility of this approach for small systems, potential complications associated with scaling this approach up to genome-scale systems remain to be determined. Nonetheless, transcriptional regulatory network matrix reconstructions for model organisms will likely be important not only in studies of regulatory network properties, but also in guiding experimental programs based upon results from these analyses.

4.4 The next big challenge

The constraint-based approach has proven immensely successful for modeling metabolic systems and, as described in this section, is showing promise for RNA and protein synthesis, cell signaling, and transcriptional regulatory networks. However, as the field currently stands, each respective framework produces models that exist as independent entities. Arguably, the ultimate goal of systems biology is to integrate data from disparate sources and generate comprehensive models that reflect biological reality for entire cells. Therefore, these constraint-based modeling strategies present an opportunity to take a significant step forward in realizing this aim through integrative modeling efforts.

To elaborate, the interconnectivity between these distinct networks is clear. For example, a simplistic, but illustrative conceptual picture (Fig. 9) can be envisioned in which system inputs are recognized by cell signaling networks that in turn stimulate regulatory processes. These regulatory processes mediate RNA and protein synthesis ultimately leading to the production of enzymes that perform metabolic processes and lead to cell growth or maintenance. Additional connectivity between the systems also exists in the form of feedback processes and shared currency metabolites such as ATP and GTP, for example. Thus, in principle, the stoichiometric and pseudo-stoichiometric representations of the networks described in

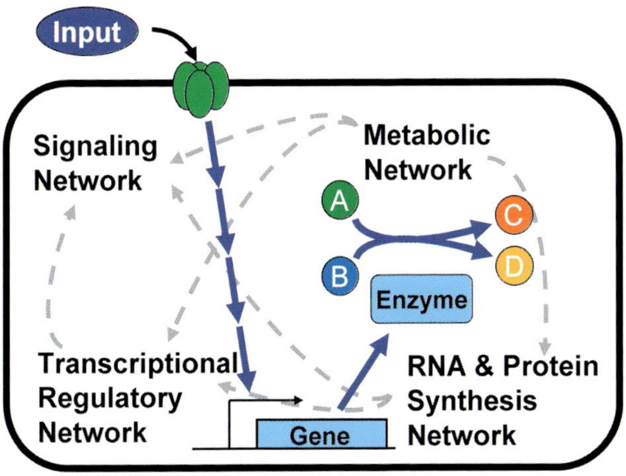

Figure 9.
The next big challenge: Model integration. This chapter has illustrated the utility of constraint-based modeling and analysis in computationally representing many cellular processes. To date, however, these models have been developed and analyzed in isolation despite the fact that these systems are all interrelated, as shown in this conceptual figure. For example, cellular signals, or inputs, are recognized by the cell signaling network, which in turn stimulate regulatory processes. These regulatory processes mediate RNA and protein synthesis ultimately leading to the production of enzymes that perform metabolic processes that result in cell growth or maintenance. The dashed arrows highlight the interconnectivity of these networks in the form of shared molecular components or feedback mechanisms. In principle, the constraint-based formalism can be used as a platform to capture these systems into a single picture. Accordingly, one of the next major challenges facing the field is to integrate these models of disparate cellular processes, thus pushing toward one of the field of systems biology's foundational goals: to computationally represent and analyze models of entire cells and biological systems.

this chapter could be integrated into a unified model of the cell. While there are certainly computational challenges that will need to be overcome in order to facilitate the development and analysis of such a model, this notion seems feasible and is sure to be tackled in the near future. Representing additional, more complicated cellular processes, such as differentiation and development, as well as accounting for multicellularity await novel research efforts and represent open problems to be addressed in the more distant future.

5 Conclusions

Despite the challenges outlined in the previous section associated with pushing the field forward, constraint-based modeling and its associated analyses are and will remain powerful tools that facilitate system-level modeling [9, 52, 88] and analysis of biological networks [56, 96–98]. Furthermore, these model-based studies can be used to help researchers prioritize experimental projects and save considerable time at the bench. Beyond its utility as a tool for basic biological research and in metabolic engineering applications [99, 100], this computational approach also has potential medical and drug development relevance. For example, in pathogenic microbial models, each gene that is predicted to be essential by constraint based modeling and analysis represents a potential drug target that could be used to develop novel antibiotics in the future. Additionally, network analysis of human systems may reveal interesting therapeutic targets and provide a platform for assessing potentially adverse pleiotropic effects of novel treatments. As more genome-scale models are developed and existing models enhanced, additional applications in a broad range of fields will likely become apparent. Consequently, the flexibility of constraint-based models will continue to be exploited to drive the exploration of countless exciting biological questions in the future.

References

1 Wheeler DL, Church DM, Edgar R, Federhen S, Helmberg W, Madden TL, Pontius JU, Schuler GD, Schriml LM, Sequeira E et al (2004) Database resources of the National Center for Biotechnology Information: update. *Nucleic Acids Res* 32 Database issue: D35–40

2 Joyce AR, Palsson BO (2006) The model organism as a system: integrating 'omics' data sets. *Nat Rev Mol Cell Biol* 7(3): 198–210

3 Arkin AP (2001) Synthetic cell biology. *Curr Opin Biotechnol* 12(6): 638–644

4 Tomita M, Hashimoto K, Takahashi K, Shimizu TS, Matsuzaki Y, Miyoshi F, Saito K, Tanida S, Yugi K, Venter JC et al (1999) E-CELL: software environment for whole-cell simulation. *Bioinformatics* 15(1): 72–84

5 Hoffmann A, Levchenko A, Scott ML, Baltimore D (2002) The IkappaB-NF-kappaB signaling module: temporal control and selective gene activation. *Science* 298(5596): 1241–1245

6 Elowitz MB, Levine AJ, Siggia ED, Swain PS (2002) Stochastic gene expression in a single cell. *Science* 297(5584): 1183–1186
7 Arkin A, Ross J, McAdams HH (1998) Stochastic kinetic analysis of developmental pathway bifurcation in phage lambda-infected *Escherichia coli* cells. *Genetics* 149(4): 1633–1648
8 Sarkar A, Franza BR (2004) A logical analysis of the process of T cell activation: different consequences depending on the state of CD28 engagement. *J Theor Biol* 226(4): 455–466
9 Reed JL, Famili I, Thiele I, Palsson BO (2006) Towards multidimensional genome annotation. *Nat Rev Genet* 7(2): 130–141
10 Price ND, Reed JL, Palsson BO (2004) Genome-scale models of microbial cells: evaluating the consequences of constraints. *Nat Rev Microbiol* 2(11): 886–897
11 Edwards JS, Covert M, Palsson B (2002) Metabolic modelling of microbes: the flux-balance approach. *Environ Microbiol* 4(3): 133–140
12 Covert MW, Famili I, Palsson BO (2003) Identifying constraints that govern cell behavior: a key to converting conceptual to computational models in biology? *Biotechnol Bioeng* 84(7): 763–772
13 Price ND, Papin JA, Schilling CH, Palsson BO (2003) Genome-scale microbial *in silico* models: the constraints-based approach. *Trends Biotechnol* 21(4): 162–169
14 Varma A, Palsson BO (1994) Stoichiometric flux balance models quantitatively predict growth and metabolic by-product secretion in wild-type *Escherichia coli* W3110. *Appl Environ Microbiol* 60(10): 3724–3731
15 Kauffman KJ, Prakash P, Edwards JS (2003) Advances in flux balance analysis. *Curr Opin Biotechnol* 14(5): 491–496
16 Price ND, Schellenberger J, Palsson BO (2004) Uniform sampling of steady-state flux spaces: means to design experiments and to interpret enzymopathies. *Biophys J* 87(4): 2172–2186
17 Thiele I, Price ND, Vo TD, Palsson BO (2005) Candidate metabolic network states in human mitochondria. Impact of diabetes, ischemia, and diet. *J Biol Chem* 280(12): 11683–11695
18 Neidhardt FC, Curtiss R (1996) *Escherichia coli and Salmonella: Cellular and molecular biology*. 2nd ed. ASM Press, Washington, DC, USA
19 Scheffler IE (1999) *Mitochondria*. Wiley-Liss, New York, USA
20 Liolios K, Tavernarakis N, Hugenholtz P, Kyrpides NC (2006) The Genomes On Line Database (GOLD) v.2: a monitor of genome projects worldwide. *Nucleic Acids Res* 34(Database issue): D332–334
21 Consortium CSAA (2005) Initial sequence of the chimpanzee genome and comparison with the human genome. *Nature* 437(7055): 69–87
22 Gibbs RA, Weinstock GM, Metzker ML, Muzny DM, Sodergren EJ, Scherer S, Scott G, Steffen D, Worley KC, Burch PE et al (2004) Genome sequence of the Brown Norway rat yields insights into mammalian evolution. *Nature* 428(6982): 493–521
23 Istrail S, Sutton GG, Florea L, Halpern AL, Mobarry CM, Lippert R, Walenz B, Shatkay H, Dew I, Miller JR et al (2004) Whole-genome shotgun assembly and

comparison of human genome assemblies. *Proc Natl Acad Sci USA* 101(7): 1916–1921

24 Kirkness EF, Bafna V, Halpern AL, Levy S, Remington K, Rusch DB, Delcher AL, Pop M, Wang W, Fraser CM et al (2003) The dog genome: survey sequencing and comparative analysis. *Science* 301(5641): 1898–1903

25 Stein L (2001) Genome annotation: from sequence to biology. *Nat Rev Genet* 2(7): 493–503

26 Brent MR (2005) Genome annotation past, present, and future: how to define an ORF at each locus. *Genome Res* 15(12): 1777–1786

27 Mao X, Cai T, Olyarchuk JG, Wei L (2005) Automated genome annotation and pathway identification using the KEGG Orthology (KO) as a controlled vocabulary. *Bioinformatics* 21(19): 3787–3793

28 Karp PD, Paley S, Romero P (2002) The Pathway Tools software. *Bioinformatics* 18 Suppl 1: S225–232

29 Cash P (2003) Proteomics of bacterial pathogens. *Adv Biochem Eng Biotechnol* 83: 93–115

30 Taylor SW, Fahy E, Ghosh SS (2003) Global organellar proteomics. *Trends Biotechnol* 21(2): 82–88

31 Kanehisa M, Goto S, Kawashima S, Okuno Y, Hattori M (2004) The KEGG resource for deciphering the genome. *Nucleic Acids Res* 32 Database issue: D277–280

32 Karp PD, Riley M, Saier M, Paulsen IT, Collado-Vides J, Paley SM, Pellegrini-Toole A, Bonavides C, Gama-Castro S (2002) The EcoCyc Database. *Nucleic Acids Res* 30(1): 56–58

33 Mewes HW, Amid C, Arnold R, Frishman D, Guldener U, Mannhaupt G, Munsterkotter M, Pagel P, Strack N, Stumpflen V et al (2004) MIPS: analysis and annotation of proteins from whole genomes. *Nucleic Acids Res* 32 Database issue: D41–44

34 Christie KR, Weng S, Balakrishnan R, Costanzo MC, Dolinski K, Dwight SS, Engel SR, Feierbach B, Fisk DG, Hirschman JE et al (2004) Saccharomyces Genome Database (SGD) provides tools to identify and analyze sequences from *Saccharomyces cerevisiae* and related sequences from other organisms. *Nucleic Acids Res* 32 Database issue: D311–314

35 Caspi R, Foerster H, Fulcher CA, Hopkinson R, Ingraham J, Kaipa P, Krummenacker M, Paley S, Pick J, Rhee SY et al (2006) MetaCyc: a multiorganism database of metabolic pathways and enzymes. *Nucleic Acids Res* 34(Database issue): D511–516

36 Karp PD, Ouzounis CA, Moore-Kochlacs C, Goldovsky L, Kaipa P, Ahren D, Tsoka S, Darzentas N, Kunin V, Lopez-Bigas N (2005) Expansion of the BioCyc collection of pathway/genome databases to 160 genomes. *Nucleic Acids Res* 33(19): 6083–6089

37 Harris MA, Clark J, Ireland A, Lomax J, Ashburner M, Foulger R, Eilbeck K, Lewis S, Marshall B, Mungall C et al (2004) The Gene Ontology (GO) database and informatics resource. *Nucleic Acids Res* 32 Database issue: D258–261

38 (2006) The Gene Ontology (GO) project in 2006. *Nucleic Acids Res* 34(Database issue): D322–326

39 Serres MH, Goswami S, Riley M (2004) GenProtEC: an updated and improved analysis of functions of *Escherichia coli* K-12 proteins. *Nucleic Acids Res* 32 Database issue: D300–302

40 Coulton G (2004) Are histochemistry and cytochemistry 'Omics'? *J Mol Histol* 35(6): 603–613

41 Arita M, Robert M, Tomita M (2005) All systems go: launching cell simulation fueled by integrated experimental biology data. *Curr Opin Biotechnol* 16(3): 344–349

42 Huh WK, Falvo JV, Gerke LC, Carroll AS, Howson RW, Weissman JS, O'Shea EK (2003) Global analysis of protein localization in budding yeast. *Nature* 425(6959): 686–691

43 Guda C, Subramaniam S (2005) pTARGET: a new method for predicting protein subcellular localization in eukaryotes. *Bioinformatics* 21(21): 3963–3969

44 Fields S (2005) High-throughput two-hybrid analysis. The promise and the peril. *Febs J* 272(21): 5391–5399

45 Deeds EJ, Ashenberg O, Shakhnovich EI (2006) A simple physical model for scaling in protein–protein interaction networks. *Proc Natl Acad Sci USA* 103(2): 311–316

46 Sprinzak E, Sattath S, Margalit H (2003) How reliable are experimental protein–protein interaction data? *J Mol Biol* 327(5): 919–923

47 Palsson B (2004) Two-dimensional annotation of genomes. *Nat Biotechnol* 22(10): 1218–1219

48 Beard DA, Liang SD, Qian H (2002) Energy balance for analysis of complex metabolic networks. *Biophys J* 83(1): 79–86

49 Covert MW, Knight EM, Reed JL, Herrgard MJ, Palsson BO (2004) Integrating high-throughput and computational data elucidates bacterial networks. *Nature* 429(6987): 92–96

50 Covert MW, Palsson BO (2003) Constraints-based models: regulation of gene expression reduces the steady-state solution space. *J Theor Biol* 221(3): 309–325

51 Covert MW, Schilling CH, Palsson B (2001) Regulation of gene expression in flux balance models of metabolism. *J Theor Biol* 213(1): 73–88

52 Covert MW, Palsson BO (2002) Transcriptional regulation in constraints-based metabolic models of *Escherichia coli*. *J Biol Chem* 277(31): 28058–28064

53 Chvatal V (1983) *Linear Programming*. WH Freeman and Company, New York, USA

54 Reed JL, Palsson BO (2004) Genome-scale *in silico* models of *E. coli* have multiple equivalent phenotypic states: assessment of correlated reaction subsets that comprise network states. *Genome Res* 14(9): 1797–1805

55 Vo TD, Greenberg HJ, Palsson BO (2004) Reconstruction and functional characterization of the human mitochondrial metabolic network based on proteomic and biochemical data. *J Biol Chem* 279(38): 39532–39540

56 Barrett CL, Herring CD, Reed JL, Palsson BO (2005) The global transcriptional regulatory network for metabolism in *Escherichia coli* exhibits few dominant functional states. *Proc Natl Acad Sci USA* 102(52): 19103–19108

57 Neidhardt FC, Ingraham JL, Schaechter M (1990) *Physiology of the bacterial cell.* Sinauer Associates, Inc., Sunderland, MA, USA
58 Reed JL, Vo TD, Schilling CH, Palsson BO (2003) An expanded genome-scale model of *Escherichia coli* K-12 (iJR904 GSM/GPR). *Genome Biol* 4(9): R54
59 Reed JL, Palsson BO (2003) Thirteen years of building constraint-based *in silico* models of *Escherichia coli. J Bacteriol* 185(9): 2692–2699
60 Edwards JS, Palsson BO (2000) The *Escherichia coli* MG1655 *in silico* metabolic genotype: its definition, characteristics, and capabilities. *Proc Natl Acad Sci USA* 97(10): 5528–5533
61 Schilling CH, Covert MW, Famili I, Church GM, Edwards JS, Palsson BO (2002) Genome-scale metabolic model of *Helicobacter pylori* 26695. *J Bacteriol* 184(16): 4582–4593
62 Thiele I, Vo TD, Price ND, Palsson B (2005) An expanded metabolic reconstruction of *Helicobacter pylori* (*i*IT341 GSM/GPR): An *in silico* genome-scale characterization of single and double deletion mutants. *J Bacteriol* 187(16): 5818–5830
63 Becker SA, Palsson BO (2005) Genome-scale reconstruction of the metabolic network in *Staphylococcus aureus* N315: an initial draft to the two-dimensional annotation. *BMC Microbiol* 5(1): 8
64 Mahadevan R, Bond DR, Butler JE, Esteve-Nunez A, Coppi MV, Palsson BO, Schilling CH, Lovley DR (2006) Characterization of metabolism in the Fe(III)-reducing organism *Geobacter sulfurreducens* by constraint-based modeling. *Appl Environ Microbiol* 72(2): 1558–1568
65 Borodina I, Krabben P, Nielsen J (2005) Genome-scale analysis of *Streptomyces coelicolor* A3(2) metabolism. *Genome Res* 15(6): 820–829
66 Feist AM, Scholten JCM, Palsson BO, Brockman FJ, Ideker T (2006) Modeling methanogenesis with a genome-scale metabolic reconstruction of *Methanosarcina barkeri. Mol Syst Biol* 2(1): msb4100046-E1-msb4100046-E14
67 Forster J, Famili I, Fu P, Palsson BO, Nielsen J (2003) Genome-scale reconstruction of the *Saccharomyces cerevisiae* metabolic network. *Genome Res* 13(2): 244–253
68 Duarte NC, Herrgard MJ, Palsson BO (2004) Reconstruction and validation of *Saccharomyces cerevisiae* iND750, a fully compartmentalized genome-scale metabolic model. *Genome Res* 14(7): 1298–1309
69 Kuepfer L, Sauer U, Blank LM (2005) Metabolic functions of duplicate genes in *Saccharomyces cerevisiae. Genome Res* 15(10): 1421–1430
70 Almaas E, Oltvai ZN, Barabasi AL (2005) The activity reaction core and plasticity of metabolic networks. *PLoS Comput Biol* 1(7): e68
71 Segre D, DeLuna A, Church GM, Kishnoy R (2005) Modular epistasis in yeast metabolism. *Nat Genet* 37(1): 77–83
72 Sheikh K, Forster J, Nielsen LK (2005) Modeling hybridoma cell metabolism using a generic genome-scale metabolic model of *Mus musculus. Biotechnol Prog* 21(1): 112–121
73 Wiback SJ, Palsson BO (2002) Extreme pathway analysis of human red blood cell metabolism. *Biophys J* 83(2): 808–818
74 Hucka M, Finney A, Sauro HM, Bolouri H, Doyle JC, Kitano H, Arkin AP, Bornstein BJ, Bray D, Cornish-Bowden A et al (2003) The systems biology markup

language (SBML): a medium for representation and exchange of biochemical network models. *Bioinformatics* 19(4): 524–531
75 Novere NL, Finney A, Hucka M, Bhalla US, Campagne F, Collado-Vides J, Crampin EJ, Halstead M, Klipp E, Mendes P et al (2005) Minimum information requested in the annotation of biochemical models (MIRIAM). *Nat Biotechnol* 23(12): 1509–1515
76 Schilling CH, Palsson BO (2000) Assessment of the metabolic capabilities of *Haemophilus influenzae* Rd through a genome-scale pathway analysis. *J Theor Biol* 203(3): 249–283
77 Forster J, Famili I, Palsson BO, Nielsen J (2003) Large-scale evaluation of *in silico* gene deletions in *Saccharomyces cerevisiae*. *Omics* 7(2): 193–202
78 Hartwell L (2004) Genetics. Robust interactions. *Science* 303(5659): 774–775
79 Tong AH, Lesage G, Bader GD, Ding H, Xu H, Xin X, Young J, Berriz GF, Brost RL, Chang M et al (2004) Global mapping of the yeast genetic interaction network. *Science* 303(5659): 808–813
80 Heinemann M, Kummel A, Ruinatscha R, Panke S (2005) *In silico* genome-scale reconstruction and validation of the *Staphylococcus aureus* metabolic network. *Biotechnol Bioeng* 92(7): 850–864
81 Baba T, Ara T, Hasegawa M, Takai Y, Okumura Y, Baba M, Datsenko KA, Tomita M, Wanner BL, Mori H (2006) Construction of *Escherichia coli* K-12 in-frame, single-gene knockout mutants: the Keio collection. 2(1): msb4100050-E1-msb4100050-E11
82 Glasner JD, Liss P, Plunkett G 3rd, Darling A, Prasad T, Rusch M, Byrnes A, Gilson M, Biehl B, Blattner FR et al (2003) ASAP, a systematic annotation package for community analysis of genomes. *Nucleic Acids Res* 31(1): 147–151
83 Salgado H, Gama-Castro S, Martinez-Antonio A, Diaz-Peredo E, Sanchez-Solano F, Peralta-Gil M, Garcia-Alonso D, Jimenez-Jacinto V, Santos-Zavaleta A, Bonavides-Martinez C et al (2004) RegulonDB (version 4.0): transcriptional regulation, operon organization and growth conditions in *Escherichia coli* K-12. *Nucleic Acids Res* 32 Database issue: D303–306
84 Palsson BO (2006) *Systems Biology: Properties of Reconstructed Networks*. Cambridge University Press, UK
85 Price ND, Thiele I, Palsson BO (2006) Candidate states of *Helicobacter pylori's* genome-scale metabolic network upon application of loop law thermodynamic constraints. *Biophys J* 90(11): 3919–3928
86 Almaas E, Kovacs B, Vicsek T, Oltvai ZN, Barabasi AL (2004) Global organization of metabolic fluxes in the bacterium *Escherichia coli*. *Nature* 427(6977): 839–843
87 Allen TE, Palsson BO (2003) Sequence-based analysis of metabolic demands for protein synthesis in prokaryotes. *J Theor Biol* 220(1): 1–18
88 Papin JA, Hunter T, Palsson BO, Subramaniam S (2005) Reconstruction of cellular signalling networks and analysis of their properties. *Nat Rev Mol Cell Biol* 6(2): 99–111
89 Varma A, Palsson BO (1993) Metabolic capabilities of *Escherichia coli*: II. Optimal growth patterns. *J Theor Biol* 165(4): 503–522

90 Papin JA, Palsson BO (2004) Topological analysis of mass-balanced signaling networks: a framework to obtain network properties including crosstalk. *J Theor Biol* 227(2): 283–297
91 Papin JA, Palsson BO (2004) The JAK-STAT signaling network in the human B-cell: an extreme signaling pathway analysis. *Biophys J* 87(1): 37–46
92 Schilling CH, Palsson BO (2000) Assessment of the metabolic capabilities of *Haemophilus influenzae* Rd through a genome-scale pathway Analysis. *J Theor Biol* 203(3): 249–283
93 Bell SL, Palsson BO (2005) Expa: a program for calculating extreme pathways in biochemical reaction networks. *Bioinformatics* 21(8): 1739–1740
94 Herrgard MJ, Lee BS, Portnoy V, Palsson BO (2006) Integrated analysis of regulatory and metabolic networks reveals novel regulatory mechanisms in *Saccharomyces cerevisiae*. *Genome Res* 16(5): 627–635
95 Gianchandani EP, Papin JA, Price ND, Joyce AR, Palsson BO (2006) Matrix formalism to describe functional states of transcriptional regulatory systems. *PLoS Comput Biol* 2(8): e101
96 Papin JA, Price ND, Palsson BO (2002) Extreme pathway lengths and reaction participation in genome-scale metabolic networks. *Genome Res* 12(12): 1889–1900
97 Price ND, Reed JL, Papin JA, Famili I, Palsson BO (2003) Analysis of metabolic capabilities using singular value decomposition of extreme pathway matrices. *Biophys J* 84(2 Pt 1): 794–804
98 Price ND, Papin JA, Palsson BO (2002) Determination of redundancy and systems properties of the metabolic network of *Helicobacter pylori* using genome-scale extreme pathway analysis. *Genome Res* 12(5): 760–769
99 Fong SS, Burgard AP, Herring CD, Knight EM, Blattner FR, Maranas CD, Palsson BO (2005) *In silico* design and adaptive evolution of *Escherichia coli* for production of lactic acid. *Biotechnol Bioeng* 91(5): 643–648
100 Burgard AP, Pharkya P, Maranas CD (2003) Optknock: a bilevel programming framework for identifying gene knockout strategies for microbial strain optimization. *Biotechnol Bioeng* 84(6): 647–657
101 Wheeler DL, Barrett T, Benson DA, Bryant SH, Canese K, Chetvernin V, Church DM, DiCuccio M, Edgar R, Federhen S et al (2006) Database resources of the National Center for Biotechnology Information. *Nucleic Acids Res* 34(Database issue): D173–180
102 Park SM, Schilling CH, Palsson BO (2003) *Compositions and methods for modeling Bacillus subtilis metabolism*. US Patent and Trademark Office, USA
103 Edwards JS, Palsson BO (1999) Systems properties of the *Haemophilus influenzae* Rd metabolic genotype. *J Biol Chem* 274(25): 17410–17416
104 Oliveira AP, Nielsen J, Forster J (2005) Modeling *Lactococcus lactis* using a genome-scale flux model. *BMC Microbiol* 5: 39
105 Hong SH, Kim JS, Lee SY, In YH, Choi SS, Rih JK, Kim CH, Jeong H, Hur CG, Kim JJ (2004) The genome sequence of the capnophilic rumen bacterium *Mannheimia succiniciproducens*. *Nat Biotechnol* 22(10): 1275–1281

106 Taylor SW, Fahy E, Zhang B, Glenn GM, Warnock DE, Wiley S, Murphy AN, Gaucher SP, Capaldi RA, Gibson BW et al (2003) Characterization of the human heart mitochondrial proteome. *Nat Biotechnol* 21(3): 281–286

Progress in Drug Research, Vol. 64
(Helena I. Boshoff and Clifton E. Barry III, Eds)

Genomics of host-pathogen interactions

By Dirk Schnappinger

Department of Microbiology and Immunology,
Weill Medical College of Cornell University,
New York, USA
<dis2003@med.cornell.edu>

Abstract

The complete sequences of hundreds of microbial genomes have provided drug discovery pipelines with thousands of new potential drug targets. Their availability has also stimulated the development of a variety of innovative approaches that allow functional studies to be performed on the entire genome of an organism. This chapter describes how these approaches have been applied to the analysis of host–pathogen interactions and discusses how such studies might facilitate the development of new antibiotics.

Abbrevations: CGHs – comparative genome hybridizations; DARQs – diarylquinolones; gDNA – genomic DNA; GWM – genome wide mutagenesis; NO – nitric oxide; NOS2 – nitric oxide synthase 2; ORF – open reading frame; PAI – pathogenicity island.

1 Introduction

In July of 1995 the first sequence of an entire genome of a free-living organism, that of the bacterium *Haemophilus influenzae* Rd, was determined [1]. About 3 months later two techniques, serial analysis of gene expression (SAGE) [2] and microarray expression profiling [3], were described that allowed to efficiently perform genome-wide expression analyses. Within the next 10 years, approximately 250 other microbial genomes were fully sequenced and genome-wide expression profiling has been applied to investigate a plethora of biological processes in numerous organisms. More recently, techniques that allow high-throughput analyses of thousands of bacterial mutants in parallel have also been developed. This chapter summarizes some of the main findings that were made by applying comparative genomics, RNA profiling and genome-wide mutagenesis to the analysis of the interactions of bacterial pathogens with their hosts and host cells.

2 Functional genomics of bacterial pathogens

2.1 Comparative genomics

Almost 250 prokaryotic genomes have been sequenced since the first complete genome sequence of a bacterium was determined in 1995 [1]. One immediate benefit of this number of completed genome sequences has been the opportunity to study not only one gene or gene family but the complete haploid genome of a species. Sequence comparisons within single genomes can be informative since horizontal gene transfer represents one of the main mechanisms that can transform commensal organisms into pathogens [4]. DNA fragments that recently entered a genome via horizontal transfer often have a G+C content that is different from the rest of the genome and are frequently flanked by DNA encoding tRNAs, sequence repeats, and/or genes encoding integrases or transposases. The role of horizontal gene acquisition for the evolution of bacterial pathogenesis is evident from the location of many virulence genes within so-called pathogenicity islands (PAIs) [5].

Because of the potential health implications, about two thirds of the sequenced genomes are from bacterial pathogens and many others are from bacteria closely related to at least one pathogen whose genome has been sequenced as well. Comparisons among these genomes have allowed the deduction of the metabolic capacities, pathogenicity-specific attributes, immune evasion mechanisms and evolution of many different pathogens [6–9]. Inter-genomic comparisons have also demonstrated that there is considerable variation in the magnitude of genetic diversity among individual isolates of different species. For example, strains of *Streptococcus, Staphylococcus aureus, Helicobacter pylori,* and *Escherichia coli* can differ in gene content by greater than 25 % [10]. In contrast, the genomes of *Chlamydia trachomatis* and *Mycobacterium tuberculosis* strains are relatively conserved.

For genetically diverse species, inter-genomic comparisons of related isolates, for example genomes of different serotypes of the same pathogen, can be informative. This was perhaps most convincingly demonstrated for group B streptococci. *S. agalactiae* is a group B streptococcus (GBS) that causes neonatal infections and invasive infections in the elderly. The *S. agalactiae* strains most frequently isolated from patients in the US and Europe belong to five different serotypes. The genome sequences of eight *S. agalactiae* strains, including representatives of all five serotypes, have recently been determined [11]. About 80 % of the genes in each individual genome have orthologs in all other genomes, almost all of which display sequence identities of >90 %. Most genes that form this core genome fulfill housekeeping functions or are involved in transport or regulatory processes. In addition, each genome contains genes that are present in only some or none of the other genomes. These strain-specific genes are enriched in genes of unknown function. Together, strain-specific and core genes form the so-called GBS pan-genome. Predictions suggest that the pan-genome is significantly bigger than that of each individual strain and that each newly sequenced genome will add on average 33 new strain-specific genes to the known pan-genome. In addition to the insights on the genetic diversity of *S. agalactiae*, these studies also provided the foundation for the development of an universal GBS vaccine [12]. For this, computer algorithms were used to identify 598 genes within the GBS pan-genome which are predicted to encode surface-associated and secreted proteins. Of these, 312 were purified and tested for their ability to protect mice from killing by *S. agalactiae*. Four antigens were identified which, if applied as a combination vaccine, are protective against many GBS strains. Only one of these antigens is encoded by the GBS core-genome, demonstrating that the development of a universal vaccine may be facilitated by the availability of several GBS genomes.

Another benefit of comparative genomics is that it allows the characterization of otherwise intractable pathogens. *Mycobacterium leprae*, for example, the causative agent of leprosy, has never been cultured axenically and can only be isolated from infected humans, armadillos or mouse foot-pads [13]. Characterization of this bacterium by traditional microbiological approaches is therefore difficult. Whole genome sequencing provided a unique opportunity to gain insights into the biology of this pathogen [14]. Comparison of the *M. leprae* genome with that of *M. tuberculosis* revealed a stunning example of genome decay in the leprosy bacillus. More than 1,100 homologs of *M. tuberculosis* genes were identified in *M. leprae* that had been inactivated by mutations leading to in-frame stop codons, frame shifts or deletions. These pseudogenes account for at least one-third of the *M. leprae* genome. Abundant inactivation of genes important for central metabolism and energy generation explains the failure of all attempts to grow this pathogen in liquid culture. Genome decay may have occurred as a consequence of the adaptation of the leprosy bacillus to a stable niche within its host. This hypothesis is supported by the highly reduced genomes found in other obligate intracellular pathogens [15–17].

While the complete genome sequence of a significant but small number of clinical isolates has been determined, it is not feasible to characterize the hundreds of bacterial pathogens isolated from patients by whole genome sequencing. For this, comparative genome hybridizations (CGHs) provide an economical alternative. CGHs employ microarrays containing hybridization targets for all open reading frames (ORFs) encoded in a sequenced reference genome. The microarray is used to compare differently labeled chromosomal DNA that has been isolated from two bacteria, usually a clinical isolate and the reference strain. Depending on the array design, this approach is limited to the detection of deletions of more than ~100 bps that occurred in the DNA segments represented on the array and cannot identify genetic diversity caused by point or frame shift mutations. However, the acquisition and deletion of genes are two of the main mechanisms leading to bacterial diversity [4]. CGHs have therefore been successfully applied to study the genomic diversity of a number of bacterial pathogens, including *M. tuberculosis* and *H. pylori*. Recent advances in comparative genome resequencing technology have allowed for detection of single nucleotid polymorphisms (SNPs) [define] and such techniques have been successfully employed in determining drug mechanism of action in *M. tuberculosis* [18, 19].

In humans, tuberculosis (TB) is most frequently caused by *Mycobacterium tuberculosis* but also by the closely related *M. bovis* and *M. africanum*. To generate a live vaccine against TB, Calmette and Guerin began to serially passage *M. bovis* in liquid cultures in 1908. By 1921 a strain, Bacillus Calmette-Guerin (BCG), was isolated that was no longer virulent in animals. In the following decades *M. bovis* BCG was distributed among medical and research centers and became one of the most widely used vaccines. Serial passaging was continued for about 40 more years and led to phenotypically heterogeneous daughter strains. In the first microarray-based CGH study, Behr et al. compared chromosomal DNA isolated from strains of *M. bovis* and *M. bovis* BCG to that of the sequenced reference strain *M. tuberculosis* H37Rv [20]. This identified 11 regions containing 91 ORFs that were deleted from all *M. bovis* and *M. bovis* BCG strains. An additional five regions containing 38 ORFs were absent from one or more of the tested BCG strains but present in *M. tuberculosis* and *M. bovis*. These results were later confirmed in a study using Affymetrix GeneChips instead of spotted microarrays [21]. A comparison of the deletion analysis with the history of 13 different *M. bovis* BCG strains revealed their genomic genealogy and, together with a previous study [22], suggested that one deletion, which occurred in the region of difference 1 (RD1) and is common to all *M. bovis* BCG strains, was the primary cause for attenuation of *M. bovis* BCG in animals. This hypothesis has since been confirmed by studies showing that (i) restoration of a functional RD1 increases the virulence of *M. bovis* BCG [23], and (ii) deletion of the entire RD1 [24, 25] or inactivation of individual genes within RD1 [26–28] decreases the virulence of *M. tuberculosis* and *M. bovis*.

In subsequent studies high-density oligonucleotide GeneChips were used to compare the genomes of more than 100 *M. tuberculosis* isolates that had recently been collected from TB patients with that of the sequenced reference strains [29, 30]. In total, 68 deletions were identified. Collectively, the deletions contain 224 ORFs corresponding to 5.5 % of all annotated *M. tuberculosis* ORFs. Certain regions of the reference genome were deleted more frequently than expected by chance, suggesting that they are of low genomic stability. Because all isolates used in this study were collected from TB patients, the deleted ORFs are not essential for causing disease in humans. However, most deletions seem to slightly reduce the fitness of the pathogen [29]. The study also provoked intriguing hypotheses regarding the function of some of the strain-specific genes. For example, genes that are part of the *M. tuberculosis* DosR regulon, which is discussed below, were found to be deleted in a group of closely related strains that may more frequently cause active disease instead of latent infections. Genotypic variability among clinical isolates is a powerful tool for assessing the value of a potential drug target: high-value targets have to be conserved in all isolates.

In contrast to *M. tuberculosis, Helicobacter pylori,* a bacterium able to persist in the human stomach, is a genetically diverse species. In most cases, this bacterium causes asymptomatic infections. However, in a small proportion of individuals, *H. pylori* causes severe diseases, such as peptic ulcer disease and gastric adenocarcinoma [31]. A comparison of the full genome sequences of two *H. pylori* strains demonstrated that many of the genes present in both strains are highly conserved, but also identified ~200 genes that are present in one genome but not the other. The full extent of the genetic diversity of clinical *H. pylori* isolates was revealed by CGHs. 362 genes that are present in one or both of the sequenced *H. pylori* genomes are missing in one or more of 15 clinical isolates analyzed by CGHs [32]. This includes 184 genes present in both sequenced genomes. Thus, less than 80% of the sequenced *H. pylori* genes is shared among the 15 isolates. The true fraction of genes shared among all *H. pylori* strains might be significantly lower because different strains are likely to have genes that are not encoded in the two sequenced genomes and were therefore not represented on the microarrays. Genes present in the core genome of all strains encode most metabolic, biosynthetic, and cellular functions. The 362 strain-specific genes are enriched in ORFs that have no sequence similarity to genes in other species and no known function. Interestingly, when strain-specific genes were analyzed with respect to their absence and presence in different strains by hierarchical clustering, some of them were identified as having a high probability to be co-inherited with the cag pathogenicity island (PAI) even though they were located elsewhere in the genome [32]. The cag-PAI encodes a bacterial secretion system that translocates the CagA protein into host cells. Within the host cell CagA interacts with host proteins and has multiple effects on host signal transduction pathways and host cell morphology [33]. Co-inherited genes often participate in common pathways, suggesting that some of the strain-specific genes are functionally connected to one of the main *H. pylori* virulence factors. As in the clinical *M. tuberculosis* isolates, strain specific genes were also found to be clustered in certain regions of the *H. pylori* chromosome [34, 35].

Two recent studies demonstrated that the development of genetic diversity in *H. pylori* can be detected during persistence within an individual host. In the first study, 30 single colony isolates of *H. pylori* were obtained from a patient six years after a duodenal ulcer had been diagnosed [36, 37]. Comparisons by PCR of these 30 strains with an archival *H. pylori* strain, which was obtained from the same patient during the initial endoscopy, revealed the recent isolates to be similar to the archival strain. This and the fact that the patient had refused antibiotic treatment suggested that the strains isolated during the second endoscopy were descendants of the archival strain. CGHs, however, revealed that the recent isolates were genetically distinct from the archival strain and also distinct from each other.

A total of 2.3% of the ORFs analyzed were not detected in at least one of the recent isolates. In this study, it was not possible to rule out that strains more similar to the recent isolates were present but not captured during the first endoscopy. However, recent studies using experimentally infected rhesus macaques, natural hosts for *H. pylori*, demonstrated that gene deletions occur *in vivo* with a frequency that may account for the genomic diversity of the strains obtained before and after persistence in the human patient [38].

The work discussed here shows how comparative genomics can (i) facilitate the development of vaccines (demonstrated by the use of a combination of strain-specific surface proteins as vaccines against Streptococci), (ii) led to insights into the importance of gene acquisition and gene decay for pathogen evolution, (iii) allow the characterization of otherwise intractable pathogens (e.g., *M. leprae*), (iv) help to identify virulence genes (e.g., the RD1 genes of *M. tuberculosis* and *M. bovis*), and (v) provide insights into the development of genetic diversity during persistence of pathogens within their natural hosts (e.g., in species with variable genomes like *H. pylori*). One of the main advantages of comparative genomics is that it analyzes the interaction of pathogen populations with humans whereas other genomic approaches usually depend on the use of animal models.

2.2 RNA profiling

In addition to their use in the comparison of genomic DNA, microarrays have been extensively applied to the analysis of complex RNA mixtures (see also Chapter 2). The analysis of RNA does, however, present additional challenges. While DNA is relatively stable, RNA degrades quickly at high pH and high temperatures and preventing its enzymatic degradation requires specific precautions that are not necessary for the preparation and storage of DNA. The biological stabilities of DNA and RNA are also fundamentally different. Bacterial genomes, while evolutionary dynamic, do not change during the time it takes to harvest cells and prepare chromosomal DNA. In contrast, bacteria can change their mRNA profiles drastically within minutes, for example in response to cooling or centrifugation for more than a few minutes. Transcription, chemical and enzymatic degradation therefore need to be inhibited as early as possibly during the preparation of RNA. Otherwise, the RNA profile analyzed may have little in common with the RNA profile one aims to characterize.

In a typical RNA profiling experiment, RNA is prepared from bacteria grown under a particular experimental condition, reverse transcribed, labeled with a fluorescent dye and co-hybridized to a microarray together with a differently labeled reference cDNA or genomic DNA (gDNA). Analysis of the microarray with a fluorescence scanner allows the determination of relative mRNA amounts for each gene represented on the microarray. A main goal of profiling the RNA of bacterial pathogens is to identify genes that are preferentially expressed within the host. Such studies are the focus of this section. For details on the experimental procedures that allow extraction of bacterial RNA from infected tissues and host cells and on other technical aspects on RNA profiling experiments, the interested reader is referred to previously published reviews [39, 40].

The first genome wide expression analysis of a bacterial pathogen obtained from human samples was performed with *Vibrio cholerae* [41]. This study was stimulated by an intriguing phenotype displayed by *V. cholerae* isolated from the stool of cholera patients. Such stool isolates were found to infect mice with a 700-fold higher efficiency than an *in vitro* grown reference strain. This phenotype was only transiently expressed and lost after cultivation of the stool isolates in broth for only 18 h. Comparisons of RNA directly isolated from stool isolates with RNA from broth-grown bacteria identified 237 differentially expressed genes. The majority of these genes (~80%) were repressed in the stool isolates. Predicted functions of regulated genes suggested that adaptations to oxygen- and iron-limited conditions occurred in the human-shed *V. cholerae*. To identify candidate genes that might be responsible for the increased infectivity of the stool isolates special attention was paid to the expression of known *V. cholerae* virulence factors. Two of the main *V. cholerae* virulence factors are the cholera toxin (CT) and the toxin co-regulated pilus (TCP). CT is essential for *V. cholerae* to cause severe diarrhea whereas the TCP is essential for host colonization [42–44]. Regulation of CT and TCP expression is complex but mainly controlled by the transcription factors ToxR, TcpP and ToxT [45–48]. Surprisingly, differential expression of these virulence factors was not observed in the stool isolates suggesting that they were not responsible for the increased infectivity of stool isolates. Instead, this phenotype might have been mediated by ORFs of unknown function that were strongly induced in the stool isolates.

That lack of regulation of the ToxR/TcpP/ToxT regulon should not be interpreted as a lack of expression was emphasized by a subsequent study, which used gDNA-cDNA hybridizations to analyze gene expression in human-shed *V. cholerae* [49]. This study demonstrated that RNA for genes associated with the ToxR regulon was indeed present in stool isolates. Other virulence-associated genes involved in motility, chemotaxis, iron transport and anaerobic metabolism were among the genes most highly expressed in stool isolates. Most of these genes were also highly expressed in *V. cholerae* isolated from infected rabbit ileal loops suggesting that the RNA profile of stool isolates is likely similar to that of *V. cholerae* growing in the upper intestine of humans [50].

To further explore *V. cholerae* gene expression in humans and to differentiate between genes expressed during early or late stages of human infections, Larocque et al. compared *V. cholerae* RNA prepared from vomitus with RNA isolated from stool [51]. This identified 35 genes as vomitus-associated and preferentially expressed during the early stage of infections. About a third of these genes were involved in DNA replication, energy production, or protein synthesis, which suggested that *V. cholerae* was more actively replicating during early infections. Three virulence genes, two putative hemolysins and *tcpA*, which encodes the main pilin subunit of the TCP, were also more highly expressed during early stage infections. Many other genes of the TCP pathogenicity island also displayed slightly elevated RNA levels, suggesting that TCP expression is one of the first steps during colonization of the human intestine.

Isolation of *V. cholerae* RNA from infected rabbits is relatively straightforward because large amounts of bacteria can be isolated from a single ileal loop. By contrast, *M. tuberculosis* only grows to approximately 10^7 CFUs in lungs of immunocompetent mice. A recent study overcame the challenge of isolating amounts of *M. tuberculosis* RNA that allow microarray analyses from infected mouse lungs by combining mycobacterial RNA isolated from 50–100 infected mice to characterize the bacterial RNA profile at individual time points post-infection [52]. Given this tremendous effort it is unfortunate that due to the way the experiments were carried out the RNA profile may have changed after the bacteria were removed from the infected animal. This study nevertheless provided some interesting observations. By comparing the expression changes that occurred during growth in broth, immunocompetent (BALB/c) mice and immunodeficient (SCID) mice, 703 genes were identified that changed expression at different growth phases. 63 % of these genes were regulated differently during growth in mice and broth. A comparison of RNA isolated from immunocompetent mice with that from immunodeficient mice suggested that activation of the host immune system had specific effects on *M. tuberculosis* that included modulation of energy and iron metabolism. The impact of the immune response of the host on bacterial gene expression was most severe at time points when activation of the immune system caused a halt of bacterial replication.

Immune-activation also had an impact on the expression of *M. tuberculosis* genes during residence in macrophages [53]. This was revealed in an analysis that compared the RNA profiles of *M. tuberculosis* in resting and IFNγ-activated macrophages. 60 genes were found to be specifically induced in *M. tuberculosis* residing in activated macrophages and eight genes were repressed. Most of these 68 genes belong to two independent regulons controlled by IdeR and DosR, respectively. IdeR is an iron-dependent transcription factor that functions as a repressor of iron acquisition genes and as an activator for genes involved in iron storage [54]. DosR (also referred to as DevR) is a transcription factor of the two-component response regulator class that directly controls expression of about 50 genes in *M. tuberculosis* [55–58]. Members of the IdeR and DosR regulons were also strongly expressed in *M. tuberculosis* isolated from infected mouse lungs [56, 59, 60]. Interestingly, induction of the DosR regulon in mouse lungs was only detected after production of IFNγ and NOS2, suggesting that regulation of the DosR regulon in the lungs of mice also depends on activation of the immune system [59]. Whereas essentiality of the IdeR regulon for virulence of *M. tuberculosis* in mice is well documented [54], the role of the DosR regulon is less clear.

Induction of the DosR regulon in liquid culture has been observed in response to multiple stresses but was strongest in response to hypoxia and chemical generators of nitric oxide (NO) [56, 58, 61–63]. The IdeR regulon can be induced by iron deprivation or treatment with NO or hydrogen peroxide. In addition, macrophage activation-dependent regulation was only observed in macrophages capable of synthesizing nitric oxide (NO) but not detected in macrophages defective in NO synthase 2 (NOS2). Together, these observations strongly suggest that activation-specific changes in the transcriptome of intraphagosomal *M. tuberculosis* were directly caused by NO produced by NOS2 in response to activation of macrophages with IFNγ. Further comparisons of the intraphagosomal RNA profile with RNA profiles of *M. tuberculosis* after exposure to diverse conditions were used to identify additional conditions encountered in the phagosomes of resting and activated macrophages. These comparisons suggested that the *M. tuberculosis*-containing phagosome of primary bone marrow derived macrophages is oxidative, protein denaturing, low in iron and carbohydrates, rich in fatty acids and capable of perturbing the pathogen's cell envelope.

In contrast to *M. tuberculosis*, which resides within phagosomes during its interaction with host cells, *Shigella flexneri* escapes from the phagosome and primarily replicates within the host cell cytoplasm. In humans, *S. flexneri* causes bacillary dysentery, a bloody diarrhea that develops as consequence of invasion of the intestinal barrier by *S. flexneri*. Invasion of the intestinal barrier involves interactions of *S. flexneri* with phagocytic and epithelial cells. Entry of *S. flexneri* into both cell types is mediated by the *ipa-mxi-spa* genes. The Ipa proteins are injected into the host cell by the Mxi-Spa type III secretion system and allow pathogen invasion by reorganizing the host cell cytoskeleton. Microarrays with specific hybridization probes for ~80 % of the genes annotated in the *S. flexneri* genome were used to profile the pathogen's RNA during growth in an epithelial cell line (HeLa) and a macrophage-like cell line (U937) [64]. About 25 % of the genome was differentially expressed in bacteria isolated from HeLa cells or U937 cells compared to broth-grown *S. flexneri*. Of the regulated genes, about two thirds were induced and one third was repressed within tissue culture cells. The repressed genes included the *ipa-mxi-spa* locus. Overall, the RNA profiles isolated from *S. flexneri* growing in HeLa and U937 cells were very similar. Expression of only 18 *S. flexneri* genes (~2 % of all regulated genes) was consistently different in HeLa and U937 cells. Among these genes were some that likely respond to acidic pH, suggesting that a lower pH is encountered within the macrophage-like cells than within HeLA cells. Genes regulated during growth in both cell lines suggested that growth in the cytosol results in downregulation of sugar catabolism, the expression of microaerobic and less energy efficient respiratory chains and the acquisition of iron, magnesium and phosphate via specific ion uptake systems.

The studies described here are only a few examples selected from a rapidly growing field. Others have characterized the RNA profiles of *Salmonella enterica* [65], *Staphylococcus aureus* [66], group A streptococcus (GAS) [67–69], *Neisseria meningitides* [70], *Pseudomonas aeruginosa* [71], enterohemorrhagic *E. coli* (EHEC) [72] and uropathogenic *E. coli* [73, 74] during the interaction with phagocytic cells, non-phagocytic cells or animals. While these RNA profiles are in part as diverse as the survival strategies of different pathogens they also reveal some common features: (i) Most pathogens induce genes involved in iron acquisition during growth within animals or host cells. Given the well documented importance of iron acquisition for the virulence of many pathogens, this finding is not surprising, but reassuring. Attachment to host cells induced iron acquisition genes in *Neisseria meningitides* [70] but repressed such genes in EHEC [72] and *Pseudomonas aeruginosa* [71], suggesting that some surface-bound pathogens can acquire iron directly from their host cell without the need for secreted siderophores. (ii) The carbon and nitrogen sources used to grow bacteria in broth are often different from those that are available to or preferred by pathogens during growth *in vivo*. This is suggested by the changes in expression of genes involved in carbon or nitrogen metabolism observed in host derived urophathogenic *E. coli* [73, 74], EHEC [72], *S. enterica* [65], GAS [68], *S. flexneri* [64] and *M. tuberculosis* [53]. (iii) Microaerobic and anaerobic respiratory chains are frequently expressed during *in vivo* growth. This can either be a consequence of low oxygen availability within the host or caused by inhibition of aerobic respiration by the host's immune system as observed for *M. tuberculosis* [53, 56]. (iv) Immune-activation and immune competence of the host can have a drastic impact on the RNA profile of bacterial pathogens as shown for uropathogenic *E. coli* [74] and *M. tuberculosis* [53]. (v) Hundreds of *in vivo* expressed genes are of unknown function, demonstrating that large aspects of the *in vivo* biology of bacterial pathogens remain to be elucidated. (vi) The regulation of known virulence genes during infections is diverse; some virulence genes are induced during growth in animals or host cells while others are repressed and many seem not to be differentially regulated. Thus, regulation during growth within the host cannot be used to define virulence genes.

2.3 Genome-wide mutagenesis (GWM)

Genome-wide mutagenesis (GWM) experiments begin with generating a large collection of bacteria each of which contain a single mutation in the genome. As a whole, the collection contains mutations in every gene within the genome. Such mutant collections have been constructed using different methods including homologous recombination [75, 76] and transposon mutagenesis [77–86]. Next, each mutant is analyzed for its ability to grow or survive under a certain experimental condition. These analyses are generally performed either with thousands of cultures each containing one mutant or with a few cultures containing thousands of mutants. The analysis of individual mutants within a mixed population depends on methods that allow the discrimination of the survival of individual bacteria each with a mutation in a different gene. This is most efficiently achieved by analyzing mixed populations of transposon mutants with microarrays. Here, the transposon serves as the mutagenizing agent and also to generate sequence labels that distinguish individual mutants [78, 79].

GWM has been widely used to identify genes essential for growth of bacteria on agar plates [78–80, 82, 83, 85, 86]. More recently this approach has also been applied to the identification of genes essential for bacterial pathogens to establish infections and to grow within animal hosts. These experiments are conceptually similar to the signature-tagged mutagenesis (STM) approach. STM has been very successful at identifying virulence genes in a number of different pathogens and for more information the interested reader is referred to recent reviews dedicated to this subject [87–89].

The first GWM analysis of a pathogen-host interaction was published by Sassetti and Rubin [81]. Mice were intravenously infected with a library of ~100,000 *M. tuberculosis* transposon mutants and bacteria were recovered from spleens 1, 2, 4 and 8 weeks post infection. Survival was analyzed in spleens instead of lungs, the primary organ of *M. tuberculosis* infections in humans, because spleens are more efficiently colonized. Even though mice can be infected intravenously with ~10^6 bacteria only a small fraction of the bacteria (typically <<1 %) colonizes the lung. Complex pools are therefore only stochastically represented in mouse lungs. In the absence of highly sensitive methods that allow the detection of a very low number of mutants this problem can only be overcome by using low complexity pools. The feasibility of using low complexity pools to interrogate a significant fraction of the *M. tuberculosis* genome for its *in vivo* essentiality was demonstrated using pools of ≤100 mutants, which were selected from an archive of defined mutants, to determine the growth of 530 *M. tuberculosis* mutants in mice [72].

Together, these two studies identified >200 genes as important for *in vivo* growth. Mutations in only ~11 % of these genes also decreased *in vitro* growth to some extent whereas the others only affected *in vivo* growth [81]. *In vivo* growth attenuating mutations were mapped to genes of a wide variety of predicted functions. Most frequent were genes involved in transport or metabolism of lipids, carbohydrates, amino acids and inorganic ions. Some mutations, for example those in genes important for disaccharide uptake, affected growth and survival during early and late stages of the infections. Others only affected survival at later stages of the infection. Mutations in the latter category demonstrated the importance of DNA repair systems for the long-term survival of *M. tuberculosis* in mice. These findings are in agreement with a recent study on the importance of *uvrB*, a gene involved in nucleotide excision repair, for virulence of *M. tuberculosis* [90].

In contrast to animal infections, pool complexity can be high in experiments that characterize the interaction of pathogens with their host cells *in vitro*. Such a study recently identified 126 genes as essential for growth of *M. tuberculosis* in bone-marrow derived murine macrophages [91]. Comparisons of these genes with those essential for growth of *M. tuberculosis* in mice revealed that about a third of the genes required in macrophages were also required in mouse spleens. This group included genes involved in carbohydrate and phosphate transport. Many genes were however only essential for survival in either macrophages or mouse spleens, demonstrating that macrophage infections only mimic some of the environments encountered *in vivo*. Another interesting finding was revealed by the comparison of genes required for survival of *M. tuberculo-*

sis in macrophages with genes differentially expressed in intraphagosomal *M. tuberculosis*. Only a small fraction of differentially expressed genes were found to be required for survival of *M. tuberculosis* in macrophages. Thus, while RNA profiling can be very informative with respect to the stimuli encountered within host environments, it does not necessarily identify genes required for virulence or *in vivo* survival of bacterial pathogens.

The procedures that allow the use of GWM to analyze the interactions of bacterial pathogens have only been recently developed and have therefore so far only been used in a small number of studies. GWM should, however, be applicable for many bacterial pathogens and might aid our understanding of host–pathogen interactions with an impact similar to that of STM.

3 RNA profiling of host cells after infections

The functional genomics approach most widely applied to explore the response of host cells to microbial infections is RNA profiling. In one of the first studies, Huang et al. showed that ~20 % of the ~6,800 genes analyzed in dendritic cells (DCs) changed their RNA level in response to infection with *E. coli, Candida albicans* or influenza virus [92]. Of the ~1,330 regulated genes, 166 genes were strongly regulated after infection with each microorganism. A comparison of the host cell RNA profiles from 77 different host-pathogen interaction studies extended this common host response to 511 host cell genes that are co-regulated in response to bacterial, fungal and viral pathogens [93]. This response includes genes that encode proinflammatory cytokines such as IL-1β, IL-6, IL-8 and TNF and chemokines (for example MIP1α, MIP1β, GRO1) and genes with roles in lymphocyte activation, antigen presentation and cell signaling [92–94]. The common host response is, therefore, crucial for the activation of an effective innate immune response and the development of adaptive immunity.

Induction of the common host response is likely mediated by a variety of pathogen receptors that include the Toll-like receptors (TLRs), the non-classical C-type lectin Dectin-1, the intracellular nucleotide-binding oligomerization domain (NOD) proteins and others [95–98]. Among these, TLRs have been most intensely studied using genomic approaches. TLRs are transmembrane proteins characterized by an NH2-terminal extracellular leucine rich domain (LLR) and a COOH-terminal intracellular tail containing the conserved Toll/IL-1 receptor (TIR) homology domain. The LLR domain is presumably involved in ligand binding and the intracellular TIR domain mediates interactions between TLRs and their downstream signal transduction components [99, 100]. Microbial recognition of TLRs facilitates TLR dimerization and triggers activation of intracellular signal transduction pathways that ultimately lead to the activation of NFκB and AP-1 transcription factors [101].

The human genome encodes at least ten different TLRs, which likely all recognize molecular patterns present on pathogens and absent from host cells, but have different ligand specificities. Cell wall components of Gram-positive and Gram-negative bacteria, for example, stimulate TLR2 and TLR4, whereas double stranded RNA stimulates TLR3 and flagellin leads to the activation of TLR5 [102]. The importance of specific TLRs for modulation of the host RNA profile in response to infections has been analyzed using two approaches. In the first, purified agonists of TLRs are used to stimulate host cells and the resulting RNA profile is compared with that obtained from cells infected with whole bacteria. This showed that the TLR4 agonist LPS is sufficient to stimulate regulation of all genes in human macrophages that are specifically regulated after infection with Gram-negative bacteria [103]. The *M. tuberculosis* 19-kDa lipoprotein, a TLR2 agonist, is sufficient to regulate ~33 % of the genes that are regulated in murine macrophages in response to *M. tuberculosis* infections [104]. A comparison of the effects of agonists for TLR1/2, TLR4, TLR2/6, TLR7 and TLR9 identified LPS as a particularly potent stimulus and revealed genes that are regulated in response to many TLR agonists as well as genes that seem to only react to activation of certain TLRs [105]. The second approach makes use of cells prepared from mice in which TLRs, or components of the TLR signaling cascades, have been genetically inactivated. Such experiments demonstrated that intact, live and virulent *M. tuberculosis* impacts the RNA profile of macrophages through TLR dependent and TLR-independent signal transduction pathways [104, 106, 107].

The functional consequences of the host cell response for the outcome of a microbial infection have been tested by experimental challenge of mice lacking pathogen recognition receptors or components of their signal transduction pathways. As expected, TLR2 and TLR4 have been proven to be critical for the control of several bacterial infections; however, the increased susceptibility of TLR deficient mice is in many cases dose dependent [108]. For example, TLR2 deficient mice are highly susceptible to infection with a high dose of *Staphylococcus aureus* yet resistant to low dose infections [109]. TLR2-dependent control of group B streptococcus (GBS) is also dose dependent [110]. Infections of TLR2-deficient mice with virulent *M. tuberculosis* led to variable results. In one study, increased susceptibility to low and intermediate doses of *M. tuberculosis* was reported [111] whereas others found a role for TLR2 only in the control of high dose *M. tuberculosis* infection [112].

Even though many of the very strongly induced host genes are part of the common response, genes regulated by specific pathogens often outnumber those that are commonly regulated. For example, expression of 1,330 genes was significantly changed after infection of DCs with *E. coli*, *C. albicans* or influenza virus but only 166 genes were part of the highly regulated common host response [92]. Results from monocyte-derived human macrophages were similar. One study reported that of 977 host genes regulated after infections with one of eight different bacteria, 191 genes were part of a shared transcriptional response [94]. A second study dedicated to the analysis of human peripheral blood mononuclear cell RNA profiles after infection with different bacteria also observed common and pathogen-specific responses [113]. In a more recent study, Chaussabel et al. identified specific expression signatures in human monocyte-derived DCs and macrophages infected with either *M. tuberculosis*, *Toxoplasma gondii*, *Leishmania major*, *Leishmania donovani* and *Brugia malayi* [114]. These studies revealed common as well as pathogen-specific and host-cell type specific responses as principal components of the adaptation of immune cells to infections.

In addition to identifying immune mechanisms, pathogen-specific changes in the RNA profiles of immune cells can also reveal how bacterial pathogens modulate their host cells. This was first shown by studies that analyzed the impact of bacterial virulence genes on the RNA profiles of host cells. *PhoP* encodes a transcription factor required for virulence of *S. typhimurium*. A comparison of the RNA profiles of macrophages after infection with *S. typhimurium* or *S. typhimurium phoP::Tn10* demonstrated that wild type *S. typhimurium* induced host genes involved in apoptosis that were not regulated by *S. typhimurium phoP::Tn10* [115]. Host cell viability assays confirmed that *phoP* is necessary to induce macrophage cell death, a process that is likely important for *S. typhimurium* to cause systemic disease [116]. Host cell RNA profiling was also applied to the analysis of *Yersinia enterocolitica* virulence genes, many of which are encoded on a plasmid called, pYV [117]. These studies suggest that a main function of pYV-encoded genes is to suppress the induction of host genes involved in inflammation. A third example for pathogen-induced manipulation of host gene expression was provided by studies of the interaction of *M. tuberculosis* human monocyte derived macrophages (hMDM) [94]. Infections of hMDMs with *M. tuberculosis* induced significantly less IL-12p40 mRNA than infections with other bacteria, e.g., *E. coli*. Furthermore, infection of hMDM with a mix of *M. tuberculosis* and *E. coli* also resulted in low levels of IL-12. In primary mouse macrophages, heat-killed *M. tuberculosis* induced significantly more IL-12p40 than live *M. tuberculosis* [118]. Taken together, these results point to an active suppression of IL-12p40 induction by live *M. tuberculosis*. IL-12 plays a fundamental role in generating a type 1 T cell response and is critical for the control of tuberculosis in mice [119, 120] and in humans [121–123]. Interference with transcriptional induction of IL-12p40 therefore likely contributes to *M. tuberculosis* virulence.

RNA profiles from epithelial cells, macrophages, neutrophils, and dendritic cells (DCs) have been obtained after infections with a plethora of pathogens. A thorough review of this field is beyond the scope of this chapter (a more extensive review has recently been published [93]). The studies presented helped to define a common transcriptional program that is important for the initial innate immune response and for the establishment of adaptive immunity but also identified numerous pathogen-specific host cell responses. RNA profiling is beginning to reveal how activation of multiple receptors through diverse microbial ligands induces common and pathogen-specific responses. And, as the studies on *S. typhimurium*, *Y. enterocolitica* and *M. tuberculosis* demonstrated, RNA profiling is also a valuable approach to identify principles and targets used by pathogens to subvert activation of an efficient immune response.

4 Functional genomics and drug discovery

A recent study identified diarylquinolones (DARQs) as promising lead structures for the development of new drugs against TB by screening chemical libraries for compounds that inhibit growth of the non-pathogenic *M. smegmatis* [18]. It thus seems that even at the beginning of the 21st century new antibacterial drugs can be identified using approaches very similar to those that led to the discovery of antibiotics in the first half of the 20th century. If this is so, who needs functional genomics to fight infectious diseases?

When discussing the potential impact of functional genomics on drug development it is helpful to distinguish between target-based and whole-cell based drug discovery strategies. The above cited study is an example of a whole-cell based strategy; its first step is the identification of a compound that inhibits bacterial growth. Such a screen can be successful without any knowledge of the pathogen's biology. The primary value of functional genomics for whole-cell based strategies therefore seems to be their usefulness in predicting molecular targets and toxicity of lead compounds [124]. For example, the genome sequences of *M. smegmatis* and *M. tuberculosis* mutants resistant to DARQs contained changes in the genes encoding the ATP synthase suggesting that inhibition of growth was caused by inactivation of this enzyme.

Functional genomics will likely have a broad impact on target-based drug discovery. The success of target-based drug discovery strategies depends on the selection of an appropriate target. For an antibiotic to be effective its target should be essential for survival or at least for growth of virtually all naturally occurring variants of a bacterial pathogen within the host during all stages of an infection. A deep understanding of the pathogen's biology is required to select such targets. However, the main biological criterion that is currently used to select bacterial targets is their essentiality for growth of bacteria in liquid broth. Most other tests performed to evaluate a target predict the likelihood that a target-specific inhibitor of low toxicity can be found. While necessary, such tests do not determine if an inhibitor will eradicate a bacterial infection from an infected individual.

The merits of using *in vitro* essentiality to select bacterial targets are, to some extent, self-evident – all current antibiotics inhibit growth of bacteria in liquid broth and they have served us well. However, it seems prudent to acknowledge the finding that bacteria growing in liquid culture differ physiologically, morphologically and in their essential gene set from bacteria of the same species isolated from infected animals or patients. For example, only 1 out of ~10 gene deletions that interfere with growth of *M. tuberculosis* in mouse spleens also affect growth in liquid broth [81]. Gene essentiality is thus conditional; genes that are essential for growth under one condition are often dispensable for growth under another. Excluding genes that are not essential for growth in liquid broth from the drug discovery process will thus eliminate targets that could lead to the development of antibiotics with high *in vivo* activities [125].

Could the focus on *in vitro* essential genes also lead to antibiotics that inhibit growth in liquid broth but do not eradicate bacterial infections? The most optimistic answer to this question seems to be that we don't know. There are certainly genes, for example those encoding the core enzyme of RNA polymerase, that are always essential for bacterial growth. However, RNA profiling demonstrates that bacterial pathogens perceive liquid broth to be vastly different from the conditioned encountered in host cells and tissues. Even though these experiments do not monitor gene essentiality, they still suggest that not all *in vitro* essential genes are also essential *in vivo*. Carbon and energy metabolism of bacterial pathogens, for example, seems to be different *in vivo* and in liquid broth suggesting that genes necessary to grow with the narrow spectrum of carbon sources provided *in vitro* might not all be essential for growth *in vivo*. Very likely, this hypothesis will soon be tested by using GWM to define essential gene sets for a variety of *in vitro* growth conditions and by combining GWM with conditional knockout approaches. Such studies will improve our ability to rationally select targets for the development of antibiotics with high *in vivo* activities.

Gene essentiality might not only be condition-specific but also strain-specific. This is suggested by comparative genomic studies that revealed a high degree of genomic diversity in some bacterial species. In addition, one of the few studies that analyzed the role of the same genes in different strains of the same species found that all of the three genes analyzed were essential for the virulence of one but dispensable for the virulence of another strain [126]. Should these findings be confirmed for a broader range of genes and pathogens, target evaluation might have to be performed using representative clinical isolates instead of a single laboratory strain.

The analysis of the interaction of *M. tuberculosis* with macrophages using RNA profiling and GWM demonstrated that genes that are preferentially expressed within host cells are not enriched in genes that are essential for survival in this environment. Expression studies will, however, be valuable to complement GWM experiments. Genes that are essential *in vitro* or in animals and are also expressed in bacteria isolated from infected humans are clearly more attractive targets than those for which expression in clinical samples cannot be detected. In addition, target-based discovery strategies are limited to genes of known function. Most *in vivo* essential genes and many *in vitro* essential genes are of unknown function. RNA profiling provides an attractive approach for assigning putative functions to such genes [127].

The areas of drug development most profoundly impacted by RNA profiling of eukaryotic cells are perhaps the toxicological evaluation of drug candidates and the identification of biomarkers that may help predicting disease progression [128, 129]. However, RNA profiles of immune cells also stimulated the identification of new targets and the re-evaluation of existing drugs. Imiquimod, for example, a drug initially approved for the treatment of genital warts [130], was recently found to stimulate murine macrophages through activation of TLR7 [131]. This drug and other TLR agonists are now being evaluated for the treatment of a variety of viral and parasitic infections and certain cancers [130, 132]. While activation of TLRs is important for a proper immune response to many infections, (over-)stimulation of TLRs can also be detrimental to the host. An uncontrolled inflammatory response to bacterial infections can, for example, lead to septic shock, a frequent cause of death in intensive care units. Mice lacking genes involved in TLR signaling are resistant to LPS-induced septic shock [133, 134] suggesting that TLR antagonists might help treating systemic bacterial infections [135, 136]. In addition, phenotypic screens are becoming more and more suitable for the identification of drug targets in eukaryotes [137]. As has been the case for prokaryotes, these screens will likely identify targets with interesting phenotypes but unknown biochemical activities. The biggest impact of genomics on drug development might therefore come from studies that increase our understanding of gene function in prokaryotes and eukaryotes and thus increase the number of targets for which high throughput screens can be developed.

Acknowledgements

I thank Drs. S. Ehrt, C. Nathan, H. Boshoff and C. Barry for critical comments. Preparation of this article and some of the work herein was supported by the NIH and the Ellison Medical Foundation. The Department of Microbiology and Immunology acknowledges the support of the William Randolph Hearst Foundation.

References

1 Fleischmann RD, Adams MD, White O, Clayton RA, Kirkness EF, Kerlavage AR, Bult CJ, Tomb JF, Dougherty BA, Merrick JM et al (1995) Whole-genome random sequencing and assembly of *Haemophilus influenzae* Rd. *Science* 269: 496–512
2 Velculescu VE, Zhang L, Vogelstein B, Kinzler KW (1995) Serial analysis of gene expression. *Science* 270: 484–487
3 Schena M, Shalon D, Davis RW, Brown PO (1995) Quantitative monitoring of gene expression patterns with a complementary DNA microarray. *Science* 270: 467–470
4 Ochman H, Moran NA (2001) Genes lost and genes found: evolution of bacterial pathogenesis and symbiosis. *Science* 292: 1096–1099
5 Hacker J, Kaper JB (2000) Pathogenicity islands and the evolution of microbes. *Annu Rev Microbiol* 54: 641–679
6 Brosch R, Pym AS, Gordon SV, Cole ST (2001) The evolution of mycobacterial pathogenicity: clues from comparative genomics. *Trends Microbiol* 9: 452–458
7 Brussow H, Canchaya C, Hardt WD (2004) Phages and the evolution of bacterial pathogens: from genomic rearrangements to lysogenic conversion. *Microbiol Mol Biol Rev* 68: 560–602, table of contents
8 Schoolnik GK (2002) Functional and comparative genomics of pathogenic bacteria. *Curr Opin Microbiol* 5: 20–26
9 Whittam TS, Bumbaugh AC (2002) Inferences from whole-genome sequences of bacterial pathogens. *Curr Opin Genet Dev* 12: 719–725
10 Fitzgerald JR, Musser JM (2001) Evolutionary genomics of pathogenic bacteria. *Trends Microbiol* 9: 547–553

11 Tettelin H, Masignani V, Cieslewicz MJ, Donati C, Medini D, Ward NL, Angiuoli SV, Crabtree J, Jones AL, Durkin AS et al (2005) Genome analysis of multiple pathogenic isolates of *Streptococcus agalactiae*: Implications for the microbial "pan-genome". *Proc Natl Acad Sci USA* 102: 13950–13955

12 Maione D, Margarit I, Rinaudo CD, Masignani V, Mora M, Scarselli M, Tettelin H, Brettoni C, Iacobini ET, Rosini R et al (2005) Identification of a universal Group B streptococcus vaccine by multiple genome screen. *Science* 309: 148–150

13 Hastings RC, Gillis TP, Krahenbuhl JL, Franzblau SG (1988) Leprosy. *Clin Microbiol Rev* 1: 330–348

14 Cole ST, Eiglmeier K, Parkhill J, James KD, Thomson NR, Wheeler PR, Honore N, Garnier T, Churcher C, Harris D et al (2001) Massive gene decay in the leprosy bacillus. *Nature* 409: 1007–1011

15 Andersson SG, Zomorodipour A, Andersson JO, Sicheritz-Ponten T, Alsmark UC, Podowski RM, Naslund AK, Eriksson AS, Winkler HH, Kurland CG (1998) The genome sequence of *Rickettsia prowazekii* and the origin of mitochondria. *Nature* 396: 133–140

16 Ogata H, Audic S, Renesto-Audiffren P, Fournier PE, Barbe V, Samson D, Roux V, Cossart P, Weissenbach J, Claverie JM et al (2001) Mechanisms of evolution in *Rickettsia conorii* and *R. prowazekii*. *Science* 293: 2093–2098

17 Stephens RS, Kalman S, Lammel C, Fan J, Marathe R, Aravind L, Mitchell W, Olinger L, Tatusov RL, Zhao Q et al (1998) Genome sequence of an obligate intracellular pathogen of humans: *Chlamydia trachomatis*. *Science* 282: 754–759

18 Andries K, Verhasselt P, Guillemont J, Gohlmann HW, Neefs JM, Winkler H, Van Gestel J, Timmerman P, Zhu M, Lee E et al (2005) A diarylquinoline drug active on the ATP synthase of *Mycobacterium tuberculosis*. *Science* 307: 223–227

19 Manjunatha UH, Boshoff H, Dowd CS, Zhang L, Albert TJ, Norton JE, Daniels L, Dick T, Pang SS, Barry CE 3rd (2006) Identification of a nitroimidazo-oxazine-specific protein involved in PA-824 resistance in *Mycobacterium tuberculosis*. *Proc Natl Acad Sci USA* 103: 431–436

20 Behr MA, Wilson MA, Gill WP, Salamon H, Schoolnik GK, Rane S, Small PM (1999) Comparative genomics of BCG vaccines by whole-genome DNA microarray. *Science* 284: 1520–1523

21 Mostowy S, Inwald J, Gordon S, Martin C, Warren R, Kremer K, Cousins D, Behr MA (2005) Revisiting the evolution of *Mycobacterium bovis*. *J Bacteriol* 187: 6386–6395

22 Mahairas GG, Sabo PJ, Hickey MJ, Singh DC, Stover CK (1996) Molecular analysis of genetic differences between *Mycobacterium bovis* BCG and virulent *M. bovis*. *J Bacteriol* 178: 1274–1282

23 Pym AS, Brodin P, Brosch R, Huerre M, Cole ST (2002) Loss of RD1 contributed to the attenuation of the live tuberculosis vaccines *Mycobacterium bovis* BCG and *Mycobacterium microti*. *Mol Microbiol* 46: 709–717

24 Hsu T, Hingley-Wilson SM, Chen B, Chen M, Dai AZ, Morin PM, Marks CB, Padiyar J, Goulding C, Gingery M et al (2003) The primary mechanism of attenuation of bacillus Calmette-Guerin is a loss of secreted lytic function required for invasion of lung interstitial tissue. *Proc Natl Acad Sci USA* 100: 12420–12425

25 Lewis KN, Liao R, Guinn KM, Hickey MJ, Smith S, Behr MA, Sherman DR (2003) Deletion of RD1 from *Mycobacterium tuberculosis* mimics bacille Calmette-Guerin attenuation. *J Infect Dis* 187: 117–123

26 Guinn KM, Hickey MJ, Mathur SK, Zakel KL, Grotzke JE, Lewinsohn DM, Smith S, Sherman DR (2004) Individual RD1-region genes are required for export of ESAT-6/CFP-10 and for virulence of *Mycobacterium tuberculosis*. *Mol Microbiol* 51: 359–370

27 Stanley SA, Raghavan S, Hwang WW, Cox JS (2003) Acute infection and macrophage subversion by *Mycobacterium tuberculosis* require a specialized secretion system. *Proc Natl Acad Sci USA* 100: 13001–13006

28 Wards BJ, de Lisle GW, Collins DM (2000) An esat6 knockout mutant of *Mycobacterium bovis* produced by homologous recombination will contribute to the development of a live tuberculosis vaccine. *Tuber Lung Dis* 80: 185–189

29 Tsolaki AG, Hirsh AE, DeRiemer K, Enciso JA, Wong MZ, Hannan M, Goguet de la Salmoniere YO, Aman K, Kato-Maeda M, Small PM (2004) Functional and evolutionary genomics of *Mycobacterium tuberculosis*: insights from genomic deletions in 100 strains. *Proc Natl Acad Sci USA* 101: 4865–4870

30 Kato-Maeda M, Rhee JT, Gingeras TR, Salamon H, Drenkow J, Smittipat N, Small PM (2001) Comparing genomes within the species *Mycobacterium tuberculosis*. *Genome Res* 11: 547–554

31 Ernst PB, Gold BD (2000) The disease spectrum of *Helicobacter pylori*: the immunopathogenesis of gastroduodenal ulcer and gastric cancer. *Annu Rev Microbiol* 54: 615–640

32 Salama N, Guillemin K, McDaniel TK, Sherlock G, Tompkins L, Falkow SA (2000) Whole-genome microarray reveals genetic diversity among *Helicobacter pylori* strains. *Proc Natl Acad Sci USA* 97: 14668–14673

33 Bourzac KM, Guillemin K (2005) *Helicobacter pylori*-host cell interactions mediated by type IV secretion. *Cell Microbiol* 7: 911–919

34 Alm RA, Ling LS, Moir DT, King BL, Brown ED, Doig PC, Smith DR, Noonan B, Guild BC, deJonge BL et al (1999) Genomic-sequence comparison of two unrelated isolates of the human gastric pathogen *Helicobacter pylori*. *Nature* 397: 176–180

35 Nilsson C, Sillen A, Eriksson L, Strand ML, Enroth H, Normark S, Falk P, Engstrand L (2003) Correlation between cag pathogenicity island composition and *Helicobacter pylori*-associated gastroduodenal disease. *Infect Immun* 71: 6573–6581

36 Israel DA, Salama N, Krishna U, Rieger UM, Atherton JC, Falkow S, Peek RM (2001) *Helicobacter pylori* genetic diversity within the gastric niche of a single human host. *Proc Natl Acad Sci USA* 98: 14625–14630

37 Joyce EA, Chan K, Salama NR, Falkow S (2002) Redefining bacterial populations: a post-genomic reformation. *Nat Rev Genet* 3: 462–473

38 Solnick JV, Hansen LM, Salama NR, Boonjakuakul JK, Syvanen M (2004) Modification of *Helicobacter pylori* outer membrane protein expression during experimental infection of rhesus macaques. *Proc Natl Acad Sci USA* 101: 2106–2111

39 Ehrt S, Voskuil M, Schnappinger D, Schoolnik G (2002) In: SHE Kaufmann, D Kabelitz (eds): *Immunology of Infection*. Academic Press, Amsterdam, The Netherlands. pp 169–180

40 Mangan JA, Monahan IM, Butcher P (2002) In: B Wren, N Dorerll (eds): *Functional microbial genomics*. Academic Press, Amsterdam, The Netherlands. pp 137–151

41 Merrell DS, Butler SM, Qadri F, Dolganov NA, Alam A, Cohen MB, Calderwood SB, Schoolnik GK, Camilli A (2002) Host-induced epidemic spread of the cholera bacterium. *Nature* 417: 642–645

42 Herrington DA, Hall RH, Losonsky G, Mekalanos JJ, Taylor RK, Levine MM (1988) Toxin, toxin-coregulated pili, and the toxR regulon are essential for *Vibrio cholerae* pathogenesis in humans. *J Exp Med* 168: 1487–1492

43 Taylor RK, Miller VL, Furlong DB, Mekalanos JJ (1987) Use of phoA gene fusions to identify a pilus colonization factor coordinately regulated with cholera toxin. *Proc Natl Acad Sci USA* 84: 2833–2837

44 Thelin KH, Taylor RK (1996) Toxin-coregulated pilus, but not mannose-sensitive hemagglutinin, is required for colonization by *Vibrio cholerae* O1 El Tor biotype and O139 strains. *Infect Immun* 64: 2853–2856

45 Carroll PA, Tashima KT, Rogers MB, DiRita VJ, Calderwood SB (1997) Phase variation in tcpH modulates expression of the ToxR regulon in *Vibrio cholerae. Mol Microbiol* 25: 1099–1111

46 DiRita VJ, Parsot C, Jander G, Mekalanos JJ (1991) Regulatory cascade controls virulence in *Vibrio cholerae. Proc Natl Acad Sci USA* 88: 5403–5407

47 Hase CC, Mekalanos JJ (1998) TcpP protein is a positive regulator of virulence gene expression in *Vibrio cholerae. Proc Natl Acad Sci USA* 95: 730–734

48 Miller VL, Mekalanos JJ (1984) Synthesis of cholera toxin is positively regulated at the transcriptional level by toxR. *Proc Natl Acad Sci USA* 81: 3471–3475

49 Bina J, Zhu J, Dziejman M, Faruque S, Calderwood S, Mekalanos J (2003) ToxR regulon of *Vibrio cholerae* and its expression in vibrios shed by cholera patients. *Proc Natl Acad Sci USA* 100: 2801–2806

50 Xu Q, Dziejman M, Mekalanos JJ (2003) Determination of the transcriptome of *Vibrio cholerae* during intraintestinal growth and midexponential phase *in vitro. Proc Natl Acad Sci USA* 100: 1286–1291

51 Larocque RC, Harris JB, Dziejman M, Li X, Khan AI, Faruque AS, Faruque SM, Nair GB, Ryan ET, Qadri F et al (2005) Transcriptional profiling of *Vibrio cholerae* recovered directly from patient specimens during early and late stages of human infection. *Infect Immun* 73: 4488–4493

52 Talaat AM, Lyons R, Howard ST, Johnston SA (2004) The temporal expression profile of *Mycobacterium tuberculosis* infection in mice. *Proc Natl Acad Sci USA* 101: 4602–4607

53 Schnappinger D, Ehrt S, Voskuil MI, Liu Y, Mangan JA, Monahan IM, Dolganov G, Efron B, Butcher PD, Nathan C et al (2003) Transcriptional adaptation of *Mycobacterium tuberculosis* within macrophages: Insights into the phagosomal environment. *J Exp Med* 198: 693–704

54 Rodriguez GM, Smith I (2003) Mechanisms of iron regulation in mycobacteria: role in physiology and virulence. *Mol Microbiol* 47: 1485–1494

55 Boon C, Dick T (2002) *Mycobacterium bovis* BCG response regulator essential for hypoxic dormancy. *J Bacteriol* 184: 6760–6767

56 Voskuil MI, Schnappinger D, Visconti KC, Harrell MI, Dolganov GM, Sherman DR, Schoolnik GK (2003) Inhibition of respiration by nitric oxide induces a *Mycobacterium tuberculosis* dormancy program. *J Exp Med* 198: 705–713

57 Dasgupta N, Kapur V, Singh KK, Das TK, Sachdeva S, Jyothisri K, Tyagi JS (2000) Characterization of a two-component system, devR-devS, of *Mycobacterium tuberculosis*. *Tuber Lung Dis* 80: 141–159

58 Sherman DR, Voskuil M, Schnappinger D, Liao R, Harrell MI, Schoolnik GK (2001) Regulation of the *Mycobacterium tuberculosis* hypoxic response gene encoding alpha-crystallin. *Proc Natl Acad Sci USA* 98: 7534–7539

59 Shi L, Jung YJ, Tyagi S, Gennaro ML, North RJ (2003) Expression of Th1-mediated immunity in mouse lungs induces a *Mycobacterium tuberculosis* transcription pattern characteristic of nonreplicating persistence. *Proc Natl Acad Sci USA* 100: 241–246

60 Timm J, Post FA, Bekker LG, Walther GB, Wainwright HC, Manganelli R, Chan WT, Tsenova L, Gold B, Smith I et al (2003) Differential expression of iron-, carbon-, and oxygen-responsive mycobacterial genes in the lungs of chronically infected mice and tuberculosis patients. *Proc Natl Acad Sci USA* 100: 14321–14326

61 Boshoff HI, Myers TG, Copp BR, McNeil MR, Wilson MA, Barry CE 3*rd* (2004) The transcriptional responses of *Mycobacterium tuberculosis* to inhibitors of metabolism: novel insights into drug mechanisms of action. *J Biol Chem* 279: 40174–40184

62 Ohno H, Zhu G, Mohan VP, Chu D, Kohno S, Jacobs WR Jr, Chan J (2003) The effects of reactive nitrogen intermediates on gene expression in *Mycobacterium tuberculosis*. *Cell Microbiol* 5: 637–648

63 Kendall SL, Movahedzadeh F, Rison SC, Wernisch L, Parish T, Duncan K, Betts JC, Stoker NG (2004) The *Mycobacterium tuberculosis* dosRS two-component system is induced by multiple stresses. *Tuberculosis (Edinb)* 84: 247–255

64 Lucchini S, Liu H, Jin Q, Hinton JC, Yu J (2005) Transcriptional adaptation of *Shigella flexneri* during infection of macrophages and epithelial cells: insights into the strategies of a cytosolic bacterial pathogen. *Infect Immun* 73: 88–102

65 Eriksson S, Lucchini S, Thompson A, Rhen M, Hinton JC (2003) Unravelling the biology of macrophage infection by gene expression profiling of intracellular *Salmonella enterica*. *Mol Microbiol* 47: 103–118

66 Voyich JM, Braughton KR, Sturdevant DE, Whitney AR, Said-Salim B, Porcella SF, Long RD, Dorward DW, Gardner DJ, Kreiswirth BN et al (2005) Insights into mechanisms used by *Staphylococcus aureus* to avoid destruction by human neutrophils. *J Immunol* 175: 3907–3919

67 Voyich JM, Braughton KR, Sturdevant DE, Vuong C, Kobayashi SD, Porcella SF, Otto M, Musser JM, DeLeo FR (2004) Engagement of the pathogen survival response used by group A Streptococcus to avert destruction by innate host defense. *J Immunol* 173: 1194–1201

68 Voyich JM, Sturdevant DE, Braughton KR, Kobayashi SD, Lei B, Virtaneva K, Dorward DW, Musser JM, DeLeo FR (2003) Genome-wide protective response used by group A Streptococcus to evade destruction by human polymorphonuclear leukocytes. *Proc Natl Acad Sci USA* 100: 1996–2001

69 Virtaneva K, Porcella SF, Graham MR, Ireland RM, Johnson CA, Ricklefs SM, Babar I, Parkins LD, Romero RA, Corn GJ et al (2005) Longitudinal analysis of the group A Streptococcus transcriptome in experimental pharyngitis in cynomolgus macaques. *Proc Natl Acad Sci USA* 102: 9014–9019

70 Dietrich G, Kurz S, Hubner C, Aepinus C, Theiss S, Guckenberger M, Panzner U, Weber J, Frosch M (2003) Transcriptome analysis of *Neisseria meningitidis* during infection. *J Bacteriol* 185: 155–164

71 Frisk A, Schurr JR, Wang G, Bertucci DC, Marrero L, Hwang SH, Hassett DJ, Schurr MJ (2004) Transcriptome analysis of *Pseudomonas aeruginosa* after interaction with human airway epithelial cells. *Infect Immun* 72: 5433–5438

72 Dahan S, Knutton S, Shaw RK, Crepin VF, Dougan G, Frankel G (2004) Transcriptome of enterohemorrhagic *Escherichia coli* O157 adhering to eukaryotic plasma membranes. *Infect Immun* 72: 5452–5459

73 Snyder JA, Haugen BJ, Buckles EL, Lockatell CV, Johnson DE, Donnenberg MS, Welch RA, Mobley HL (2004) Transcriptome of uropathogenic *Escherichia coli* during urinary tract infection. *Infect Immun* 72: 6373–6381

74 Staudinger BJ, Oberdoerster MA, Lewis PJ, Rosen H (2002) mRNA expression profiles for *Escherichia coli* ingested by normal and phagocyte oxidase-deficient human neutrophils. *J Clin Invest* 110: 1151–1163

75 Knuth K, Niesalla H, Hueck CJ, Fuchs TM (2004) Large-scale identification of essential *Salmonella* genes by trapping lethal insertions. *Mol Microbiol* 51: 1729–1744

76 Kobayashi K, Ehrlich SD, Albertini A, Amati G, Andersen KK, Arnaud M, Asai K, Ashikaga S, Aymerich S, Bessieres P et al (2003) Essential *Bacillus subtilis* genes. *Proc Natl Acad Sci USA* 100: 4678–4683

77 Lamichhane G, Tyagi S, Bishai WR (2005) Designer arrays for defined mutant analysis to detect genes essential for survival of *Mycobacterium tuberculosis* in mouse lungs. *Infect Immun* 73: 2533–2540

78 Lamichhane G, Zignol M, Blades NJ, Geiman DE, Dougherty A, Grosset J, Broman KW, Bishai WR (2003) A postgenomic method for predicting essential genes at subsaturation levels of mutagenesis: application to *Mycobacterium tuberculosis*. *Proc Natl Acad Sci USA* 100: 7213–7218

79 Sassetti CM, Boyd DH, Rubin EJ (2001) Comprehensive identification of conditionally essential genes in mycobacteria. *Proc Natl Acad Sci USA* 98: 12712–12717

80 Sassetti CM, Boyd DH, Rubin EJ (2003) Genes required for mycobacterial growth defined by high density mutagenesis. *Mol Microbiol* 48: 77–84

81 Sassetti CM, Rubin EJ (2003) Genetic requirements for mycobacterial survival during infection. *Proc Natl Acad Sci USA* 100: 12989–12994
82 Akerley BJ, Rubin EJ, Novick VL, Amaya K, Judson N, Mekalanos JJ (2002) A genome-scale analysis for identification of genes required for growth or survival of *Haemophilus influenzae*. *Proc Natl Acad Sci USA* 99: 966–971
83 Gerdes SY, Scholle MD, Campbell JW, Balazsi G, Ravasz E, Daugherty MD, Somera AL, Kyrpides NC, Anderson I, Gelfand MS et al (2003) Experimental determination and system level analysis of essential genes in *Escherichia coli* MG1655. *J Bacteriol* 185: 5673–5684
84 Hutchison CA, Peterson SN, Gill SR, Cline RT, White O, Fraser CM, Smith HO, Venter JC (1999) Global transposon mutagenesis and a minimal Mycoplasma genome. *Science* 286: 2165–2169
85 Salama NR, Shepherd B, Falkow S (2004) Global transposon mutagenesis and essential gene analysis of *Helicobacter pylori*. *J Bacteriol* 186: 7926–7935
86 Winterberg KM, Luecke J, Bruegl AS, Reznikoff WS (2005) Phenotypic screening of *Escherichia coli* K-12 Tn5 insertion libraries, using whole-genome oligonucleotide microarrays. *Appl Environ Microbiol* 71: 451–459
87 Autret N, Charbit A (2005) Lessons from signature-tagged mutagenesis on the infectious mechanisms of pathogenic bacteria. *FEMS Microbiol Rev* 29: 703–717
88 Mecsas J (2002) Use of signature-tagged mutagenesis in pathogenesis studies. *Curr Opin Microbiol* 5: 33–37
89 Shea JE, Santangelo JD, Feldman RG (2000) Signature-tagged mutagenesis in the identification of virulence genes in pathogens. *Curr Opin Microbiol* 3: 451–458
90 Darwin KH, Nathan CF (2005) Role for nucleotide excision repair in virulence of *Mycobacterium tuberculosis*. *Infect Immun* 73: 4581–4587
91 Rengarajan J, Bloom BR, Rubin EJ (2005) Genome-wide requirements for *Mycobacterium tuberculosis* adaptation and survival in macrophages. *Proc Natl Acad Sci USA* 102: 8327–8332
92 Huang Q, Liu D, Majewski P, Schulte LC, Korn JM, Young RA, Lander ES, Hacohen N (2001) The plasticity of dendritic cell responses to pathogens and their components. *Science* 294: 870–875
93 Jenner RG, Young RA (2005) Insights into host responses against pathogens from transcriptional profiling. *Nat Rev Microbiol* 3: 281–294
94 Nau GJ, Richmond JF, Schlesinger A, Jennings EG, Lander ES, Young RA (2002) Human macrophage activation programs induced by bacterial pathogens. *Proc Natl Acad Sci USA* 99: 1503–1508
95 Brown GD (2006) Dectin-1: a signalling non-TLR pattern-recognition receptor. *Nat Rev Immunol* 6: 33-43
96 Mukhopadhyay S, Herre J, Brown GD, Gordon S (2004) The potential for Toll-like receptors to collaborate with other innate immune receptors. *Immunology* 112: 521–530
97 Sabroe I, Read RC, Whyte MK, Dockrell DH, Vogel SN, Dower SK (2003) Toll-like receptors in health and disease: complex questions remain. *J Immunol* 171: 1630–1635

98 Triantafilou M, Triantafilou K (2002) Lipopolysaccharide recognition: CD14, TLRs and the LPS-activation cluster. *Trends Immunol* 23: 301–304

99 Matsumoto M, Funami K, Tanabe M, Oshiumi H, Shingai M, Seto Y, Yamamoto A, Seya T (2003) Subcellular localization of Toll-like receptor 3 in human dendritic cells. *J Immunol* 171: 3154–3162

100 Underhill DM, Ozinsky A (2002) Phagocytosis of microbes: complexity in action. *Annu Rev Immunol* 20: 825–852

101 Akira S, Takeda K (2004) Toll-like receptor signalling. *Nat Rev Immunol* 4: 499–511

102 Takeda K, Akira S (2005) Toll-like receptors in innate immunity. *Int Immunol* 17: 1–14

103 Nau GJ, Schlesinger A, Richmond JF, Young RA (2003) Cumulative Toll-like receptor activation in human macrophages treated with whole bacteria. *J Immunol* 170: 5203–5209

104 Pai RK, Pennini ME, Tobian AA, Canaday DH, Boom WH, Harding CV (2004) Prolonged toll-like receptor signaling by *Mycobacterium tuberculosis* and its 19-kilodalton lipoprotein inhibits gamma interferon-induced regulation of selected genes in macrophages. *Infect Immun* 72: 6603–6614

105 Schmitz F, Mages J, Heit A, Lang R, Wagner H (2004) Transcriptional activation induced in macrophages by Toll-like receptor (TLR) ligands: from expression profiling to a model of TLR signaling. *Eur J Immunol* 34: 2863–2873

106 Shi S, Blumenthal A, Hickey CM, Gandotra S, Levy D, Ehrt S (2005) Expression of many immunologically important genes in *Mycobacterium tuberculosis*-infected macrophages is independent of both TLR2 and TLR4 but dependent on IFN-alphabeta receptor and STAT1. *J Immunol* 175: 3318–3328

107 Shi S, Nathan C, Schnappinger D, Drenkow J, Fuortes M, Block E, Ding A, Gingeras TR, Schoolnik G, Akira S et al (2003) MyD88 primes macrophages for full-scale activation by interferon-gamma yet mediates few responses to *Mycobacterium tuberculosis*. *J Exp Med* 198: 987–997

108 Schnare M, Rollinghoff M, Qureshi S (2005) Toll-like receptors: Sentinels of host defence against bacterial infection. *Int Arch Allergy Immunol* 139: 75–85

109 Takeuchi O, Hoshino K, Akira S (2000) Cutting edge: TLR2-deficient and MyD88-deficient mice are highly susceptible to *Staphylococcus aureus* infection. *J Immunol* 165: 5392–5396

110 Mancuso G, Midiri A, Beninati C, Biondo C, Galbo R, Akira S, Henneke P, Golenbock D, Teti G (2004) Dual role of TLR2 and myeloid differentiation factor 88 in a mouse model of invasive group B streptococcal disease. *J Immunol* 172: 6324–6349

111 Drennan MB, Nicolle D, Quesniaux VJ, Jacobs M, Allie N, Mpagi J, Fremond C, Wagner H, Kirschning C, Ryffel B (2004) Toll-like receptor 2-deficient mice succumb to *Mycobacterium tuberculosis* infection. *Am J Pathol* 164: 49–57

112 Reiling N, Holscher C, Fehrenbach A, Kroger S, Kirschning CJ, Goyert S, Ehlers S (2002) Cutting edge: Toll-like receptor (TLR)2- and TLR4-mediated pathogen recognition in resistance to airborne infection with *Mycobacterium tuberculosis*. *J Immunol* 169: 3480–3484

113 Boldrick JC, Alizadeh AA, Diehn M, Dudoit S, Liu CL, Belcher CE, Botstein D, Staudt LM, Brown PO, Relman DA (2002) Stereotyped and specific gene expression programs in human innate immune responses to bacteria. *Proc Natl Acad Sci USA* 99: 972–977

114 Chaussabel D, Semnani RT, McDowell MA, Sacks D, Sher A, Nutman TB (2003) Unique gene expression profiles of human macrophages and dendritic cells to phylogenetically distinct parasites. *Blood* 102: 672–681

115 Detweiler CS, Cunanan DB, Falkow S (2001) Host microarray analysis reveals a role for the *Salmonella* response regulator phoP in human macrophage cell death. *Proc Natl Acad Sci USA* 98: 5850–5855

116 Monack DM, Hersh D, Ghori N, Bouley D, Zychlinsky A, Falkow S (2000) *Salmonella* exploits caspase-1 to colonize Peyer's patches in a murine typhoid model. *J Exp Med* 192: 249–258

117 Sauvonnet N, Pradet-Balade B, Garcia-Sanz JA, Cornelis GR (2002) Regulation of mRNA expression in macrophages after *Yersinia enterocolitica* infection. Role of different Yop effectors. *J Biol Chem* 277: 25133–25142

118 Ehrt S, Schnappinger D, Bekiranov S, Drenkow J, Shi S, Gingeras TR, Gaasterland T, Schoolnik G, Nathan C (2001) Reprogramming of the macrophage transcriptome in response to interferon-gamma and *Mycobacterium tuberculosis*: signaling roles of nitric oxide synthase-2 and phagocyte oxidase. *J Exp Med* 194: 1123–1140

119 Cooper AM, Magram J, Ferrante J, Orme IM (1997) Interleukin 12 (IL-12) is crucial to the development of protective immunity in mice intravenously infected with *Mycobacterium tuberculosis*. *J Exp Med* 186: 39–45

120 Flynn JL, Goldstein MM, Triebold KJ, Sypek J, Wolf S, Bloom BR (1995) IL-12 increases resistance of BALB/c mice to *Mycobacterium tuberculosis* infection. *J Immunol* 155: 2515–2524

121 Altare F, Durandy A, Lammas D, Emile JF, Lamhamedi S, Le Deist F, Drysdale P, Jouanguy E, Doffinger R, Bernaudin F et al (1998) Impairment of mycobacterial immunity in human interleukin-12 receptor deficiency. *Science* 280: 1432–1435

122 Altare F, Lammas D, Revy P, Jouanguy E, Doffinger R, Lamhamedi S, Drysdale P, Scheel-Toellner D, Girdlestone J, Darbyshire P et al (1998) Inherited interleukin 12 deficiency in a child with bacille Calmette-Guerin and *Salmonella enteritidis* disseminated infection. *J Clin Invest* 102: 2035–2040

123 de Jong R, Altare F, Haagen IA, Elferink DG, Boer T, van Breda Vriesman PJ, Kabel PJ, Draaisma JM, van Dissel JT, Kroon FP et al (1998) Severe mycobacterial and *Salmonella* infections in interleukin-12 receptor-deficient patients. *Science* 280: 1435–1438

124 Lord PG (2004) Progress in applying genomics in drug development. *Toxicol Lett* 149: 371–375

125 Nathan C (2004) Antibiotics at the crossroads. *Nature* 431: 899–902

126 Orihuela CJ, Radin JN, Sublett JE, Gao G, Kaushal D, Tuomanen EI (2004) Microarray analysis of pneumococcal gene expression during invasive disease. *Infect Immun* 72: 5582–5596

127 Hughes TR, Marton MJ, Jones AR, Roberts CJ, Stoughton R, Armour CD, Bennett HA, Coffey E, Dai H, He YD et al (2000) Functional discovery via a compendium of expression profiles. *Cell* 102: 109–126

128 Seo D, Ginsburg GS (2005) Genomic medicine: bringing biomarkers to clinical medicine. *Curr Opin Chem Biol* 9: 381–386

129 Waters MD, Fostel JM (2004) Toxicogenomics and systems toxicology: aims and prospects. *Nat Rev Genet* 5: 936–948

130 Hoffman ES, Smith RE, Renaud RC Jr (2005) From the analyst's couch: TLR-targeted therapeutics. *Nat Rev Drug Discov* 4: 879–880

131 Hemmi H, Kaisho T, Takeuchi O, Sato S, Sanjo H, Hoshino K, Horiuchi T, Tomizawa H, Takeda K, Akira S (2002) Small anti-viral compounds activate immune cells via the TLR7 MyD88-dependent signaling pathway. *Nat Immunol* 3: 196–200

132 Skinner RB Jr (2003) Imiquimod. *Dermatol Clin* 21: 291–300

133 Suzuki N, Suzuki S, Duncan GS, Millar DG, Wada T, Mirtsos C, Takada H, Wakeham A, Itie A, Li S et al (2002) Severe impairment of interleukin-1 and Toll-like receptor signalling in mice lacking IRAK-4. *Nature* 416: 750–756

134 Takaoka A, Yanai H, Kondo S, Duncan G, Negishi H, Mizutani T, Kano S, Honda K, Ohba Y, Mak TW et al (2005) Integral role of IRF-5 in the gene induction programme activated by Toll-like receptors. *Nature* 434: 243–249

135 Lawton JA, Ghosh P (2003) Novel therapeutic strategies based on toll-like receptor signaling. *Curr Opin Chem Biol* 7: 446–451

136 Zuany-Amorim C, Hastewell J, Walker C (2002) Toll-like receptors as potential therapeutic targets for multiple diseases. *Nat Rev Drug Discov* 1: 797–807

137 Austen M, Dohrmann C (2005) Phenotype-first screening for the identification of novel drug targets. *Drug Discov Today* 10: 275–282

The PDR-Series
Progress in Drug Research

Progress in Drug Research is a prestigious book series which provides extensive expert-written reviews on highly topical areas in current pharmaceutical and pharmacological research.

Founded in 1959 by Ernst Jucker, the series moved from its initial focus on medicinal chemistry to a much wider scope. Today it encompasses all fields concerned with the development of new therapeutic drugs and the elucidation of their mechanisms of action, reflecting the increasingly complex nature of modern drug research. Invited authors present their biological, chemical, biochemical, physiological, immunological, pharmaceutical, toxicological, pharmacological and clinical expertise in carefully written reviews and provide the newcomer and the specialist alike with an up-to-date list of prime references.

Starting with volume 61, *Progress in Drug Research* is continued as a series of monographs.

Available volumes:

Advances in Targeted Cancer Therapy (PDR 63), R.M. Schultz (Editor), 2005
Imaging in Drug Discovery and Early Clinical Trials (PDR 62), M. Rudin (Editor), 2005
Peptide Transport and Delivery into the Central Nervous System (PDR 61), L. Prokai, K. Prokai-Tatrai (Editors), 2003
Progress in Drug Research, volumes 1–60, E. Jucker (Editor), 1959–2003